Creative Resources for the
Early Childhood Classroom

CREATIVE RESOURCES FOR THE EARLY CHILDHOOD CLASSROOM

Judith Herr
Yvonne Libby

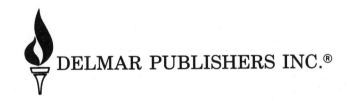

DELMAR PUBLISHERS INC.®

NOTICE TO THE READER

Delmar Staff
  Associate Editor: Jay Whitney
  Managing Editor: Gerry East
  Project Editor: Carol Micheli
  Production Coordinator: Sandra Woods
  Design Coordinator: Susan Mathews

Printed in the United States of America
Published simultaneously in Canada
by Nelson Canada,
a division of The Thomson Corporation

10 9 8 7 6 5 4 3 2 1

Library of Congress Cataloging-in-Publication Data

Herr, Judith.
    Creative resources for the early childhood classroom / Judy Herr,
  Yvonne Libby.
      p.   cm.
    ISBN 0-8273-3603-9
    1. Education, Preschool — Curricula. 2. Unit method of teaching.
I. Libby, Yvonne.   II. Title
LB1140.4H47   1990
372.10—dc20   89-17020
                                                                    CIP

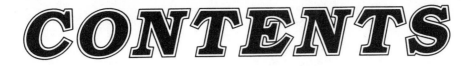

CONTENTS

Table of Contents by Subjects

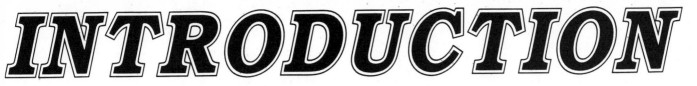

INTRODUCTION

The purpose of this introduction is to explain the process involved in curriculum planning for young children using the thematic, or unit approach. To support each theme, planning and construction ideas are included for bulletin boards, name and cubby tags, as well as parent letters and a wide variety of classroom learning experiences.

As you use this guide, remember that children learn best when they can control and act upon their environment. Many opportunities should be available for seeing, touching, tasting, learning, and self expression. To provide these opportunities, the teacher's primary role is to set the stage by offering many experiences that stimulate the children's senses and curiosity; children learn by doing and play is their work. As a result, it is the authors' intention that you will use this book as a resource. Specifically the ideas in this book should help you to enrich the children's environment, providing them an opportunity to make choices among a wide variety of activities that stimulate their natural curiosity.

Play in the classroom should be child-centered and self-initiated. To provide an environment that promotes these types of play, it is the adult's role to provide unstructured time, space and materials. Using a theme approach to plan curriculum is one way to ensure that a wide variety of classroom experiences are provided.

It is important that all curriculum be adapted to match the developmental needs of children. An activity that is appropriate for one group of children may be inappropriate for another. To develop an appropriate curriculum, knowledge of the typical development of children is needed. For this reason, the inside covers of this book contain such information. Review these developmental norms before selecting a theme or specific activities.

Theme Planning

A developmentally appropriate curriculum for young children integrates the children's needs, interests and abilities. Before planning curriculum, observe the children's development.

Record notes of what you see. At the same time, note the children's interests and listen carefully. Children's conversations provide clues; this information is vital in theme selection. After this, review your observations by discussing them with other staff members. An appropriate curriculum for young children cannot be planned without understanding their development.

There are many methods for planning a curriculum other than using themes. In fact, you may prefer not to use a theme during parts of the year. If this is your choice, you may wish to use the book as a source of ideas, integrating activities and experiences from a variety of the themes outlined in the book.

Planning a curriculum using a theme approach involves several steps. The first step involves selecting a theme that is appropriate for the developmental level and interests of your group of children. After selecting a theme, the next step is developing a flowchart. From the flowchart, goals, conceptual understandings and vocabulary words can easily be extracted. The final steps in curriculum planning is selecting activities based upon the children's stages of development as well as available resources. While doing this, the covers of this book should be used as a reference to review development characteristics for children of different ages.

To help you understand the theme approach to curriculum development, each step of the process will be discussed. Included are developing flowcharts, theme goals, concepts, vocabulary and activities. In addition, suggestions are given for writing parent letters, designing bulletin boards and selecting children's books.

Flowcharts. The flowchart is a simple way to record all possible subconcepts that relate to the major concept or theme. To illustrate, plan a theme on apples. In the center of a piece of paper, write the word "apple." Then using an encyclopedia as a resource, record the subconcepts that are related. Include origin, parts, colors, tastes, sizes, textures, food preparation and nutrition. The following flowchart includes these concepts. In addition, under each subconcept list content that could be included. For example, apples may be colored green, yellow or red.

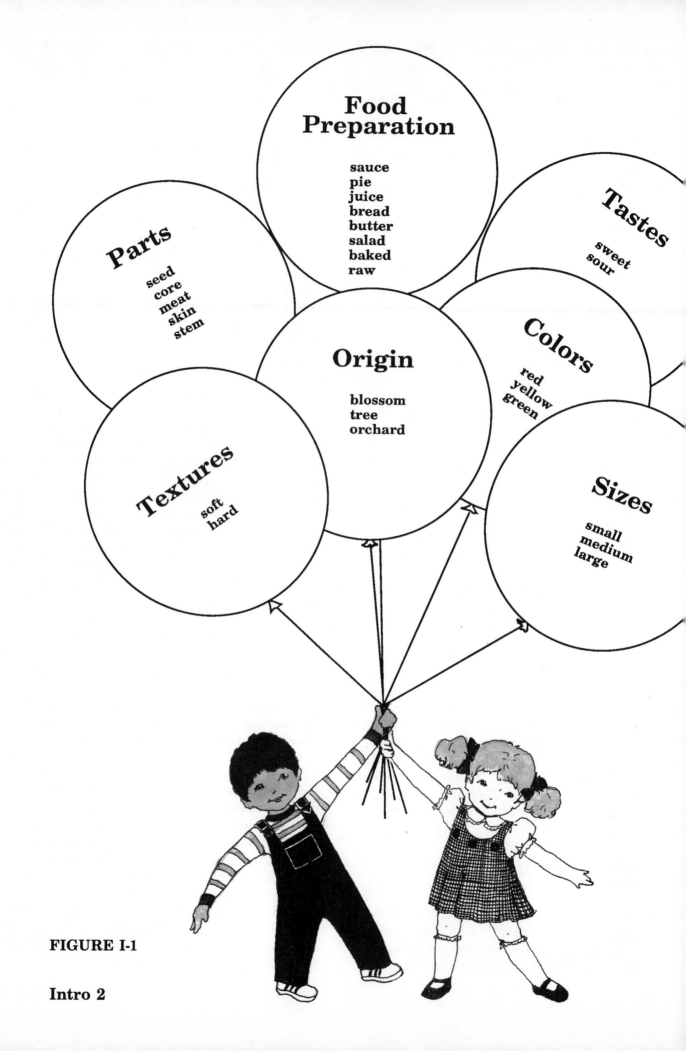

Food Preparation

sauce
pie
juice
bread
butter
salad
baked
raw

Parts

seed
core
meat
skin
stem

Tastes

sweet
sour

Origin

blossom
tree
orchard

Colors

red
yellow
green

Textures

soft
hard

Sizes

small
medium
large

FIGURE I-1

Intro 2

Theme goals. Once you have prepared a flowchart, abstracting theme goals is a simple process. Begin by reviewing the chart. Notice the subheadings listed. For the unit on apples, the subheadings include: parts, food preparation, tastes, textures, colors, size, and origin. Writing each of these subheadings as a goal is the next step of the process.

Since there were eight subheadings, each of these can be included as a goal. In some cases, subheadings may be combined. For example, note the fourth goal listed. It combines several subheadings. Included are textures, sizes and colors.

Through participation in the experiences provided by using apples as a curriculum theme, the children may learn:

1. Parts of an apple.
2. Preparation of apples for eating.
3. Apple tastes.
4. Textures, sizes, and colors of apples.
5. The origin of an apple.

Concepts. The concepts must be related to the goal; however, they are more specific. To write the concepts, study the goals. Then prepare sentences that are written in a simple form that children can understand. Examples of concepts for a unit on apples may include:

1. An apple is a fruit.
2. An apple has five parts: seed, core, meat, skin and stem.
3. Apples grow on trees.
4. A group of apple trees is called an orchard.
5. Bread, butter, pies, puddings, applesauce, dumplings, butter and jellies can be prepared from apples.
6. Some apples are sweet; others are sour.
7. Apples can be colored green, yellow or red.
8. Apples can be large or small.
9. Apples may be hard or soft.
10. Apples can be eaten raw.
11. Seeds from an apple can grow into a tree.

Vocabulary. The vocabulary should include new words that you want to informally introduce to the children. Vocabulary words need to be tailored to meet the specific needs of your group of children. The number of vocabulary words will vary, depending upon the theme and the developmental level of the children. For example, it might be assumed that the children know the word sweet but not tart. So the definition of the word tart is included. Collectively, the following words could be introduced in this unit: apple, texture, core, blossom and apple butter. Definitions for these words could include:

1. apple—a fruit that is grown on a tree.
2. texture—how something feels.
3. core—the part of the apple that contains the seeds.
4. apple blossom—a flower on the apple tree.
5. apple butter—a spread for bread made from apples.

Activities. Now that you have learned how to develop goals related to a theme using a flowchart, you will need to learn how to select appropriate activities. You will find that many theme goals can be accomplished by additions to the environment, bulletin boards, field trips and stories or resource people at large group time. Your major role as an adult, or teacher, is that of a facilitator, planning and preparing the environment to stimulate the child's natural curiosity.

To begin this process, review each goal and determine how it can be introduced in the classroom. For example, if you were going to develop a theme on apples, review the goals. A bulletin board or game could introduce the three colors of apples. The children could also learn these colors through cooking experiences. The third vehicle for teaching the colors of apples would be placing the three colors of apples on a science table.

The five parts of an apple could also be introduced through participation in a tasting or cooking experience, bulletin board or even discussion on a field trip or at the snack table. Always remember that children need to observe and manipulate the concrete object while engaged in child-initiated or child-directed play that is teacher supported. For that reason, fresh apples could be cut horizontally and placed on the science table with a magnifying glass. Likewise, simultaneously, apple seeds and paper could be available on the art table to construct a collage. Always remember that the best activities for young children are hands on and open ended. That is: focus on the process, rather than the product. As a teacher, you should take the ideas in this book and use and adapt them for planning and preparing the environment.

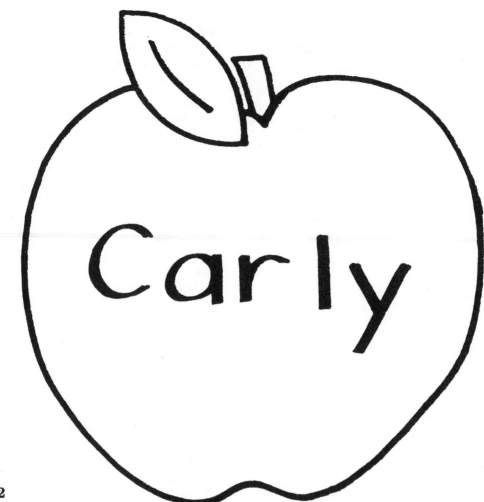

FIGURE I-2

Name and Cubby Tags

Representative tags for each theme appear in Appendix A. They may be reproduced to be used in conjunction with the theme or the children can make their own.

Making Name Tags

"Who is that child? Is it Tommy or Teddy?" These questions are echoed over and over again after new children, staff or volunteers are introduced to a group. Parents will also appreciate the use of name tags to identify staff members and their children's playmates. To assist in learning names, simple name tags can be made, although they need not be prepared for every unit. In some centers, when there isn't a high turnover of children, name tags are worn, if at all, only at the beginning of the year or on field trips.

Some center personnel prepare two sets of name tags. One set, containing the child's first name, is primarily for classroom use. Another set of name tags is used for the children to wear on field trips. Printed on these tags, in addition to the child's first name, is the name, address and telephone number of the center. This information may be useful if a child accidentally strays from the group. Also, the availability of the child's first name can be useful tool for a tour director. Personal examples can be included to help direct and maintain the child's attention.

Roll call is another purpose for using name tags in many preschool settings and kindergarten classrooms. These tags can be kept on a bulletin board, or in a small basket at the entrance to a classroom. As children arrive, they put on their name tags. By reviewing the remaining tags, the teacher can determine who is absent at any given time.

Considerations. Preplanning is necessary. Consideration needs to be given to the size of the

CUBBY TAG

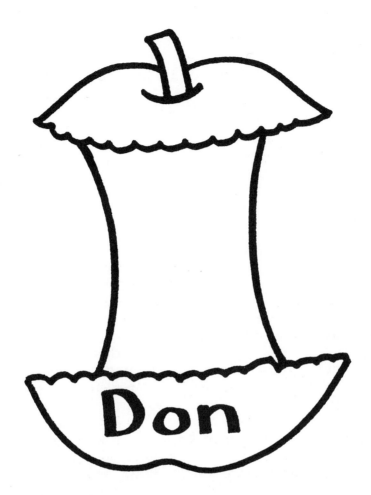

FIGURE I-3

name tag. Tags must be large enough so that the child's name can be easily seen from a distance. On the other hand, name tags can be made too large. When this happens, the name tag can be cumbersome, interfering with the child's comfort and play.

Durability is also important. So it is important to select materials on the basis of durability. In addition, name tags in some centers are planned to coordinate with curriculum themes. For example, the shape of a name tag used during a unit on farm animals may resemble a lamb. Color also needs to be considered. Light colored materials are preferable. They allow legibility when a dark felt-tip marker is used for recording the child's name.

Name tags can be worn either on the front or back of the body. Most teachers prefer the front of the body, allowing the child's name to be visible during group time. This is a particularly important aid for substitute teachers or classroom volunteers.

Attachment of the name tag must be considered. Traditionally, teachers have used a variety of methods. Shoestrings, yarn, thin rope, safety pins and masking tape have all been used. Name tag attachment, like curriculum, should be planned by considering the developmental skills of the children. Consequently, a thin rope, shoestring or yarn allows young children an opportunity to independently put on their own name tag.

There are drawbacks to all types of attachments. Children can independently place over their heads name tags that are attached by shoestrings, yarn and thin rope. However, when displayed by these methods, name tags can be easily pulled and twisted. This could cause a possible irritation or even injury. The drawback of using safety pins is that assistance by adults is required. If the child's clothing is damaged by the pin, parents may complain. While masking tape is probably the safest, it is not permanent; consequently, the tape may have to be replaced

Intro 5

several times per day causing frustration for the child and staff.

Materials. Name tags can be constructed from a wide variety of materials. Disposable identification tags and construction paper are the least durable. Felt, fabric, interfacing, leather, press board and wood are more permanent. You may even prefer using badges or buttons as name tags.

Preparation. The materials selected for the name tags will determine the preparation. A woodburning set can be used for engraving the child's name on leather or wood. Permanent felt-tip markers can be used on felt, fabric, interfacing, paper and press board. A protective spray such as Scotchgard can be applied to fabric to repel dirt and other stains.

Parent Letters

Communications between the child's home and school is important. It builds mutual understanding and cooperation. With the efficiency of modern technology, parent letters are a form of written communication that can be shared on a weekly basis. The most interesting parent letters are written in the active voice. It states the subject did something. To illustrate, "Mark played with blocks and read books today."

When writing the parent letter, consider the parent's educational level. Then write the letter in a clear, friendly, concise style. To do this, eliminate all words that are not needed. Limit the length of the letter to a page or two. To assist you with the process, an example of a parent letter is included for each theme.

Parent letters can be divided into three sections. Included should be a general introduction, school activities and home activities. One way to begin the letter is by introducing new children, staff, or sharing something that happened the previous week. After this, introduce the theme for the coming week by explaining why it was chosen.

The second section of the parent letter could include some of the goals and special activities for the week. Share with the parents all of the interesting things you will be doing at school throughout the week. By having this information, the parent can initiate verbal interaction with their child.

The third section of the parent letter should be related to home activities. Suggest developmentally appropriate activities that the parents can provide in the home. These activities may or may not relate to the theme. Include the words of new songs and fingerplays. This section can also be used to provide parenting information such as the developmental value of specific activities for young children.

Bulletin Boards

Bulletin boards add color, decoration and interest to the classroom. They also communicate what is happening in the classroom to parents and other visitors. The most effective bulletin boards involve the child. That is, the child will manipulate some pieces of the board. As a result, they are called involvement bulletin boards. Through the concrete experience of interacting with the bulletin board materials, children learn a variety of concepts and skills. Included may be size, shape, color, visual discrimination, eye-hand coordination, etc.

Carefully study the bulletin boards included for each theme in this book. They are simple, containing a replica of objects from the child's immediate environment. Each bulletin board has a purpose. It teaches a skill or concept.

As you prepare the bulletin boards provided in this book, you will become more creative. Gradually, you will combine ideas from several bulletin boards as you develop new themes for curriculum.

An opaque projector is a useful tool for individuals who feel uncomfortable with their drawing skills. Using the opaque projector, you can enlarge images from storybooks, coloring books, greeting cards, wrapping paper, etc. To do this, simply place the image to be copied in the projector. Then tape paper or tagboard on the wall. Turn on the projector. Using a pencil, color marker or crayon, trace the outline of the image onto the paper or tagboard.

Another useful tool for preparing bulletin boards is the overhead projector. Place a clear sheet of acetate on the picture desired for enlargement. This may include figures from a coloring or storybook. Trace around the image using a washable marker designed for tranparencies. Project the image onto a wall and follow the same procedures as with the opaque projector.

To make your bulletin board pieces more durable, laminate them. If your center does not have a laminating machine, use clear contact paper. This process works just as well, but it can be more expensive.

Finally, the materials you choose to use on a bulletin board should be safe and durable. Careful attention should be given when selecting attachments. For two-, three- and four-year-old children, adhesive velcro and staples are preferred attachments. Push pins may be used with older children under careful supervision.

Selecting Books

Books for young children need to be selected with care. Before selecting books, once again, refer to the covers and review the typical development for your group of young children. This information can provide a framework for selecting appropriate books.

There are some general guidelines for selecting books. First, children enjoy books that relate to their experiences. They also enjoy action. The words written in the book should be simple, descriptive and within the child's understanding. The pictures should be large, colorful and closely represent the actions.

A book that is good for one group of children may be inappropriate for another. You must know the child or group of children for whom the story is being selected. Consider their interests, attention span and developmental level.

Developmental considerations are important. Two-year-olds enjoy stories about they things they do, know and enjoy. Commonplace adventure is a preference for three-year-olds. They like to listen to things that could happen to them, including stories about community helpers. Four-year-old children are not as self-centered. These children do not have to be part of every situation that they hear about. Many are ready for short and simple fantasy stories. Five-year-olds like stories that add to their knowledge. That is, books that contain new information.

We hope you find this book to be a valuable guide in planning curriculum. The ideas should help you build curriculum based upon the children's natural interests. The book should also give you ideas so that your program will provide a wide variety of choices for children.

In planning a developmentally valid curriculum, consult the table of contents by subject. It has been prepared to allow you easy selection from all the themes. So pick and choose and make it your own! The contents is arranged as follows:

— Art
— Cooking
— Dramatic Play
— Features (by Theme)
— Field Trips/Resource People
— Fingerplays
— Group Time
— Large Muscle
— Math
— Rain Day
— Science
— Sensory
— Songs

Other Sources

Early childhood educators, select from these other Delmar publications for the 1990s.

The World of Child Development: Conception to Adolescence, by George S. Morrison

Early Childhood Experiences in Language Arts: Emerging Literacy, 4th edition, by Jeanne M. Machado

Creative Activities for Young Children, 4th edition, by Mary E. Mayesky, PhD

Math and Science for Young Children, by Rosiland Charlesworth and Karen K. Lind

Growing Up with Literature, by Diana E. Comer

Infants and Toddlers: Curriculum and Teaching, 2nd edition, by Eva Essa, PhD

Administration of Schools for Young Children, 3rd edition, by Phyllis and Donald Click

Developing and Administering a Child Care Center, 2nd edition, by Dorothy June Sciarra and Anne G. Dorsey

Positive Child Guidance, by Darla Ferris Miller

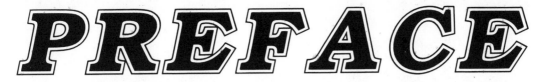

PREFACE

While reviewing early childhood curriculum resources, it becomes apparent that few books are available using a thematic or unit approach for teaching young children. As a result, our university students, colleagues and alumni convinced us of the importance of such a book. Likewise, they convinced us of the contribution the book could make to early childhood teachers and, subsequently, the lives of young children.

Before preparing the manuscript, we surveyed hundreds of day care, preschool and kindergarten teachers. Specifically, we wanted them to share their curriculum problems and concerns. Our response has been to design and write a book tailored to their teaching needs using a thematic approach. Each theme or unit contains a flow-chart, theme goals, concepts for the children to learn, theme related vocabulary words, music, fingerplays, science, dramatic play, arts and crafts, sensory, mathematics, cooking experiences, books and puzzles. Additionally, creative ideas for designing child-involvement bulletin boards, name and cubby tags as well as parent letters have been included. All of these resources were identified, by the teachers included in our survey, as being critical components that have been lacking in other curriculum guides.

In addition to the themes included in this book, many others can be developed for teaching young children. Due to limitations of space, only the most popular themes have been developed. The authors, however, wish to caution the readers that it is the classroom teacher's responsibility to select, plan and introduce developmentally appropriate themes and learning experiences for his group of children. Specifically, the adult must tailor the curriculum to meet the individual needs of the children. Consequently, we encourage all teachers to carefully select, adapt or change any of the activities in this book to meet the needs, abilities and interests of their group of children to ensure developmental appropriateness. The inside covers of this book can be used as handy references for checking developmental norms.

As you study this guide, you will note that some themes readily lend themselves to particular curriculum areas. As a result, the number of activities listed under each curriculum area will vary from theme to theme.

The detailed introduction is designed to help teachers use the book most effectively. It includes:

1. a discussion on how to develop the curriculum using a thematic approach;
2. a list of possible themes;
3. techniques for making name tags;
4. suggestions for writing parent letters;
5. methods for constructing and evaluating creative involvement bulletin boards; and
6. criteria for selecting children's books.

This book would not have been possible without the constant encouragement provided by our families, the laboratory teachers in the Child and Family Study Center, and the faculty, students and alumni of the University of Wisconsin-Stout. Our thanks to all of these people and especially to Carla Ahmann, Candy Aruthur, Mary Babula, Grace Bahr, Terry Bloomberg, Margaret Braun, Renee Bruce, Anne Budde, Diane Carriveau, Michelle Case, Thelma Caturia, Patti Coker, Bruce Cunningham, Jeanette Daines, Carol Davenport, Jill Davis, Linda DeMoe, Rita Pittman Devery, Donna Dixon, Paulette Fontaine, Lisa Fuerst, Shirley Gebhart, Judy Gifford, Nancy Graese, Barbara Grundleger, Patti Herman, John Herr, Mark Herr, Joan Herwig, Priscilla Huffman, Margy Ingram, Paula Iverson, Judy Jax, Brenda Johnson, Angela LaBonne Kaiser, Julia Lorenz, Beth Libby, Janet Maffet, Janet Massa, Nancy McCarthy, Julie Meyers, Teresa Mitchell, Laura Moran, LaVonne Mueller, Gerri Mundschau, Paula Noll, Mary Pugmire, Kelli Railton, Pat Resinger, Lori Singerhouse Register, Melba Rolland, Peg Saienga, J. Anthony Samenfink, Kathy Rucker Schaeffer, Mary Selkey, Cheryl Smith, Sue Smith, Mary Ann Spangler, Amy Sprengler, Karen Stephens, Barbara Suihkonen, Judy Teske, Connie Weber, Mary Eileen Zenk and Karen Zimmerman. We are also grateful to our reviewers: Jane L. French, Catherine L. Carnavos, Ruth Steinbrunner, Alice P. Eyman, Carole Newkirk, Patti C. Issacs, M. C. Pugmire-Stoy, and Marjorie J. Kosatelnik. Finally, our special thanks to two individuals whose assistance made this book possible. Jay Whitney, our editor from Delmar, provided continous encouragement, support, and creative suggestions. Also, special thanks to Robin Muza, our typist and research assistant.

APPLES

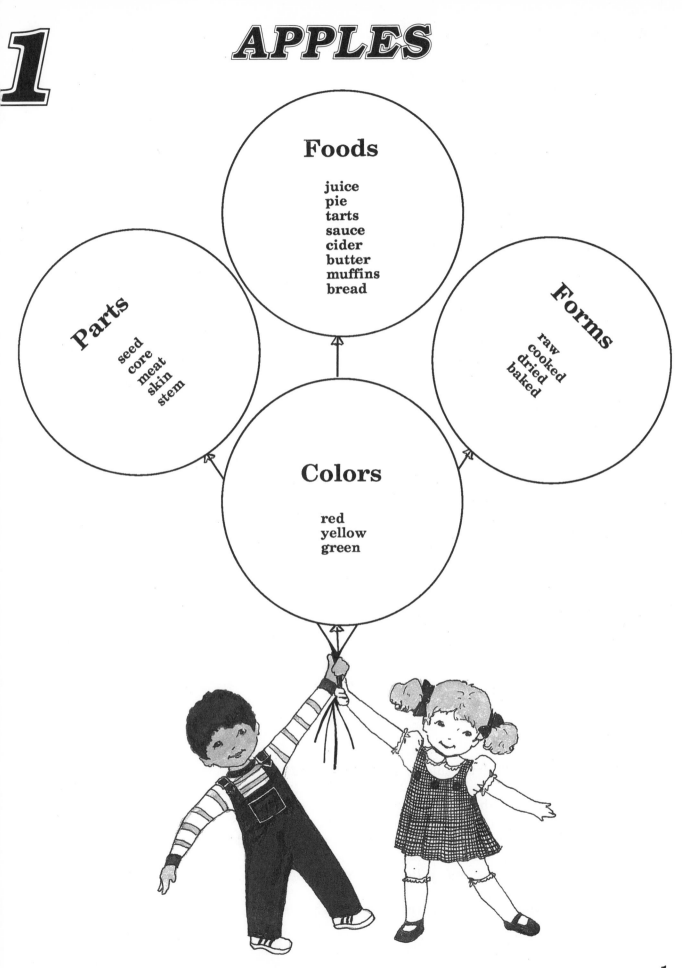

Foods

juice
pie
tarts
sauce
cider
butter
muffins
bread

Parts

seed
core
meat
skin
stem

Forms

raw
cooked
dried
baked

Colors

red
yellow
green

Theme Goals:

Through participating in the experiences provided by this theme, the children may learn:

1. Parts of an apple.

2. Preparation of apples for eating.

3. Apple tastes.

4. Textures, sizes and colors of apples.

5. The origin of an apple.

Concepts for the Children to Learn:

1. An apple is a fruit.

2. An apple has five parts: seed, core, meat, skin, and stem.

3. Apples grow on trees.

4. A group of apple trees is an orchard.

5. Bread, butter, pies, pudding, applesauce, dumplings, butter and jelly can be prepared from apples.

6. Some apples are sweet; others are sour.

7. Apples can be green, yellow or red.

8. Apples can be large or small.

9. Apples can be hard or soft.

10. Seeds from an apple can grow into a tree.

Vocabulary:

1. **apple**—a fruit that is grown on a tree.

2. **texture**—how something feels.

3. **core**—the part of the apple that contains seeds.

4. **apple blossom**—a flower on the apple tree.

5. **apple butter**—a spread for bread made from apples.

Bulletin Board

The purpose of this bulletin board is to develop the mathematical skill of sets, as well as to identify written numerals. Construct red apples. The number will depend upon the developmental level of the children. Laminate the apples. Collect containers for baskets, such as large cottage cheese or pint berry containers. Cover the containers with paper if necessary. Affix numerals on baskets, beginning with the numeral 1. Staple the baskets to the bulletin board. The object is for the children to place the appropriate number of apples in each basket.

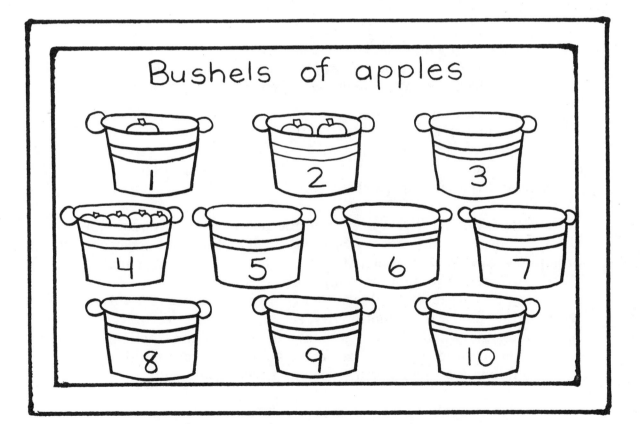

Parent Letter

Dear Parents,

Is it true that "an apple a day keeps the doctor away?" I'm not sure, but the children will make many discoveries as we begin a new unit on apples this week at school. Through active exploration and interaction, they will become more aware of the different flavors of apples, colors of apples, and ways apples can be prepared and eaten.

At School This Week

Some of this week's classroom activities include:

* preparing applesauce for Thursday's snack.
* drying apples in the sun.
* creating apple prints in the art area.
* visiting the apple orchard! Arrangements have been made for a tour of the apple orchard on Wednesday morning. We will be leaving the center at 10:00 a.m. Feel free to join us.

At Home

Apples are a tasty and nutritious food—and most children enjoy eating them. This week try a variety of apples for meals or snacks. You might also enjoy preparing caramel apples with your child. A recipe is as follows:

1 pound of vanilla caramels
2 tablespoons of water
dash of salt
6 crisp apples
6 wooden skewers or popsicle sticks

Melt the caramels with water in a microwave oven or double boiler, stirring frequently until smooth. Stir in the salt and stick a wooden skewer or popsicle stick in each apple. Dip the apple into the syrup, turning until the surface of the apple is completely covered.

Cooking is a great way to learn by experience because it involves the whole child—physically, emotionally, socially and intellectually. It also builds vocabulary and involves amounts, measuring and fractions which are mathematical concepts. When a recipe is used, your child will also learn to follow a sequence. Enjoy cooking with your child.

Have a good week!

Music:

1. "If I Had an Apple"
(Sing to the tune of "If I Had a Hammer")

If I had an apple
I'd eat it in the morning,
I'd eat it in the evening,
All over this land.
I'd eat it for breakfast,
I'd eat it for supper,
I'd eat it with all my friends and sisters
and brothers
All, all over this land.

Source: *Creative Activities for Young Children*. Mimi Brodsky Chenfeld.

2. "Little Apples"
(Sing to the tune of "Ten Little Indians")

One little, two little, three little apples,
Four little, five little, six little apples,
Seven little, eight little, nine little apples,
All fell to the ground.

A variation for older children would be to give each child a number card (with a numeral from 1 through 9). When that number is sung, that child stands up. At the end of the fingerplay all the children fall down.

3. "Apples Off My Tree"
(Sing to the tune of "Skip to My Lou")

Pick some apples off my tree,
Pick some apples off my tree,
Pick some apples off my tree,
Pick them all for you and me.

4. "My Apple Tree"
(Sing to the tune of "The Muffin Man")

Did you see my apple tree,
Did you see my apple tree,
Did you see my apple tree,
Full of apples red?

Fingerplays:

APPLE TREE

Way up high in the apple tree
  (stretch arm up high)
Two little apples smiled at me.
  (hold up 2 fingers)
I shook that tree as hard as I could
  (make shaking motion)
Down came the apples.
  (make downward motions)
Mmmm—they were good.
  (smile and rub stomach)

PICKING APPLES

Here's a little apple tree.
  (left arm up, fingers spread)
I look up and I can see
  (look at fingers)
Big red apples, ripe and sweet,
  (cup hands to hold apple)
Big red apples, good to eat!
  (raise hands to mouth)
Shake the little apple tree.
  (shake tree with hands)
See the apples fall on me.
  (raise cupped hands and let fall)
Here's a basket, big and round.
  (make circle with arms)
Pick the apples from the ground.
  (pick and put in basket)
Here's an apple I can see.
  (look up to the tree)
I'll reach up. It's ripe and sweet.
  (reach up to upper hand)
That's the apple I will eat!
  (hands to mouth)

AN APPLE

An apple is what I'd like to be.
My shape would be round.
  (fingers in circular shape)
My color would be green
  (point to something green)
Children could eat me each and every day.
I'm good in tarts and pies and cakes
  (make these foodshapes)
An apple is good to eat or to bake
  (make stirring motion)

5

THE APPLE

Within its polished universe
The apple holds a star.
  (draw design of star with index finger)
A secret constellation
To scatter near and far.
  (point near and far)
Let a knife discover
Where the five points hide.
Split the shiny ruby
And find the star inside.

After introducing the fingerplay the
teacher can cut an apple crosswise to find
a star.

APPLE TREE

This is the tree
With leaves so green.
  (make leaves with fingers outstretched)
Here are the apples
That hang inbetween.
  (make fist)
When the wind blows
  (blow)
The apples will fall.
  (falling motion with hand)
Here is the basket to gather them all.
  (use arms to form basket)

Sensory:

1. Cut different varieties of apples for a
tasting party. This activity can easily be
extended. On another day provide the
children applesauce, apple pie, apple juice, or
apple cider to taste during snack or lunch.

2. Place several different kinds of seeds on the
sensory table. In addition, to create interest
provide scoops, bowls, and bottles to fill.

Math:

1. Cut apple shapes of various sizes from construction paper. Let the children sequence
the shapes from smallest to largest.

2. Place a scale and various sized apples on
the math table. The children can experiment by weighing the apples.

Science:

1. **Solar Baked Apple Slices**

   Materials: 4 styrofoam cups
              black paper
              scissors
              masking tape
              apple
              knife
              plastic wrap
              rubber bands
              white paper
              foil
              newspaper

   Line 2 cups with black paper. Place 2
   equal-sized slices of apple inside each cup.
   Cover with plastic wrap held by rubber
   band. With paper and tape make a cone.
   Place one apple cup into it. Cover the
   inside of another paper cone with
   aluminum foil and place second apple cup
   into it. Place both in a sunny window
   facing the sun on crumpled newspaper.
   Which one cooks faster? The apple baked
   in the aluminum foil.

   Source: *Nature With Children of All Ages.*
   Edith A. Sisson.

2. **Dried Apples**

   Peel, core, and cut apples into slices or
   rings about 1/8 inch thick. Prepare a salt
   water solution by mixing a tablespoon of
   salt in a gallon of water for several minutes.
   Place the apples in this solution. Place the
   apples in 180-degree oven for 3 to 4 hours
   or until dry. Turn the apples occasionally.

3. **Oxidation of an Apple**

   Cut and core an apple into sections. Dip
   half the apple into lemon juice and place it
   on a plate. Place the remaining sections of
   apple on another plate. What happens to
   each plate of apples? Discuss the effects of
   the lemon juice coating which keeps
   oxygen from the apples. As a result, they
   do not discolor as rapidly.

4. **Explore an Apple**

   Discuss the color, size, and shape of an
   apple. Then discuss the parts of an apple.

Include the skin, stem, core, meat, etc. Feel the apple. Then cut the apple in half. Observe the core and seeds. An apple is a fruit because it contains seeds.

Dramatic Play:

Set Up an Apple Stand

Prepare an apple stand by providing the children with bags, plastic apples, cash register, money, stand, bushels. Encourage buying, selling, and packaging.

Arts and Crafts:

1. Apple Printing

Cut apples in half. Place them in individual shallow pans of red, yellow, and green tempera paint. Provide paper. The apple can be used as a painting tool. To illustrate, the children can place an apple half in the paint. After shaving off the excess paint, the apple can be placed on paper creating a print.

2. Seed Pictures

Collect: apple seeds along with other seeds
    paper
    colors
    glue

Each child who chooses to participate should be provided a small amount of seeds. As they are distributed, discuss the seeds' similarities and differences. Provide uninterrupted time for the children to glue seeds onto paper and create pictures.

3. Shakers

Collect: appleseeds
    paper plates (2 per child)
    glue or stapler
    color crayons or felt-tip markers

The children can decorate the paper plates with color crayons or felt-tip markers. After this, the seeds can be placed between the two plates. To create the shakers, staple or glue the two plates together by securing the outer edges of the plates. The children can use the shakers as a means of self expression during music or self-directed play.

Field Trips/Resource People:

1. Visit an Apple Orchard

Observe the workers picking, sorting, and/or selling the apples. Call attention to the colors and types of apples.

2. Visit a Grocery Store

Observe all the forms of apples sold in a grocery store. Also, in the produce department, observe the different colors and sizes of apples. To show children differences in weight, take a large apple and place on a scale. Note the weight. Then take a small apple and repeat the process.

Group Time (games, language):

1. What Is It?

Collect a variety of fruits such as an apple, banana and orange. Begin by placing one fruit in a bag. Choose a child to touch the fruit, describe it and name it. Repeat with each fruit, discussing the characteristics. During the activity each child should have an opportunity to participate.

2. Transition Activity

The children should stand in a circle. As a record is played, the children pass an apple. When the record stops, the child holding the apple can get up to get a snack, put on outdoor clothes, clean up, etc. Continue until all children have a turn. For older children, more than one apple may be successfully passed at a time.

Cooking:

1. Caramel Apple Slices

Prepare the following recipe which should serve 12 to 14 children.

1 pound caramels
2 tablespoons water
dash of salt
6 crisp apples

Melt caramels with water in the microwave oven or double boiler, stirring frequently until melted. Stir in the salt. Pour the melted caramel over the sliced apples and cool before serving.

2. Applesauce

30 large apples
2 1/2 cups water
1 1/2 cups sugar
1 tablespoon red hots

1. Clean apples by peeling, coring, and cutting into small pieces.
2. Place the apples in a large kettle containing water.
3. Simmer the apples on low heat, stirring occasionally until soft.
4. Add the remaining ingredients.
5. Stir and simmer a few minutes.
6. Cool prior to eating.

3. Persian Apple Dessert

3 medium apples, cut up
2 to 3 tablespoons sugar
2 tablespoons lemon juice
dash of salt

Place half the apples and the remaining ingredients in a blender. Cover and blend until coarsely chopped, about 20 to 30 seconds. Add remaining apples and repeat. Makes 3 servings.

4. Charoses

6 medium apples
1/2 cup raisins
1/2 teaspoon cinnamon
1/2 cup chopped nuts
1/4 cup white grape juice

Chop the peeled or unpeeled apples. Add the remaining ingredients. Mix well and serve.

5. Fruit Leather

2 cups applesauce
vegetable shortening or oil

Preheat oven to 400 degrees. Pour applesauce onto greased shallow pan. Spread to 1/8 inch in thickness. Place pan in oven and lower temperature to 180-degrees. Cook for approximately 3 hours until the leather can be peeled from the pan. Cut with scissors to serve.

6. Dried Apples

5 or 6 apples
2 tablespoons salt
water

Peel, core, and cut apples into slices or rings 1/8 inch thick. Place apple slices in salt-water solution (2 tablespoons per 1 gallon water) for several minutes. Place in 180-degree oven for 3 to 4 hours until dry. Turn apples occasionally.

Books and Stories:

The following books and stories can be used to complement this theme:

1. **The Story of Johnny Appleseed.** Aliki. (Englewood Cliffs, NJ: Prentice Hall, 1963).

2. **Apple.** Nonny Hogrogian. (New York: Macmillan, 1972).

3. **Rain Makes Apple Sauce.** Julian Scheer. (New York: Holiday House, 1968).

4. **Ten Apples Up On Top.** Theodore LeSieg. (New York: Beginner Books, 1961).

5. **Apple Orchard.** Irmengarde Eberle. (New York: Henry Z. Walck, Inc., 1962).

6. **Apples, How They Grow.** Bruce McMillan (Boston: Houghton Mifflin, 1979).

7. **The Apple and the Moth.** Iela Maria and Enzo Mari. (New York: Pantheon, 1970).

Puzzles:

The following puzzles can be found in preschool educational catalogs:

1. **"Fruits"** Judy/Instructo.

2. **"Familiar Things"** Lauri.

3. **"Knobbed Fruit Puzzle"** 4 pieces. Constructive Playthings.

4. **"Apple"** 5 pieces. Constructive Playthings.

5. **"Eating An Apple"** 4 pieces. Puzzle People.

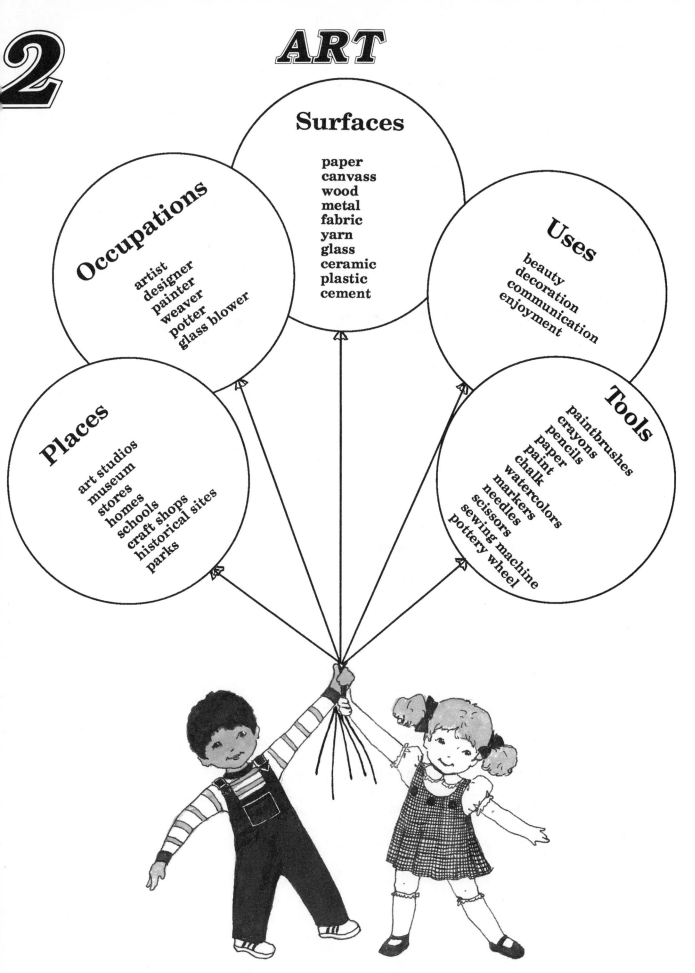

ART

Surfaces

paper
canvass
wood
metal
fabric
yarn
glass
ceramic
plastic
cement

Occupations

artist
designer
painter
weaver
potter
glass blower

Uses

beauty
decoration
communication
enjoyment

Places

art studios
museum
stores
homes
schools
craft shops
historical sites
parks

Tools

paintbrushes
crayons
pencils
paper
paint
chalk
watercolors
markers
needles
scissors
sewing machine
pottery wheel

11

Theme Goals:

Through participating in the experiences provided by this theme, the children may learn:

1. The uses of art.

2. Places where works of art can be found.

3. Art tools.

4. Surfaces used for art.

5. Occupations associated with art.

Concepts for the Children to Learn:

1. Art is an expression of feelings and thoughts.

2. Brushes, paints, pencils, felt-tip markers, crayons, chalk and paper are all art tools.

3. An artist uses art tools to make designs, pictures or sculptures.

4. Art is a form of communication.

5. A museum has art objects.

6. An art gallery sells art objects.

7. Paper, canvas and wood can all be painted.

Vocabulary:

1. **art**—a form of beauty.

2. **crayon**—an art tool made of wax.

3. **paint**—a colored liquid used for decoration.

4. **paintbrush**—a tool for applying paint.

5. **chalk**—a soft stone used for writing or drawing.

6. **artist**—a person who creates art.

7. **gallery**—a place to display works of art.

Bulletin Board

The purpose of this bulletin board is to reinforce color matching skills. Construct a crayon match bulletin board by drawing sixteen crayons on white tagboard. Divide the crayons into pairs. Color each pair of crayons a different color. Include the colors pink, red, blue, yellow, purple, orange, brown and green. Hang one from each pair on the top of the bulletin board and attach a corresponding colored string from the crayons. Hang the second set of crayons on the lower end of the bulletin board. A push pin can be added to the bottom set of crayons and the children can match the top crayons to their corresponding match on the bottom of the bulletin board.

Adjust the bulletin board to match the developmental needs and level of the children. For younger children, use fewer color choices. Let the children use the bulletin board during self-directed and self-initiated play periods. Repetition of this activity is important for assimilation providing it is child initiated.

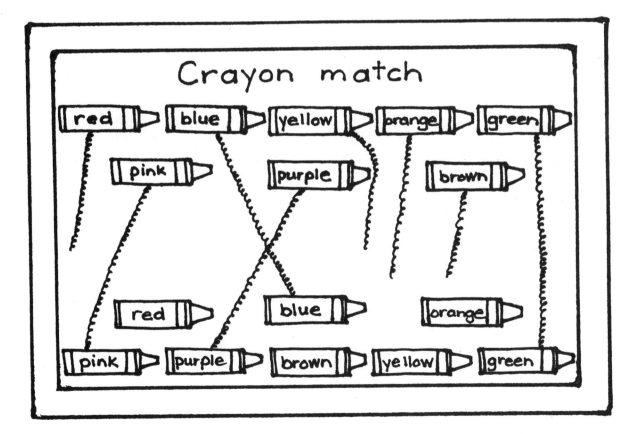

Parent Letter

Dear Parents,

Art is an expressive and aesthetic activity. It is also the theme that we will be focusing on this week. The children will be exploring many different types of art tools and supplies. In addition they will learn where works of art can be found. Throughout the week the works of art produced by the children will be saved to display in an outdoor art gallery on Thursday. You are invited to browse when you pick up your child from the center.

At School This Week

Some of the artistic experiences planned for the week include:

* creating chalk murals on the sidewalk.
* staging an art gallery in the dramatic play area.
* visiting on Tuesday with Bob Jones, a tour guide at the city museum. Mr. Jones will be sharing several art objects with us in our classroom.
* sorting art tools.
* participating in a wide variety of art activities.

At Home:

You can introduce the concepts of this unit into your home by collecting art tools and exploring them together. A fun art idea is to paint on paper using kitchen tools as applicators. Forks, potato mashers and slotted spoons all work well for this activity. Through this and other art activities your child will discover interesting and creative ways to use materials. Art also provides opportunities to experiment with color.

Have a great week!

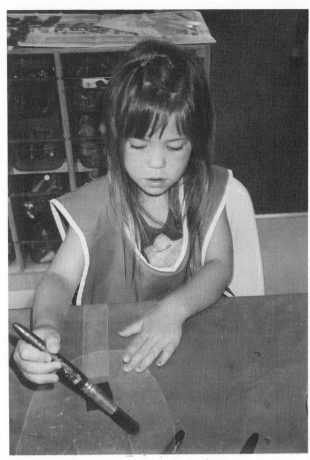

FIGURE 2 Art is a fun activity.

Music:

"Let's Pretend"
(Sing to the tune of "Here We Are Together")

Let's pretend that we are artists,
are artists, are artists.
Let's pretend that we are artists
How happy we'll be.
We'll paint with our brushes,
and draw with our crayons.
Let's pretend that we are artists
How happy we'll be.

Fingerplays:

CLAY

I stretch it.
  (pulling motion)
I pound it.
  (pounding motion)
I make it firm.
  (pushing motion)

I roll it.
  (rolling motion)
I pinch it.
  (pinching motion)
I make a worm.
  (wiggling motion)

PAINTING

Hands are blue.
  (look at outstretched hands)
Hands are green.
Fingers are red,
Inbetween.
  (wiggle fingers)
Paint on my face.
  (touch face)
Paint on my smock.
  (touch smock)
Paint on my shoes.
  (touch shoes)
Paint on my socks.
  (touch socks)

Social Studies:

The Feel of Color

This activity can be introduced at large group time. Begin by collecting colored construction paper. Individually hold each color up and ask the children how that particular color makes them feel. Adjectives that may be used include: hot, cold, cheerful, warm, sad, tired, happy, clean.

Group Time (games, language):

Towards the end of the unit, collect all art projects and display them in an art gallery at your center. The children can help hang their own projects and decide where to have the gallery. If weather permits, the art gallery can be set up on the playground using low clotheslines and easels to display the art. If weather does not permit, a gallery can be set up in the classroom or center lobby, using walls and tables to display the art.

Cooking:

GRAHAM CRACKER TREAT

Give each child a graham cracker, honey and a brush to spread the honey. Top with grated cheese, raisins or coconut.

COOKIE DECORATING

Sugar cookies can be purchased commercially or baked and decorated. Recipes for the cookies and frosting are as follows:

1. Drop Sugar Cookies

2 eggs
2/3 cup vegetable oil
2 teaspoons vanilla
3/4 cup sugar
2 cups flour
2 teaspoons baking powder
1/2 teaspoon salt

Beat eggs with fork. Stir in oil and vanilla. Blend in sugar until mixture thickens. Add flour, baking powder and salt. Mix well. Drop dough by teaspoons about 2 inches apart on an ungreased baking sheet. Flatten with the bottom of a plastic glass dipped in sugar. Bake 8 to 10 minutes or until delicate brown. Remove from baking sheet immediately. Makes about 4 dozen cookies that are 2 1/2 inches in diameter.

2. Favorite Icing

1 cup sifted confectioner's sugar
1/4 teaspoon salt
1/2 teaspoon vanilla
1 tablespoon water
food coloring

Blend salt, sugar and vanilla. Add enough water to make frosting easy to spread. Tint with food coloring. Allow children to spread on cookie with spatula or paintbrush.

Science:

1. Art Tools

A variety of art tools can be placed on the science table. Included may be brushes, pencils, felt-tip markers, crayons and chalk. The children can observe, smell and feel the difference in the tools.

2. Charcoal

Place charcoal pieces and magnifying glasses on the science table.

3. Rock Writing

Provide the children with a variety of soft rocks. The children can experiment drawing on the sidewalks with them.

Dramatic Play:

1. Artist

Artist's hats, smocks, easels, and paint tables can be placed in the dramatic play area. The children can use the materials to pretend they are artists.

2. Art Gallery

Mount pictures from magazines on sheets of tagboard. Let the children hang the pictures around the classroom. A cash register and play money for buying and selling the paintings can extend the play.

Arts and Crafts:

1. Frames

During the course of this unit, the children can frame, with your assistance, their works of art by mounting them on sheets of colored tagboard and trimming it to a frame-like border. Older children may be able to do this unassisted. Display the works of art in the lobby, classroom—or outdoors, if weather permits.

2. Experimenting

In a unit on art, many kinds of art media need to be explored. Include the following art experiences:

* markers (both jumbo and skinny)
* chalk (both wet and dry)
* charcoal
* pencils (both colored and lead)
* crayons (jumbo, regular sized and shavings)
* paint (watercolors, tempera, fingerpaint)
* paper (colored construction, white, typing, tissue, newsprint, fingerpaint, tagboard)
* other (tinfoil, cotton, glitter, glue and paste, lace, scraps, crepe paper, bags, waxed paper, yarn and string)
* tools for painting (marbles, string, fingers, brushes of all sizes, straws, sponges)
* playdough and clay
* printing tools (stamps and ink pads, kitchen tools, sponges, potatoes, apples and carrot ends)
* seeds

Sensory:

Additions to the Sensory Table

1. goop

Mix together food coloring, 1 cup cornstarch and 1 cup water in the sensory table. If a larger quantity is desired, double or triple the recipe.

2. silly putty

Mix food coloring, 1 cup liquid starch and 2 cups of glue together. Stir constantly until the ingredients are well mixed. Add more starch as needed.

3. wet sand and sand mold containers

Large Muscle:

1. Sidewalk Chalk

Washable colored chalk can be provided for the children to use outside on the sidewalk. After the activity the designs can be removed with a hose. The children may even enjoy using scrub brushes to remove the design.

2. Painting

Provide large paintbrushes and buckets of water for the children to paint the sidewalks, walls and fences surrounding your center or school.

3. Foot Art

Prepare a thick tempera paint and pour a small amount in a shallow pan. Roll out long sheets of paper. The children can take off their shoes and socks, step into the tempera paint, and walk or dance across the sheets of paper. Provide buckets with soapy water and towels at the end of the paper for the children to wash their feet. Dry the foot paintings and send them home with the children.

Field Trips/Resource People:

1. Museum

Take a field trip to a museum, if one is available. Observe art objects. Point out and discuss color and form.

2. Art Store

Take a walk to a nearby art store. Observe the many kinds of pencils, markers, crayons, paints and other art supplies that are available.

3. Resource People

Invite the following people to show the children their artwork.

* painter
* potter
* weaver
* glass blower
* sculptor

Math:

1. Counting Cans

Counting cans for this unit can be made from empty soup cans with filed edges. On each can write a numeral. The number prepared will depend upon the developmental needs of the children. Then provide an equal number of the following objects: pencils, pens, markers, paintbrushes, crayons, chalk sticks, sponges, etc. The object is for the children to relate the number of objects to numerals on the can.

2. Measuring Art Tools

Art tools come in all different lengths. Provide a variety of art tools and rulers, or a tape measure that has been taped to the table. The children can measure the objects to find which one is the longest. Make a chart showing the longest tool and continuing to the shortest.

3. Sorting Art Supplies

A large ice cream pail can be used to hold pencils, pens, markers, crayons, glue bottles, etc. that can be sorted into shoeboxes.

PAINTING SURFACES

There are many types of interesting surfaces that children can successfully use for painting. The list of possibilities are only limited by ones' imagination. Included are:

construction paper	shelf paper	mirror
newsprint (plain/printed)	paper table cloths	plexi-glass
tissue paper	paper place mats	paper bags
tracing paper	waxed paper	cookie sheets
tin foil	boxes	meat trays—plastic,
clear/colored acetate	leather scrap	cardboard, styrofoam
wood	sand paper	table surfaces
cardboard	paper toweling	

Records:

The following records can be found in preschool educational catalogs:

1. **Color a Song.** Linda Tsuruoka and Jacqueline Pliskin.

2. **I Know the Colors in the Rainbow.** Ella Jenkins.

3. **There's Music in the Colors.** Kimbo Records.

Books and Stories:

The following books and stories can be used to complement this theme:

1. **Harold and the Purple Crayon.** Crockett Johnson. (New York: Harper and Row, 1955).

3. **Picasso.** Elizabeth Ripley. (New York: J.B. Lippincott Co., 1959).

4. **I Want to Paint My Bathroom Blue.** Ruth Krauss. (New York: Harper and Row, 1956).

5. **This Thumbprint.** Ruth Krauss. (New York: Harper and Row, 1967).

6. **Harold's Circus.** Crockett Johnson. (New York: Scholastic, 1959).

7. **Spence Makes Circles.** Christa Chevalier. (Niles, IL: Albert Whitman and Co., 1982).

8. **Cherries and Cherry Pits.** Vera B. Williams. (New York: Scholastic, 1986).

9. **A Ball of Clay.** John Hawkinson. (Niles, IL: Albert Whitman and Co., 1974).

10. **Arts of Clay.** Christine Price. (New York: Charles Scribner's Sons, 1977).

11. **Emma.** Wendy Kesselman. (New York: Doubleday, 1980).

12. **The Penquin's Paint.** Valerie Tripp. (Chicago: Childrens Press, 1987).

13. **What Can You Make of It?** F. Brandenburg. (New York: Greenwillow Books, 1977).

14. **Chalk Box Story.** D. Freeman (New York: J. B. Lippincott, 1976).

15. **Mystery of the Stolen Blue Paint.** S. Kellogg. (New York: Dial, 1982).

Puzzles:

The following puzzles can be found in preschool educational catalogs:

1. **"Crayons"** Judy/Instructo.

2. **"School"** Judy/Instructo.

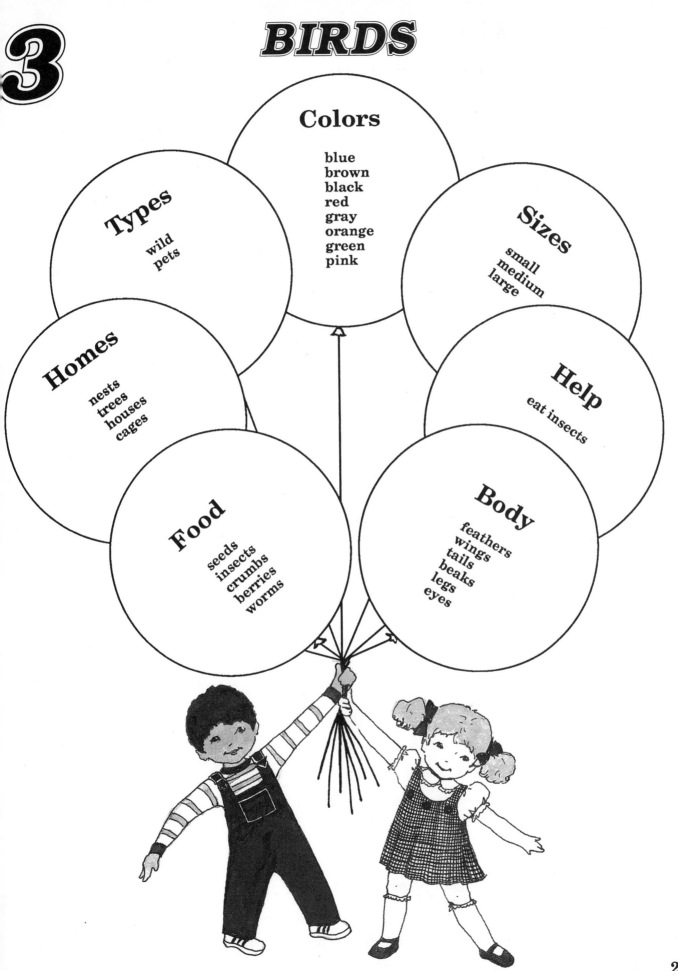

3 BIRDS

Colors

blue
brown
black
red
gray
orange
green
pink

Types

wild
pets

Sizes

small
medium
large

Homes

nests
trees
houses
cages

Help

eat insects

Food

seeds
insects
crumbs
berries
worms

Body

feathers
wings
tails
beaks
legs
eyes

Theme Goals:

Through participating in the experiences provided by this theme, the children may learn:

1. The bird's body parts.
2. Types of birds.
3. Bird homes.
4. Foods that birds eat.
5. Ways birds help.
6. Sizes of birds.
7. Colors of birds.

Concepts for the Children to Learn:

1. There are many kinds of birds.
2. Birds hatch from eggs.
3. Birds have feathers, wings and beaks.
4. Most birds fly.
5. Birds live in nests, trees, houses and cages.
6. Some birds are pets.
7. Many birds make sounds.
8. Birds eat seeds, insects, crumbs and worms.
9. Some birds eat fish.
10. Some birds help us by eating insects.

Vocabulary:

1. **beak**—the part around a bird's mouth.
2. **bird watching**—watching birds.
3. **bird feeder**—a container for bird food.
4. **feathers**—covers skin of a bird.
5. **hatch**—to come from an egg.
6. **nest**—bed or home prepared by a bird.
7. **perch**—a pole for a bird to stand on.
8. **wing**—movable body part that helps most birds fly.

Bulletin Board

The purpose of this bulletin board is to develop skills in matching a set to its corresponding numeral. To construct the board, cut ten bird nests out of brown colored tagboard. Draw a set of dots, beginning with one on each bird nest. Tack the nest on the bulletin board. Next, construct the same number of birds out of tagboard. On each bird, write a numeral beginning with one. By matching the numeral on each bird to the number of dots on the nests, the children can help each bird find a home. The number of birds and nests on this bulletin board should match the children's developmental needs.

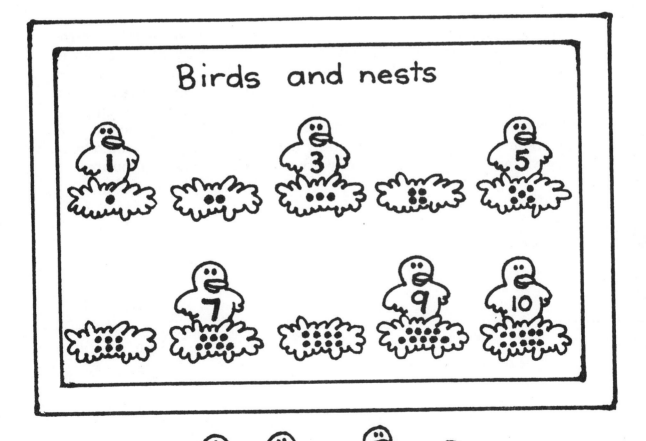

Parent Letter

Dear Parents,

This week our class will be discussing our "feathered friends"—birds! The children will be introduced to birds kept as pets and birds in the wild. In addition they will discover the unique body parts of birds and the homes in which they live.

At School This Week

Some of the activities planned for the unit on birds include:

* observing different types of bird nests with a magnifying glass at the science table.
* visiting with Jodi's pet canary on Wednesday.
* creating collages using birdseed and glue in the art area.
* making bird feeders to hang outdoors in our play yard.

At Home

Whether you live in the city or country, chances are there are birds nearby. The following game may be fun to play with your child. Set an egg or kitchen timer for three to five minutes. Then look out the window and see how many birds you can see. For each bird, drop a button in a jar. When the timer goes off, count how many buttons are in the jar. This game will strengthen your child's observation skills and increase his understanding of number concepts. Variations of this game would be to observe for cars, squirrels, or any other object that can be counted.

Happy bird watching!

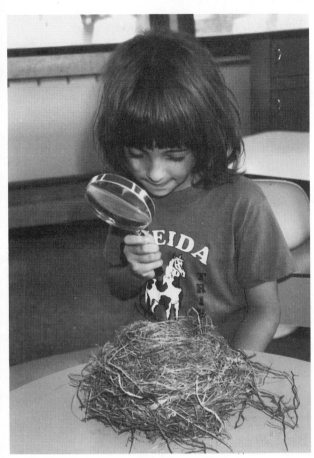

FIGURE 3 Investigating a bird's nest.

Music:

1. **"Birds"**
   (Sing to the tune of "Here We Go Round the Mulberry Bush")
   The first verse remains the same, with the children walking around in a circle holding hands.

   This is the way we scratch for worms.
     (children move foot in a scratching motion like a chicken)
   This is the way we peck our food.
     (children peck)
   This is the way we sit on our eggs.
     (children squat down)
   This is the way we flap our wings.
     (bend arms at elbows, and put thumbs under armpit, flap)
   This is the way we fly away.
     (children can "fly" anywhere they want, but return to the circle at the end of the verse)

2. **"Pretty Birds"**
   (Sing to the tune of "Ten Little Indians")

   One pretty, two pretty
   Three pretty birdies.
   Four pretty, five pretty,
   Six pretty birdies.
   Seven pretty, eight pretty,
   Nine pretty birdies,
   All sitting in a tree.

Fingerplays:

THE DUCK

   I waddle when I walk.
     (hold arms and elbows high and twist trunk side to side or squat down)
   I quack when I walk
     (place palm together and open and close)
   And I have webbed toes on my feet.
     (spread fingers wide)
   Rain coming down, makes me smile, not frown
     (smile)
   And I dive for something to eat.
     (put hands together and make diving motion)

   Source: *Action Verse for Early Childhood.* Hillert, Margaret. (Minneapolis, T.S. Denison and Co. Inc., 1982).

THE OWL

   There's a wide-eyed owl
     (encircle each eye with thumb and forefinger)
   With a pointed nose.
     (direct forefingers to a point down side of nose)
   And two pointed ears
     (extend forefingers up from top of head)
   And claws for toes.
     (curve fingers like claws)
   He lives high in a tree.
     (point overhead)
   When he looks at you.
     (point to another child)
   He flaps his wings
     (bend elbows and flap arms like wings)
   And says "whoo, whoo, whoo."

   Source: *Action Verse for Early Childhood.* Hillert, Margaret. (Minneapolis; T.S. Denison and Co. Inc., 1982).

HOUSES

Here is a nest for a robin.
  (cup both hands)
Here is a hive for a bee.
  (fists together)
Here is a hole for the bunny;
  (finger and thumb make circle)
And here is a house for me!
  (fingertips together to make roof)

TWO LITTLE BLACKBIRDS

Two little blackbirds sitting on a hill,
  (close fists, extend index fingers)
One named Jack. One named Jill.
  (talk to one finger; talk to other finger)
Fly away Jack. Fly away Jill.
  (toss index fingers over shoulder separately)
Come back, Jack. Come back Jill.
  (bring back hands separately with index
  fingers extended)

BIRD FEEDER

Here is the bird feeder. Here, seeds and
crumbs.
  (left hand out flat, right hand cupped)
Sprinkle them on and see what comes.
  (sprinkling motion with right hand over
  left hand)
One cardinal, one chickadee, one junco,
one jay,
  (join fingers of right hand and peck at
  the bird feeder once for each bird)
Four of my bird friends are eating today.
  (hold up four fingers of left hand)

IF I WERE A BIRD

If I were a bird, I'd sing a song
And fly about the whole day long
  (twine thumbs together and move hands
  like wings)
And when the night comes, go to rest,
  (tilt head and close eyes)
Up in my cozy little nest.
  (cup hands together to form nest)

TAP TAP TAP

Tap, tap, tap goes the woodpecker
  (tap with right pointer finger on inside
  of left wrist)
As he pecks a hole in a tree.
  (make hole with pointer finger and thumb)
He is making a house with a window
To peep at you and me.
  (hold circle made with finger and thumb
  in front of eye)

STRETCH, STRETCH

Stretch, stretch away up high:
On your tiptoes, reach the sky.
See the bluebirds flying high.
  (wave hands)
Now bend down and touch your toes.
Now sway as the North Wind blows.
Waddle as the gander goes!

Science:

1. **Bird Feeders**

   Make bird feeders. Suet can be purchased
   from a butcher shop or meat department
   of a supermarket. For each feeder, purchase 1/2 pound of suet, a 12" x 12" piece
   of netting and birdseed. Begin by rolling
   the suet in birdseed. Place the seeded suet
   in the netting. Tie the four corners of the
   netting together and hang in tree or set
   outside on window ledge for children to
   observe.

2. **Grapefruit Cup Feeders**

   Place seeds in an empty grapefruit half. If
   possible, place the feeder in an observable
   location for the children. Some children
   may wish to take their feeders home.

3. **Science Table**

   On the science table, provide magnifying
   glasses and the following items:

   * feathers
   * eggs
   * nests

4. Observing a Bird

Arrange for a caged parakeet to visit the classroom. A parent may volunteer or a pet store may lend a bird for a week. Encourage the children to note the structure of the cage, the beauty of the bird, food eaten and the behavior of the bird.

Dramatic Play:

1. Birdhouse

Construct a large birdhouse out of cardboard. Place in the dramatic play area, allowing the children to imitate birds. Unless adequate room is available, this may be more appropriate for an outdoor activity. Bird accessories such as teacher-made beaks and wings may be supplied to stimulate interest.

2. Bird Nest

Place several hay bales in the corner of a play yard, confining the materials to one area. Let the child rearrange the straw to simulate a bird nest.

3. Hatching

Here is a general idea of what you can say to create the hatching experience with young children. Say, "Close your eyes. Curl up very small; as small as you can. Lie on your side. Think of how dark it is inside your egg. Yes, you're in an egg! You're tiny and curled up and quiet. It's very dark. Very warm. But now, try to wiggle a little—just a little! Remember, your eggshell is all around you. You can wiggle your wingtips a little, and maybe your toes. You can shake your head just a little. Hey! Your beak is touching something. I think your beak is touching the eggshell. Tap the shell gently with your beak. Hear that? Yes, that's you making that noise. Keep tapping. A little harder. Something is happening. The shell has cracked—oh, close your eyes. It's bright out there. Now you can wiggle a little more. The shell is falling away. You can stretch out, stretch to be as long as

you can make yourself. Stretch your feet. Stretch your wings. Doesn't that feel good, after being in that little egg? Stretch! You're brand new—can you stand up, slowly? Can you see other new baby birds?"

Arts and Crafts:

1. Feather Painting

On the art table, place feathers, thin paper and paint. Let the children experiment with different paint consistencies and types of feathers.

2. Birdseed Collages

Birdseed, paper and white glue are needed for this activity. Apply glue to paper and sprinkle birdseed over the glue. For a variation, use additional types of seeds such as corn and sunflower seeds.

3. Eggshell Collage

Save eggshells and dye them. Crush the dyed shells into small pieces. Using glue, apply the eggshells to paper.

4. Robin's Eggs

Cut easel paper into the shape of an egg. Provide light blue paint with sand for speckles.

5. Dying Eggs

Boil an egg for each child. Then let the children paint the eggs with easel brushes. The eggs can be eaten at snack time or taken home.

Sensory:

Additions to the Sensory Table

* feathers and sand
* eggshells
* sticks and twigs for nests
* worms and soil
* water, ducks and other water toys
* birdseed and measuring tools

Field Trips/Resource People:

1. Pet Store

Take a field trip to a pet store. Arrange to have the manager show the children birds and bird cages. Ask the manager how to care for birds.

2. Bird Sanctuary

Take a field trip to a bird sanctuary, nature area, pond, or park. Observe where birds live.

3. Museum

Arrange a visit a nature museum or taxidermy studio to look at stuffed birds. Extend the activity by providing magnifying glasses.

4. Zoo

Visit the bird house. Observe the color and sizes of birds.

5. Resource People

Invite resource people to visit the classroom. Suggestions include:

* wildlife management people
* ornithologists
* veterinarian
* bird owners
* bird watchers
* pet store owners

Math:

1. Feather Sorting

During the self-directed activity period, place a variety of feathers on a table. Encourage the children to sort them according to attributes such as color, size, and/or texture. This activity can be followed with other sorting activities including egg shapes and pictures of birds.

2. Cracked Eggs

Cut tagboard egg shapes. Using scissors, cut the eggs in half making a jagged line. Record a numeral on one side of the egg and corresponding dots on the other side. The number of eggs prepared should reflect the children's developmental level.

Social Studies:

1. Caring for Birds

Arrange for a pet canary to visit the classroom. The children can take turns feeding and caring for the bird. Responsibilities include cleaning the cage, providing water and birdseed. Also a cuttlebone should be inserted in the bars of the cage within reach of the bird's bill. This bone will help keep the bird's bill sharp and clean, providing the bird uses it.

2. Bird Feeders

Purchase birdseed and small paper cups. The children can fill a cup with a small amount of seed. After this the teacher can attach a small string to the cup for use as a handle. The bird feeders can then be hung in bushes outdoors. If bushes are not available, they can be placed on window sills.

Group Time (games, language):

1. Little Birds

This is a movement game that allows for activity. To add interest, the teacher may use a tambourine for rhythm. One child can be the mother bird and the remainder of the children can act out the story.

All the little birds are asleep in their nest.
All the little birds are taking a rest.
They do not even twitter, they do not even tweet.
Everything is quiet up and down the street.
Then came the mother bird and tapped them on the head.

They opened up one little eye and this is what was said,
"Come little birdies, it's time to learn to fly,
Come little birdies, fly way up in the sky."
Fly fly, oh fly away, fly, fly, fly
Fly fly, oh fly away, fly away so high.
Fly fly, oh, fly away, birds, can fly the best.
Fly fly, oh, fly away, now fly back to your nest.

2. Who Is Inside?

The purpose of this game is to encourage the child to develop listening skills. To prepare for the activity, find a piece of large muscle equipment such as a jungle gym to serve as the bird house. Cover it with a large blanket. To play the game one child looks away from the group or covers his eyes. A second child should go into the bird house. The first child says, "Who is inside?" The second child replies, "I am inside the bird house." Then the first child tries to guess who is in the bird house by recognizing the voice. Other clues may be asked for, if voice alone does not work.

3. Little Red Hen

Tell the story of the *Little Red Hen*. After listening to the story, let the children help make bread.

Cooking:

1. Egg Salad Sandwiches

eggs
bread
mayonnaise
dry mustard (just a pinch)
salt
pepper

Boil, shell, and mash the eggs, adding enough mayonnaise to provide a consistent texture. Add salt, pepper, and dry mustard to flavor. Spread on the bread.

2. French Bread Recipe

1/2 cup water
2 packages rapid rise yeast
1 tablespoon salt
2 cups lukewarm water
7 to 7 1/2 cups all purpose flour

Soften the yeast in 1/2 cup lukewarm water. Be careful that the water isn't too warm or the activity of the yeast will be destroyed. Add salt to 2 cups of lukewarm warm in a large bowl. Gradually add 2 cups of flour and beat well. Add the softened yeast and gradually add the remaining flour, beating well after each addition. Turn the soft dough out on a lightly floured surface and knead until elastic. Lightly grease a bowl and place the dough into it, turning once to grease surface. Let rise until double. Divide into 2 portions. Bake in a 375-degree oven until light brown, about 35 minutes.

3. Bird's Nest Salad

1 grated carrot
1/2 cup canned Chinese noodles
mayonnaise to moisten
peas or grapes

Have the children grate a carrot. Next have them mix the carrot with 1/2 cup canned Chinese noodles and mayonnaise to moisten. Put a mound of this salad on a plate and push in the middle with a spoon to form a nest. Peas or grapes can be added to the nest to represent bird's eggs. The nest could also be set on top of a lettuce leaf. Makes 2 salads.

Source: *Super Snacks*. Jean Warren. (Alderwood Manor, WA: Warren Publishing, 1982).

4. Egg Foo Young

12 eggs
1/2 cup finely chopped onion
1/3 cup chopped green pepper
3/4 teaspoon salt
dash of pepper
2-16 ounce cans bean sprouts, drained

Sauce:
2 tablespoons cornstarch
2 teaspoons sugar
2 cubes or 2 teaspoons chicken bouillon
dash of ginger
2 cups of water
3 tablespoons soy sauce

Heat oven to 300 degrees. Beat eggs in a large bowl. Add remaining ingredients, except sauce ingredients; mix well. Heat 2 tablespoons of oil in a large skillet. Drop egg mixture by tablespoons into skillet and fry until golden. Turn and brown other side. Drain on a paper towel. Continue to cook the remaining egg mixture, adding oil to skillet if necessary. Keep warm in 300-degree oven while preparing sauce. Combine the first four sauce ingredients in a saucepan. Add water and soy sauce. Cook until mixture boils and thickens, stirring constantly.

Records:

The following records can be found in preschool educational catalogs:

1. **The Animal Fair** January Productions. Fair Lawn, NJ.

   * Six Little Ducks
   * Three Crows
   * Bird's Courting Song
   * I Bought Me A Rooster
   * Cluck Old Hen
   * The Old Grey Hen
   * Listen to the Mockingbird
   * Animal Fair

2. **Folk Song Carnival** by Hap Palmer. Activity Records, Inc.

   * Going to the Zoo
   * Blue Bird
   * Hush Little Baby

3. **Fourteen Numbers, Letters and Animal Songs** by Alan Mills, Folkways Records.

   * Animal Alphabet
   * Six Little Ducks

Books and Stories:

The following books and stories may be used to complement this theme:

1. **What's Inside the Egg?** May Garelick. (Reading, MA: Addison-Wesley Publishing Co., 1955).

2. **The Remarkable Egg.** Adelaide Holl. (New York: Lothrop, Lee and Shepard Co., 1968).

3. **It's Nesting Time.** Roma Gans. (New York: Thomas Y. Crowell Co., 1964).

4. **Birds in the Sky.** Lucy and John Hawkinson. (Chicago: Childrens Press, 1965).

5. **What Makes a Bird a Bird.** May Garelick. (Chicago: Follett Publishing Co., 1969).

6. **Birds Eat and Eat and Eat.** Roma Gans. (New York: Thomas Y. Crowell Co., 1963).

7. **The Nest.** Bethany Tudor. (New York: Harvey House Press Inc., 1972).

8. **The Happy Egg.** Ruth Krause. (Chicago: Phillip O'Hara Inc., 1967).

9. **Birds.** Brian Wildsmith. (New York: Franklin Watts, 1968).

10. **Flap Your Wings.** P.D. Eastman. (New York: Random House, 1977).

11. **What is a Bird?** Jennifer W. Day. (New York: Golden Press, 1975).

12. **Birds.** Rosamund K. Cox and Barbara Cork. (London: Usborne Publishing, Ltd., 1980).

13. **Birds.** (Los Angeles: Price/Stern/Sloan, Inc. 1984).

14. **Have You Seen Birds?** Joanne Oppenheim. (New York: Scholastic Books, 1986).

15. **What's Inside?** May Garelick. (New York: Scholastic Books, 1968).

16. **Why Can't I Fly?** Rita Golden Gelman. (New York: Scholastic Books, 1976).

17. **A First Look at Birds.** Millicent Selsam. (New York: Scholastic Books, 1981).

18. **From Egg to Bird.** Marlene Reidel. (Minneapolis, MN: Carolrhoda, 1981).

Puzzles:

The following puzzles can be found in preschool educational catalogs:

1. **"Bird"** Lauri.

2. **"Rainbow and Bird"** Lauri.

3. **"Rooster"** 15 pieces. Judy/Instructo.

4. **"Robin"** 4 pieces. Judy/Instructo.

5. **"Meadowlark"** 15 pieces. Judy/Instructo.

6. **"Chicken and Chicks"** 9 pieces. Judy/Instructo.

7. **"Owl"** 11 pieces. Judy/Instructo.

8. **"Duck"** 8 pieces. Judy/Instructo.

9. **"Birds"** 6 pieces. Judy/Instructo.

10. **"Penguin Family"** 8 pieces. Judy/Instructo.

BLUE

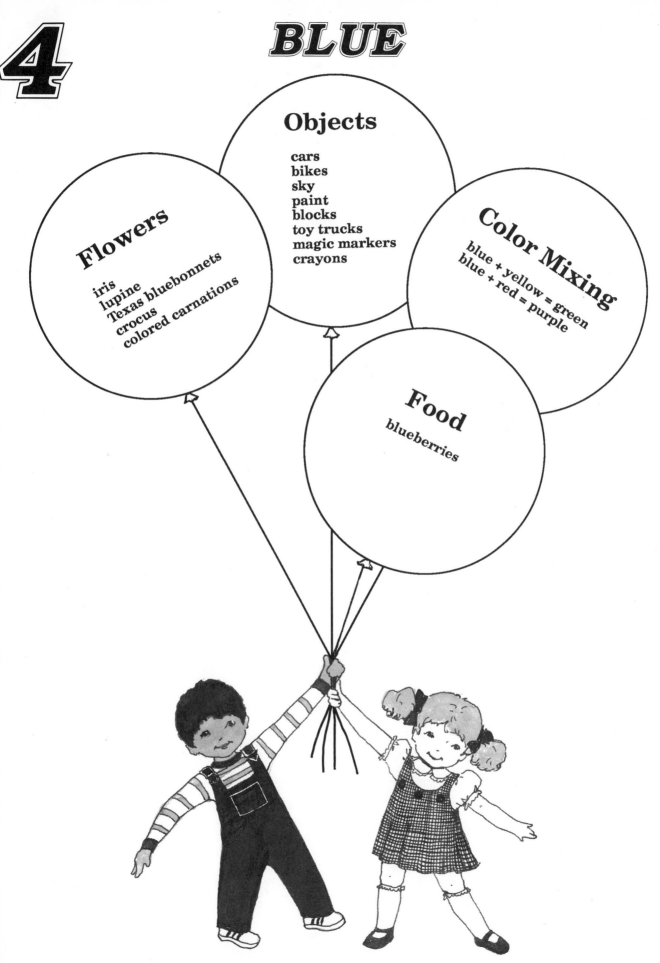

4

Objects

cars
bikes
sky
paint
blocks
toy trucks
magic markers
crayons

Flowers

iris
lupine
Texas bluebonnets
crocus
colored carnations

Color Mixing

blue + yellow = green
blue + red = purple

Food

blueberries

Theme Goals:

Through participating in the experiences provided by this theme, the children may learn:

1. Blue is the color of many objects.

2. A type of berry is colored blue.

3. Some flowers are colored blue.

4. Blue can be mixed with other colors.

Concepts for the Children to Learn:

1. Blue is the name of a color.

2. Mixing blue with yellow makes green.

3. Blue mixed with red makes purple.

4. Some cars and bikes are a blue color.

5. On sunny, clear days the sky is a blue color.

6. Blueberries are a blue colored food.

7. White carnations can be colored blue.

8. An iris is a blue flower.

Vocabulary:

1. **blue**—a primary color.

2. **primary colors**—red, yellow and blue.

Bulletin Board

The purpose of this bulletin board is to develop visual discrimination skills. A blue bulletin board can be constructed by focusing on familiar objects. Draw pictures of many familiar objects on tagboard. Color them various shades of blue. Cut the objects out and laminate. Next, trace the pictures, allowing ¼-inch borders, on black construction paper. Cut out shadow pieces and hang on the bulletin board. Add a magnet piece to each shadow and picture. The children can match each picture to its corresponding shadow.

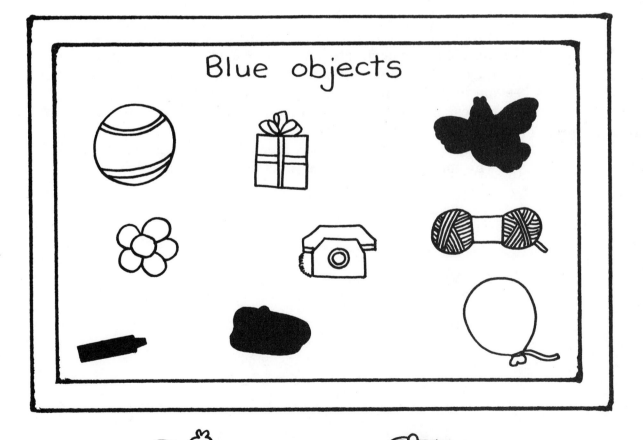

Parent Letter

Dear Parents,

Colors! Colors! Colors! This week we will be focusing our activities on the color blue. The children will learn that blue can be mixed with red to make purple. Yellow mixed with blue makes green. The children will also become aware that many familiar objects are blue in color.

At School This Week

Some of the learning experiences planned for the week include:

* singing a song called "Two Little Bluejays."
* looking out our blue windows in the classroom.
* playing in a paint store in the dramatic play area.
* fingerpainting with blue paint.
* eating blueberries for snack.

At Home

You can make almost any meal entertaining by occasionally adding a small amount of food coloring to one of your food items. Children often find this amusing. The food coloring adds interest to your food and meal times become fun! Try adding a drop or two to milk, vanilla pudding, mashed potatoes, scrambled eggs or cottage cheese. Does the color of a food affect its taste? (Try drinking green milk!) You be the judge! To further develop an awareness of color, identify foods that are red, blue, yellow, etc. This improves memory, classification, and expressive language skills.

Have a great week!

Music:

1. "Two Little Bluejays"
(Sing to the tune of "Two Little Blackbirds")

Two little bluejays
sitting on a hill
One named Sue
One named Bill.

Fly away Sue
Fly away Bill.
Come back Sue
Come back Bill.

Two little bluejays
sitting on a hill
One named Sue
One named Bill.

To add interest, you can substitute names after the song has been sung several times. The children will enjoy hearing their names.

2. "Finding Colors"
(Sing to the tune of "The Muffin Man")

Oh, can you find the color blue,
The color blue, the color blue?
Oh, can you find the color blue,
Somewhere in this room?

Science:

1. Just One Drop

Each child will need a smock for this activity. Also provide a glass of water and blue food coloring. Encourage the children to add a drop of blue food coloring to the water. Watch as the water becomes a light blue. Add a few more drops of food coloring, observing as the blue water turns a darker shade.

2. Blue Color Paddles

Construct blue color paddles out of stiff tagboard and blue overhead transparency sheets. Make a form for the paddle out of tagboard, leaving the inside empty. Put the sheet of blue transparency paper on the back, glue and trim. The children can hold the paddle up to their eyes and see how the colors have changed.

3. Blue Windows

Place blue colored cellophane or acetate sheets over some of the windows in the classroom. It is fun to look out the windows and see the blue world.

4. Dying Carnations

Place the stem of a white carnation in a bottle of water with blue food coloring added on the science table. Observe the change of the petal colors.

Dramatic Play:

Paint Store

Provide paintbrushes, buckets and paint sample books. The addition of a cash register, play money and pads of paper will extend the children's play.

Arts and Crafts:

1. Arm Dancing

Provide each child with two blue crayons and a large sheet of paper. Play music encouraging the children to color, using both arms. Because of the structure of this activity, it should be limited to older children.

2. Sponge Painting

Collect sponge pieces, thick blue tempera paint and sheets of light blue paper. If desired, clothespins can be clipped on the sponges and used as handles. To use as a tool, dip the sponge into blue paint and print on light blue paper.

3. Easel Ideas

* Feature different shades of blue paint at the easel.

* Use blue paint on aluminum foil.
* Add whipped soap flakes to blue paint.
* Add a container of yellow paint to the easel. Allow the children to mix the yellow and blue paints at the easel. This activity can be extended by providing red and blue tempera paint.

4. **Fingerpainting**

Blue fingerpaint and large sheets of paper should be placed in the art area.

5. **Melted Crayon Design**

Grate broken blue crayons. Place the shreddings on one square of waxed paper 6 inches x 6 inches. On top of the shreddings, place another 6 inch x 6 inch piece of waxed paper. Cover with a dishtowel or old cloth. Apply heat with a warm iron for about 30 seconds. Let the sheets cool, and the child can trim them with scissors. These melted crayon designs can be used as nice sun catchers on the windows. (This activity needs to be closely supervised. Only the teacher should handle the hot iron.)

Sensory:

Additions to the Sensory Table

1. **water with blue food coloring**

2. **blue goop**

Mix together blue food coloring, 1 cup cornstarch and 1 cup of water.

Large Muscle:

1. **Painting**

Provide a bucket of blue colored water and large paintbrushes. Encourage the children to paint the sidewalks, building, fence, sandbox, etc.

2. **Blue Ribbon Dance**

Make blue streamer ribbons by attaching blue crepe paper to unsharpened pencils. Play lively music and encourage the children to move to the music.

Field Trips/Resource People:

1. **"Blue" Watching**

Walk around your center's neighborhood and observe blue items. Things to look for include cars, bikes, birds, houses, flowers, etc. When you return, have the children dictate a list. Record your responses.

2. **Paint Store**

Visit a local paint store. Observe all the different shades of blue paint. Look carefully to see if they look similar. Ask the store manager for discarded sample cards. These cards can be added to the materials to use in the art area.

Social Studies:

Eye Color

Prepare an eye color chart with the children. Colors on the chart should include blue, brown and green. Under each category, record the children's names who have that particular eye color. Extend the activity by adding the number of children with each color.

Group Time (games, language):

1. **Bluebird, Bluebird**

The children should join hands and stand in a circle. Construct one bluebird necklace out of yarn and construction paper. Choose one child to be the first bluebird. This bluebird weaves in and out of the children's arms while the remainder of the children chant:

"Bluebird, Bluebird Through My Window
Bluebird, Bluebird Through My Window
Bluebird, Bluebird Through My Window
Who will be the next bluebird?"

At this time the child takes off the necklace and hands it to a child he would like to be the next bluebird.

2. I Spy

The teacher says, "I spy something blue that is sitting on the piano bench," or other such statements. The children will look around and try to figure out what the teacher has spied. Older children may enjoy taking turns repeating, "I spy something on the _____."

Cooking:

1. Blueberries

Wash and prepare fresh or frozen blueberries for snack. Blueberry muffins are also appropriate for this theme.

2. Blueberry Muffins

2 tablespoons sugar
1 3/4 cups flour
2 1/2 teaspoons baking powder
3/4 teaspoon salt
1 egg
1/2 cup milk
1/3 cup salad oil

Mix all of the ingredients together. Add 2 tablespoons of sugar to 1 cup frozen or fresh blueberries. Mix slightly and gently add to the batter. Bake at 400 degrees for approximately 25 minutes.

3. Cream Cheese and Crackers

Tint cream cheese blue with food coloring and spread on crackers.

4. Cupcakes

Add blue food coloring to a white cake mix. Fill paper cupcake holders with the batter and bake as directed.

TRANSITIONS: DISMISSAL OF CHILDREN

* colors of clothing/types of clothing/patterns of fabrics (stripes, polka dots, plaid)
* shoes (boots, shoes with buckles, shoes with ties, shoes with velcro, slip-on shoes, jelly shoes) Also, number of eyelets on shoes, number of buckles
* ages in years
* number of brothers/sisters
* hair/eye color
* birthdays in certain months
* name cards
* first letter of names
* last names
* rhyming names
* animal or word that starts with same sound as your name (Tiger-Tom)

* give each child a turn at something while putting rugs away (blowing a bubble, strumming a guitar, hugging puppet)
* play "I Spy" by saying "I spy someone wearing blue pants and a Mickey Mouse sweatshirt."
* play a quick game of "Simon Says" and then have Simon tell where the children are to go next.

* "Two Little Blackbirds"
Two little blackbirds
    sitting on a hill
One named Jack, one
    named Jill
Fly away Jack, fly away
    Jill,
Come back Jack, come

back Jill.
Two little blackbirds
    sitting on a hill,
One named Jack, one
    named Jill.

* "I Have a Very Special Friend"
(Sing to the Tune of "Bingo")
I have a very special friend,
Can you guess his name-o?
J-A-R-E-D, J-A-R-E-D, J-A-R-E-D,
And Jared is his name-o.

*"I'm Looking For Someone"
I'm looking for someone named Kristen,
I'm looking for someone named Kristen,
If there is someone named Kristen here now,

Stand up and take a bow. (Or, Stand up and go to lunch.)

*"Where, Oh, Where is My Friend"
Where, oh, where is my friend Travis?
Where, oh, where is my friend Travis?
Where, oh, where is my friend Travis?
Please come to the door.

*"How Did You Come To School Today?"
How did you come to school today,
How did you come on Monday? (Child responds)
He came in a blue car,
Came in a blue car on Monday.

*"One Elephant Went Out To Play"
One elephant went out to play
Upon a spider's web one day.
He had such enormous fun
That he called for another elephant to come.

Group Dismissal

* hop like a bunny
* walk as quiet as a mouse
* tiptoe
* walk backwards
* count steps as you walk
* have footsteps for group to walk on or a winding trail to follow

*"This Train" (Tune: "This Train is Bound for Glory")
This train is bound for the lunchroom,
This train is bound for the lunchroom,
This train is bound for the lunchroom,
Katie, get on board.
Matthew, get on board.
Zachary, get on board.
Afton, get on board.
*Change lunchroom to fit situation.

Fillers

*"One Potato"
One potato, two potato, three potato, four
Five potato, six potato, seven potato, more.

*"And One and Two"
And one and two and three and four,
And five and six and seven and eight.
(Repeat faster)

*"Colors Here and There"
Colors here and there,
Colors everywhere.
What's the name of this color here?

*"This is What I Can Do"
This is what I can do,
Everybody do it, too.
This is what I can do,
Now I pass it on to you.

*"A Peanut Sat On a Railroad Track"
A peanut sat on a railroad track,
It's heart was all a-flutter.
Engine Nine came down the track,
Toot! Toot! Peanut butter!

*apple-applesauce
*banana-banana split
*orange-orange juice

*"Lickety Lick"
Lickety lick, lickety lick,
The batter is getting all thickety thick.
What shall we bake?
What shall we bake?
A great, big beautiful carrot cake.

Change "carrot" to any kind of cake

*"I Clap My Hands"
I clap my hands. (Echo)
I stamp my feet. (Echo)
I turn around. (Echo)
And it's really neat. (Echo)
I touch my shoulders. (Echo)
I touch my nose. (Echo)
I touch my knees. (Echo)
And that's how it goes. (Echo)

Records:

The following records can be found in preschool educational catalogs:

1. **Color Me a Rainbow.** Melody House Records.

2. **There's Music in the Colors.** Kimbo Records.

3. **Learning Basic Skills Through Music.** Hap Palmer. "Colors"

Books and Stories:

The following books and stories can be used to complement this theme:

1. **I Want To Paint My Bathroom Blue.** Ruth Krauss. (New York: Harper and Row, 1956).

2. **Little Blue and Little Yellow.** Leo Lionni. (New York: Astor-Honor, 1959).

3. **A Blue Seed.** Rieko Nakagawa. (New York: Hastings House, 1967).

4. **Andy's Square Blue Animal.** Jane Thayer. (New York: William Morrow, 1962).

5. **The Sky Was Blue.** Charlotte Zolotow. (New York: Harper and Row, 1963).

6. **Is It Red? Is It Yellow? Is It Blue?** Tana Hoban. (New York: William Morrow, 1978).

7. **Blue Ribbon Puppies.** Crockett Johnson. (New York: Harper and Row, 1958).

8. **The Red Horse and the Bluebird.** Sandy Rabinowitz. (New York: Harper and Row, 1975).

9. **New Blue Shoes.** Eve Rice. (New York: Macmillan, 1975).

10. **Mystery of the Stolen Blue Paint.** S. Kellogg. (New York: Dial, 1982).

11. **Feeling Blue.** R.J. Wolff. (New York: Charles Scribner's Sons, 1968).

Puzzles:

The following puzzles can be found in preschool educational catalogs:

1. **"Great Big Blue Tugboat"** Judy/Instructo.

2. **"Color Puzzles"** 8 pieces. Judy/Instructo.

3. **"Great Big Blue Choo Choo"** Judy/Instructo.

4. **"Little Boy Blue"** Judy/Instructo.

5 BRUSHES

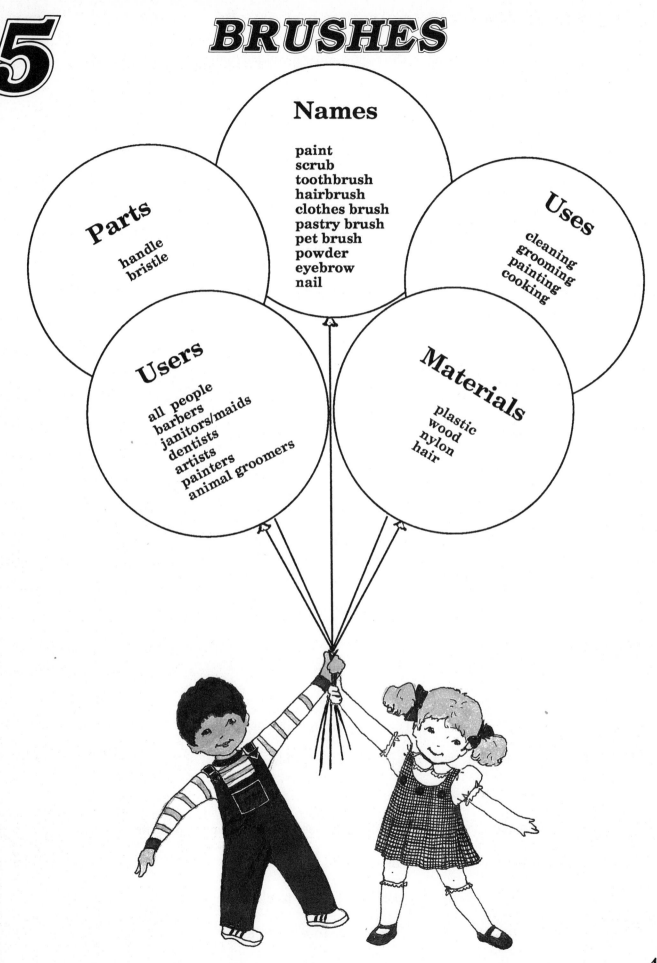

Names

paint
scrub
toothbrush
hairbrush
clothes brush
pastry brush
pet brush
powder
eyebrow
nail

Parts

handle
bristle

Uses

cleaning
grooming
painting
cooking

Users

all people
barbers
janitors/maids
dentists
artists
painters
animal groomers

Materials

plastic
wood
nylon
hair

Theme Goals:

Through participating in the experiences provided by this theme, the children may learn:

1. Parts of a brush.

2. Kinds of brushes.

3. Uses of brushes.

4. Materials used to make brushes.

5. Community helpers who need brushes for their work.

Concepts for the Children to Learn:

1. A brush is a tool.

2. Brushes come in many sizes.

3. Brushes have handles.

4. Some brushes are used in cleaning in our home.

5. Toothbrushes help clean our teeth.

6. Hair brushes are used for grooming.

7. A pastry brush is used for cooking.

8. Brushes can be made of plastic, wood, or nylon.

9. Some people use brushes while working.

Vocabulary:

1. **brush**—a tool made of bristles or wires attached to a handle.

2. **bristle**—a short, stiff hair or thread like objects.

3. **handle**—the part of a brush that is held.

4. **groom**—to clean.

5. **powder brush**—a brush that is used to apply facial powder.

6. **toothbrush**—a small brush used to clean teeth.

7. **vegetable brush**—a stiff brush used to clean vegetables.

8. **dog brush**—a brush used to clean a dog's hair.

Bulletin Board

The purpose of this bulletin board is to promote the development of color identification and matching skills. Construct and paint pallets and brushes out
of tagboard. Use a different colored marker to draw paint spots on each pallet
and to "paint" the bristles of each brush. Laminate all the pieces. Attach the
pallets to the bulletin board. Map tacks, putty or velcro may be used to place
the brushes next to the corresponding color of paint pallet.

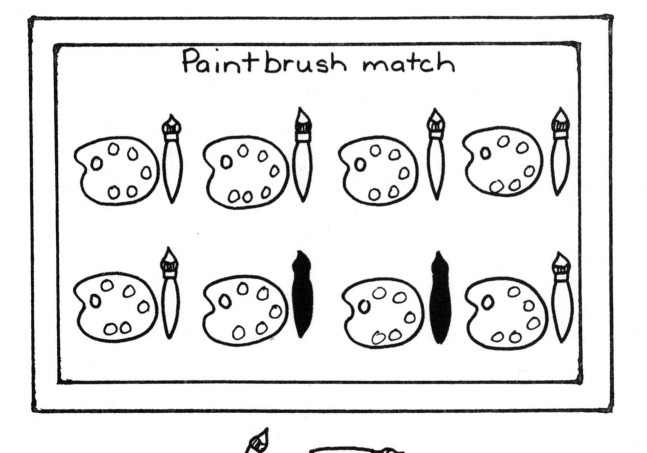

Parent Letter

Dear Parents,

Did you ever stop to think about the number and types of brushes we use in a day? Brushes will be the subject that we will explore this week. Each one has a different function and helps us do a different job. Through the activities related to the theme, the children will become aware of the many types and uses of brushes. In addition they will be exposed to materials used in constructing brushes.

At School This Week

Some of the learning experiences this week will include:

* setting up a hair stylist shop in the dramatic play area.
* "painting" outside with buckets of water and brushes.
* observing teeth being cleaned with electric and hand held brushes as we visit Dr. Smith's dental office on Thursday morning.
* painting with a variety of brushes at the easel each day.

At Home

With your child, go through your home and locate brushes. Examples include: toothbrushes, hair brushes, paintbrushes, fingernail polish brushes, pastry brushes and makeup brushes. Compare and sort the various brushes. This will help your child discriminate between weights, colors, sizes, textures and shapes. The brushes can also be counted and it can be determined which room contains the most and which the least amount of brushes, which will promote the understanding of number concepts.

Have a good week!

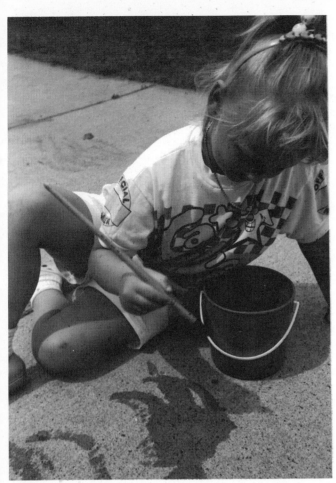

FIGURE 5 Brushes are handy and fun to use.

Music:

"Using Brushes"
(Sing to the tune of "Mulberry Bush")

This is the way we brush our teeth,
brush our teeth, brush our teeth.
This is the way we brush our teeth
So early in the morning.

Variations:
* This is the way we brush our hair....
* This is the way we polish our nails....
* This is the way we paint the house....

Act out each verse, and allow the children
to make up more verses.

Fingerplays:

BRUSHES IN MY HOME

These brushes in my home
Are simply everywhere.
I use them for my teeth each day,
(brushing teeth motion)
And also for my hair.
(hair brushing motion)

We use them in the kitchen sink
(scrubbing motion)
And in the toilet bowls
(scrubbing motion)
For putting polish on my shoes
(touch shoes and rub)
And to waterproof the soles.

Brushes are used to polish the floors
(polishing motions)
And also paint the wall,
(painting motion)
To clean the charcoal barbecue,
(brushing motion)
It's hard to name them all.

MY TOOTHBRUSH

I have a little toothbrush.
(use pointer for toothbrush)
I hold it very tightly.
(make tight fist)
I brush my teeth each morning
(pretend to brush teeth)
And then again at night.

SHINY SHOES

First I loosen mud and dirt,
My shoes I then rub clean.
For shoes in such a dreadful sight,
Never should be seen.

I spread the polish on the shoes.
And then I let it dry.
I brush the shoes until they shine.
And sparkle in my eye.

Science:

1. Identifying Brushes

Inside the feely box place various small
brushes. The children can reach into the
box, feel the object and try to identify it
by name.

2. Exploring Bristles

Add to the science table a variety of brushes and magnifying glasses. Allow the children to observe the bristles up close, noting similarities and differences.

Dramatic Play:

1. Hair Stylist

Collect hair spray bottles, brushes, empty shampoo bottles, chairs, mirrors, hair dryers, curling irons and place in the dramatic play area. If possible, cut the cords off the electrical appliances.

2. Water Painting

Outdoors provide children with buckets of water and house paintbrushes. They can pretend to "paint" the building, sidewalks, equipment and fence.

3. Shining Shoes

In the dramatic play area place clear shoe polish, shoes, brushes and shining cloths for the children to polish.

Arts and Crafts:

1. Brush Painting

Place various brushes such as hair, makeup, toothbrushes, clothes brushes on a table in the art area. In addition, thin tempera paint and paper should be provided. Let the children explore the painting process with a variety of brushes.

2. Easel Ideas

Each day change the type of brushes the children can use while painting at the easel. Variations may include: sponge brushes, discarded toothbrushes, nail polish brushes, vegetable brushes and makeup brushes.

3. Box House Painting

Place a large cardboard box outside. To decorate it provide smocks, house painting brushes and tempera paint for the children.

Large Muscle:

Sidewalk Brushing

Place buckets of water and paintbrushes for use outdoors on sidewalks, fences and buildings.

Field Trips/Resource People:

1. The Street Sweeper

Contact the city maintenance department. Invite them to clean the street in front of the center or school for the children to observe.

2. Artist's Studio

Visit a local artist's studio. Observe the various brushes used.

3. Dentist's Office

Visit a dentist's office. Ask the dentist to demonstrate and explain the use of various brushes.

4. Animal Groomer

Invite an animal groomer to school. Ask the groomer to show the equipment, emphasizing the importance of brushes.

Math:

1. Sequencing

Collect various sized paintbrushes. Encourage the children to sequence them by height and width.

2. Weighing Brushes

Place a balance scale and several brushes in the math area. Encourage the children to weigh and balance the brushes.

3. Toothbrush Counting

Collect toothbrushes and cans. Label each can with a numeral. The children can place the corresponding number of brushes into each labeled can. If desired, the toothbrushes can be constructed out of tagboard.

Social Studies:

1. Brushes Chart

Design a "Brushes in our Classroom" chart. Encourage the children to find all that are used in the classroom.

2. Helper Chart

Design a helper chart. Include tasks such as sweeping floors, cleaning paintbrushes, putting brushes and brooms away. This chart can encourage the children to use brushes everyday in the classroom.

Group Time (games, language):

1. Brush Hunt

Hide several brushes in the classroom. Have one child search for the brushes. When he gets close to them, clap loudly. When he is further away, clap quietly.

2. Brush of the Day

At group time each day introduce a new brush. Discuss the shape, color, materials, and uses. Then allow the children to use the brush in the classroom during self-selected play period.

Cooking:

1. Cleaning Vegetables

Place several washtubs filled with water in the cooking area. Then provide children with fresh carrots and brushes. Encourage the children to clean the carrots using a vegetable brush. The carrots can be used to make carrot cake, muffins or can be added to soup.

2. Pretzels

1 1/2 cups warm water
1 envelope yeast
4 cups flour
1 teaspoon salt
1 tablespoon sugar
1 egg
coarse salt (optional)

Mix water, yeast, sugar. Let stand for 5 minutes. Place salt and flour in a bowl. Add the yeast and stir to prepare dough mixture. Shape the dough. Beat egg and apply the egg glaze with a pastry brush. Sprinkle with salt if desired. Bake at 425 degrees for approximately 12 minutes.

PAINT APPLICATORS

There are many ways to apply paint. The size and shape of the following applicators produce unique results. While some are recycleable, others are disposable.

Recycleable Examples

paintbrushes, varying
    sizes and widths
wisk brooms
fingers and hands
tongue depressors or
    popsicle sticks
potato mashers
forks and spoons
toothbrushes
aerosol can lids
cookie cutters

spray bottles
string/yarn
roll-on deodorant bottles
squeeze bottles (plastic
    ketchup containers)
marbles and beads
styrofoam shapes
sponges
feet
spools
rollers

**Disposable Applicators
to Use with Paint**

twigs and sticks
string/yarn
feathers
pine cones
rocks
cloth
cardboard tubes
straws
leaves
cotton balls
cotton swabs

Books and Stories:

The following books and stories can be used to complement the theme:

1. **Straight Hair, Curly Hair.** Augusta Goldin. (New York: Thomas Y. Crowell, 1966).

2. **My Dentist.** Harlow Rockwell. (New York: Greenwillow Books, 1975).

3. **Oh! Were They Ever Happy.** Peter Spier. (New York: Doubleday, 1978).

4. **The Color Kittens.** Margaret Wise Brown. (New York: Golden Press, 1967).

5. **I Can Be A Beautician.** Dee Lillegard. (Chicago: Childrens Press, 1987).

6. **The Penguins Paint.** Valerie Tripp. (Chicago: Childrens Press, 1987).

7. **Peter's Chair.** Ezra Jack Keats. (New York: Harper and Row, 1967).

Puzzles:

The following puzzles can be found in a preschool educational catalog:

1. **"Dentist"** 12 pieces. Judy/Instructo.

2. **"Lavatory Puzzle"** 7 pieces. The Preschool Source.

BUILDINGS

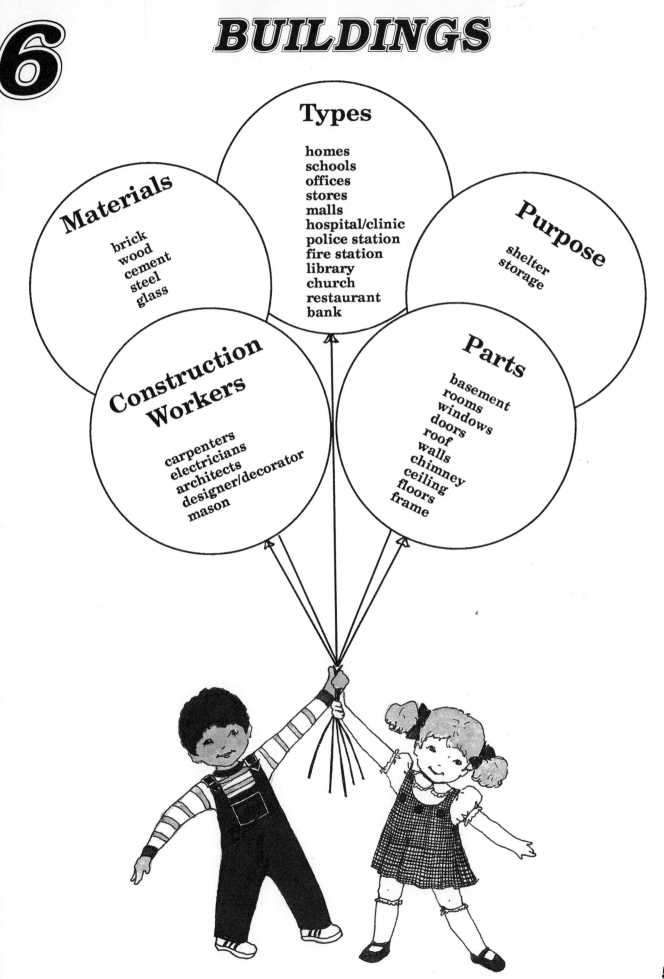

6

Materials

brick
wood
cement
steel
glass

Types

homes
schools
offices
stores
malls
hospital/clinic
police station
fire station
library
church
restaurant
bank

Purpose

shelter
storage

Construction Workers

carpenters
electricians
architects
designer/decorator
mason

Parts

basement
rooms
windows
doors
roof
walls
chimney
ceiling
floors
frame

Theme Goals:

Through participating in the experiences provided by this theme, the children may learn:

1. Types of buildings.

2. Purposes of buildings.

3. Materials used to make buildings.

4. Parts of a building.

Concepts for the Children to Learn:

1. There are many types of buildings: homes, offices, stores, hospitals, malls, etc.

2. Buildings can be made of brick, wood, cement, steel and glass.

3. Many workers help construct buildings: architects, carpenters, electricians, plumbers and masons.

4. Buildings can be used for shelter and storage.

5. Most buildings have a roof, walls, windows and a floor.

Vocabulary:

1. **building**—a structure.

2. **mall**—a building containing many stores.

3. **skyscraper**—a very tall building.

4. **carpenter**—a person who builds.

5. **electrician**—a person who wires a building for light, heat and cooking.

6. **architect**—a person who designs a building.

7. **room**—a part of a building set off by walls.

8. **ceiling**—the top "wall" of a room.

9. **roof**—the top covering of a building.

Bulletin Board

The purpose of this bulletin board is to develop awareness of size as well as visual discrimination skills. Construct house shapes out of tagboard ranging in size from small to large. Color the shapes and laminate. Punch a hole in the top of each house. Trace each house shape on black construction paper and cut out. Hang the shadow pieces on the bulletin board with a push pin inserted in the top of each. During self-directed and self-initiated play, the children match each colored house to the corresponding shadow piece by hanging it on the push pin.

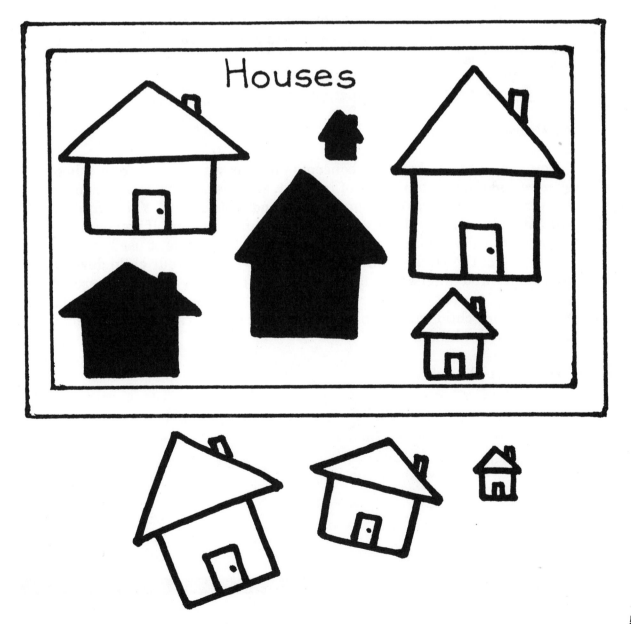

Parent Letter

Dear Parents,

Your home, the library, our school...these are all buildings with which your child is familiar. Buildings will be the theme that we will focus on this week. Discoveries will be made regarding different kinds and parts of buildings, materials used to make buildings, and the people who construct buildings.

At School This Week

A sampling of this week's learning experiences include:

* building with various materials—such as boxes and milk cartons.
* working at the woodworking bench to practice hammering, drilling and sawing.
* weighing and balancing bricks.
* taking a walk to a construction site.

At Home

You can reinforce building concepts on your way to and from school by pointing out any buildings of interest, such as the fire station, police station, hospital, library, shopping mall and restaurants. Your children are naturally curious about why and how things happen. If you pass any construction sites, point out the materials and equipment used, as well as the jobs of the workers on the sites. This will help your child develop vocabulary and language skills. Concepts of time can also be fostered if you are able to visit the construction site over an extended period of time. You and your child will be able to keep track of progress in the development of the building.

Have a good week!

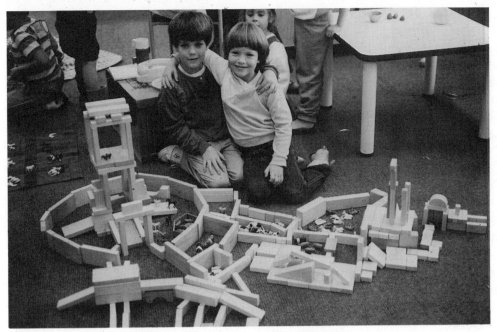

FIGURE 6 Creating a village out of buildings.

Music:

"Go In and Out the Window"

Form a circle with the children and hold hands. While holding hands have the children raise their arms up to form windows. Let each child have a turn weaving in and out the windows. Use the following chant as you play.

_____ goes in and out the window,
In and out the windows,
In and out the windows.
_____ goes in and out the windows,
As we did before.

Fill in child's name in the _____.

Fingerplays:

THE CARPENTER'S TOOLS

The carpenter's hammer goes rap, rap, rap
  (make hammering motion with fist)
And his saw goes see, saw, see.
  (make sawing motion with arm and hand)
He planes and hammers and saws
  (make motions for each)
While he builds a building for me.
  (point to yourself)

CARPENTER

This is the way he saws the wood
  (make sawing motion)
Sawing, sawing, sawing.

This is the way he nails a nail
  (make hammering motion)
Nailing, nailing, nailing.

This is the way he paints a building
  (make brushing motion)
Painting, painting, painting.

MY HOUSE

I'm going to build a little house.
  (draw house with fingers by outlining in
  the air)
With windows big and bright,
  (spread out arms)
With chimney tall and curling smoke
  (show tall chimney with hands)
Drifting out of sight.
  (shade eyes with hands to look)
In winter when the snowflakes fall
  (use fingers to make the motion of snow
  falling downward)
Or when I hear a storm,
  (place hand to ear)
I'll go sit in my little house
  (draw house again)
Where I'll be snug and warm.
  (hug self)

Science:

1. Building Materials

Collect materials such as wood, brick, cement, metal and magnifying glasses and place on the science table. Encourage the children to observe the various materials up close.

2. Mixing Cement

Make cement using a small amount of cement and water. Mix materials together in a large plastic ice cream bucket. Allow the children to help. The children can also observe and feel the wet cement.

3. Building Tools

Collect and place various tools such as a hammer, level, wedge, and screwdriver on the science table for the children to examine. Discuss each tool and demonstrate how it is used. Then place the tools in the woodworking area. Provide wood and styrofoam so that the children are encouraged to use the tools as a self-selected activity with close adult supervision.

Dramatic Play:

1. Library

Rearrange the dramatic play area to resemble a library. Include books, library cards, book markers, tables, and chairs for the children's use.

2. Buildings

Collect large cardboard boxes from an appliance dealer. The children can construct their own buildings and paint them with tempera paint.

3. Construction Site

Place cardboard boxes, blocks, plastic pipes, wheelbarrows, hard hats, paper and pencils in the dramatic play area to represent a construction site.

Arts and Crafts:

1. Our Home

Provide paper, crayons and markers for each child to draw his home. Collect all of the drawings and place them in mural fashion on a large piece of paper to create a town. To extend this activity, have the children also draw buildings in the town to extend the mural. (This activity may be limited to kindergarten children or children who have reached the representational stage of art development.)

2. Blueprints

Blueprint paper, pencils and markers should be placed in the art area. The children will enjoy marking on it. Older children may also enjoy using rulers and straight edges.

3. Building Shapes

Cut out building shapes from easel paper. Place at the easel, allowing children to paint their buildings.

4. Building Collages

Collect magazines with pictures of houses. Encourage children to cut or tear out pictures of buildings. The pictures can be glued on paper to create a mural.

5. Creating Structures

Save half pint milk cartons. Rinse well and allow the children to paint, color and decorate the cartons to look like buildings.

Sensory:

1. Wet Sand

Fill the sensory table with sand and add water. Provide cups, square plastic containers, bowls, etc. for children to create molds with the sand.

2. Wood Shavings

Place wood shavings in the sensory table.

3. Scented Playdough

Prepare scented playdough and place in the sensory table.

Large Muscle:

Workbench

Call attention during group time to the woodworking bench explaining the activities that can occur there. Try to encourage the children to practice pounding nails, sawing, drilling, etc. during self-initiated play.

Field Trips/Resource People:

1. Building Site

Visit a local building site if available. Observe and discuss the people who are working, how buildings look and safety. Take pictures. When the pictures are developed, post them in the classroom.

2. Neighborhood Walk

Take a walk around the neighborhood. Observe the various kinds of buildings. Talk about the different sizes and colors of the buildings.

3. Library

Visit a library. Observe how books are stored. Read the children a story while there. If possible, allow the children to check out books.

4. Browsing at the Mall

Visit the shopping mall. Talk about the mall being a large building that houses a variety of stores. Visit a few of the stores that may be of special interest to the children. Included may be a toy store, pet store, and a sporting goods store.

5. Classroom Visitors

Invite people to visit the classroom such as:

* construction worker
* carpenter
* electrician
* architect
* decorator/designer
* plumber

Math:

1. Weighing Bricks

Set out balance scale and small bricks. The children can weigh and balance the bricks.

2. Wipe-off Windows

Cut out and laminate a variety of buildings with varying amounts of windows. Provide children with grease markers or watercolor markers. Encourage the children to count the number of windows of each building and print the corresponding numeral on the building. The numerals can be wiped off with a damp cloth. (This activity would be most appropriate for kindergarten children.)

3. Blocks

Set out blocks of various shapes including triangles, rectangles and squares for the children to build with.

Social Studies:

1. Buildings in Our Town

Make a chart with the children's names listed vertically on the right-hand side. Across the top of the chart draw buildings or glue pictures of buildings that the children have visited. Suggestions include a theater, supermarket, clinic, museum, post office, fire station, etc. At group time, ask the children what buildings they have visited. Mark the sites for each child.

2. Unusual Buildings

Show pictures of unusual buildings cut from various magazines, travel guides, etc. Allow the children to use their creative thinking by asking them the use of each building. All answers and possibilities should be acknowledged.

3. Occupation Match

Cut out pictures of buildings and the people who work in them. Examples would include: hospital—nurse, fire station—fire fighter. Glue these pictures to tagboard and laminate. The children should be encouraged to match each worker to the appropriate building.

Group Time (games, language):

1. Identifying Buildings

Collect several pictures of buildings that are easily identified such as school, fire station, hospital, home. Talk about each picture. Ask, "How do you know this is a school?" Discuss the function of each building. To help the children, pictures of buildings in their community can be used.

2. Exploring our Center

Explore your center. Walk around the outside and observe walls, windows, roof, etc.

Explore the inside also. Check out the rooms, floor, walls, ceiling, stairs... Colors, materials and size are some things you can discuss with each. Allow the children to help make an, "Our Center Has...." chart.

Cooking:

Sugar Cookies

1 1/2 cups powdered sugar
1 cup margarine or butter
1 egg
1 teaspoon vanilla
2 1/2 cups all purpose flour
1 teaspoon baking soda
1 teaspoon cream of tartar
granulated sugar

Mix the powdered sugar, margarine, egg, and vanilla together. Stir in the flour, baking soda, and cream of tartar. Chill, to prevent sticking while rolling the dough out. Heat the oven to 375 degrees. Roll out the dough. Cut into squares, triangles, diamonds, rectangles, circles. Sprinkle with sugar. Place on a lightly greased cookie sheet. Bake until lightly brown, about 7 to 8 minutes. Give each child 3 to 5 cookies. Allow them to make buildings with their shapes before eating.

Record:

The following record can be found in preschool educational catalogs:

My Street Begins At My House. Ella Jenkins. (Kaplan)

Books and Stories:

The following books and stories can be used to complement the theme:

1. **The House That Jack Built.** Paul Galdone. (New York: McGraw Hill Book Company, 1961).

2. **Tool Book.** Gail Gibbons. (New York: Holiday House, 1982).

3. **The Lonely Skyscraper.** Jenny Hawkesworth. (New York: Doubleday, 1980).

4. **The Post Office Book.** Gail Gibbons. (New York: Thomas Y. Crowell, 1982).

5. **Apt. 3.** Ezra Jack Keats. (New York: Macmillan, 1971).

6. **Around the Neighborhood.** Robert Durham. (Chicago: Childrens Press, 1987).

7. **Department Store.** Gail Gibbons. (New York: Thomas Y. Crowell, 1984).

Puzzles:

The following puzzles can be found in preschool educational catalogs:

1. **"House"** Lauri.

2. **"Carpenter"** Judy/Instructo.

3. **"Architect"** Judy/Instructo.

4. **"Construction Worker"** Judy/Instructo.

5. **"The City"** Judy/Instructo.

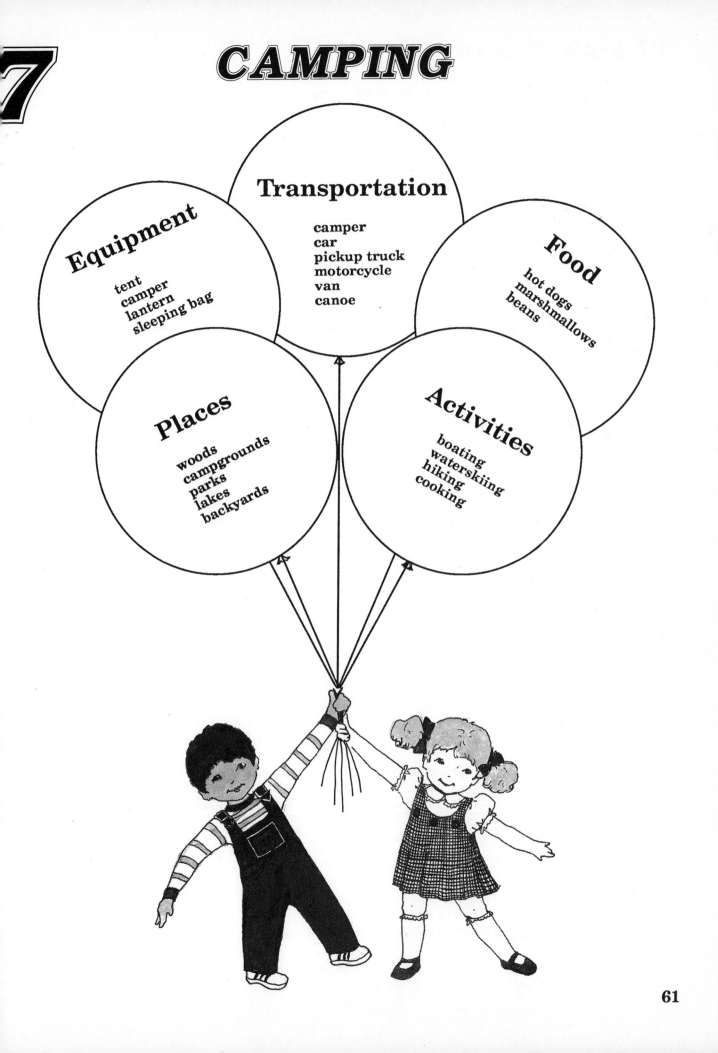

CAMPING

7

Equipment

tent
camper
lantern
sleeping bag

Transportation

camper
car
pickup truck
motorcycle
van
canoe

Food

hot dogs
marshmallows
beans

Places

woods
campgrounds
parks
lakes
backyards

Activities

boating
waterskiing
hiking
cooking

Theme Goals:

Through participating in the experiences provided by this theme, the children may learn:

1. Places where people camp.

2. Equipment used for camping.

3. Camping transportation.

4. Camping activities.

5. Foods we eat while camping.

Concepts for the Children to Learn:

1. A tent is a shelter used for camping.

2. We can camp in the woods or at a campground.

3. We can also camp in a park, at a lake or in our backyard.

4. Hot dogs, marshmallows and beans are all camping foods.

5. A camper can be driven or attached to the back of a car or pickup truck.

6. Lanterns and flashlights are sources of light used for camping.

7. A sleeping bag is a blanket used for camping.

8. Some people camp by a lake to waterski and go boating and fishing.

Vocabulary:

1. **backpack**—a zippered bag worn on one's back to carry objects.

2. **recreational vehicle**—a living and sleeping area on wheels.

3. **campfire**—a controlled fire that is made at a campground.

4. **campsite**—a place for tents and campers to park.

5. **camping**—living outdoors in sleeping bags, tents, cabins or campers.

6. **woods**—an area with many trees.

7. **hiking**—taking a long walk.

8. **sleeping bag**—a zippered blanket.

9. **tent**—a movable shelter made out of material.

10. **lantern**—a covered light used for camping.

Bulletin Board

The purpose of this bulletin board is to develop recognition of colors and color words. Construct several tents out of tagboard. Make an identical set out of white tagboard. Color the first set of tents using the primary colors. Print the color names using corresponding colored markers onto the second set of tents. Laminate the materials. Staple the tents with color names to bulletin board. Punch holes in colored tents. Children can attach the tent to a push pin on the corresponding color word tent.

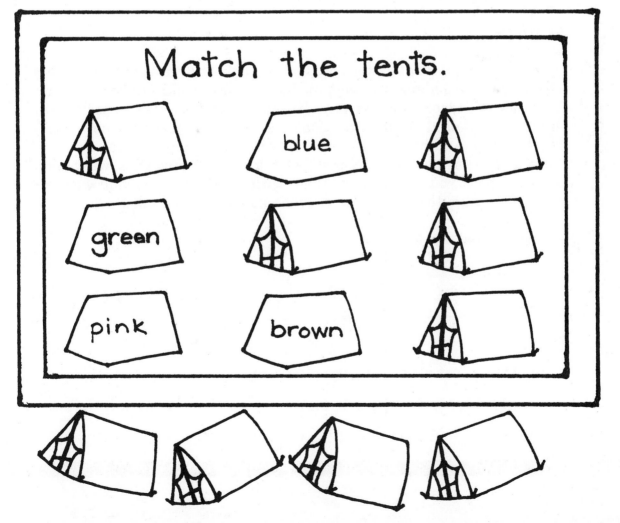

Parent Letter

Dear Parents,

With summer approaching, this week we will be focusing on a fun family activity — camping! The children will become aware of items and equipment that are commonly used while camping. From listening to the children's conversations, it sounds as if many have already been camping with their family. It should be fun to hear the camping stories they will share!

At School This Week

Some of the learning experiences planned for the week include:

* setting up the dramatic play area with a tent, sleeping bags and other camping items.
* singing songs around a pretend campfire.
* going on a "bear hunt" (a rhythmic chant).
* preparing foods that are eaten while camping.

At Home

Help your child create a tent by draping a sheet over a table. Provide a flashlight and a blanket or sleeping bag and your child will be prepared for hours of indoor camping fun! Through dramatic play experiences children relive and clarify situations and roles. They act out how they see the world and how they view relationships among people.

If you have any photographs or slides of family camping trips, we would be delighted if you would share them with us. Contact me and we can work out a time that would be convenient for you. Thanks!

Have a great week!

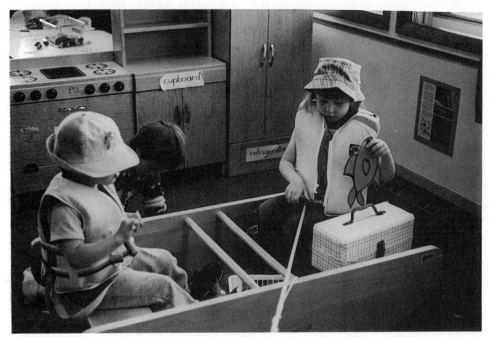

FIGURE 7 "Fishing" is one activity that can be done while "camping."

Music:

1. **"A Camping We Will Go"**
(Sing to the tune of "The Farmer and The Dell")

A camping we will go.
A camping we will go.
Hi ho we're off to the woods.
A camping we will go.

Sue will bring the tent.
Oh Sue will bring the tent.
Hi ho we're off to the woods.
A camping we will go.

Tom will bring the food.
Oh Tom will bring the food.
Hi ho we're off to the woods.
A camping we will go.

The names in the song can be changed to children's names.

2. **Two Little Black Bears**
(Sing to the tune of "Two Little Blackbirds")

Two little black bears sitting on a hill
One named Jack, one named Jill
Run away Jack
Run away Jill

Come back Jack
Come back Jill.
Two little black bears sitting on a hill
One named Jack, one named Jill.

3. **Campfire Songs**

Pretend that you are sitting around a campfire. Explain to the children that often people sing their favorite songs around a campfire. Encourage the children to name their favorite songs, and then sing some of them.

Fingerplays:

BY THE CAMPFIRE

We sat around the campfire
On a chilly night
  (hug self)
Telling spooky stories
In the pale moonlight
  (look up to the sky)

Then we added some more logs,
To make the fire bright,
And sang some favorite camp songs
Together with all our might.
  (extend arms outward)

And when the fire flickered
and embers began to form.
We snuggled in our sleeping bags
all cozy, tired and warm.
　　(lay on ground, hug self)

Source: *Everyday Circle Times*. Liz and
Dick Wilmes. Building Block Publications.

FIVE LITTLE BEAR CUBS

Five little bear cubs
Eating an apple core.
One had a sore tummy
And then there were four.

Four little bear cubs
Climbing in a tree.
One fell out
And then there were three.

Three little bear cubs
Playing peek-a-boo.
One was afraid
And then there were two.

Two little bear cubs
Sitting in the sun.
One ran away
And then there was one.

One little bear cub
Sitting all alone.
He saw his mommy
And then he ran home.

Science:

1. **Scavenger Hunt**

   While outside, have the children find
   plants growing, insects crawling, insects
   flying, a plant growing on a tree, a vine, a
   flower, bird feathers, a root, a seed, etc.

2. **Sink/Float**

   Collect various pieces of camping equipment. Fill the water table with water and
   let the children test which objects sink or
   float. If desired make a chart.

3. **Magnifying Glasses**

   Provide magnifying glasses for looking at
   objects seen on a camping trip.

Dramatic Play:

1. **Camping**

   Collect various types of clothing and camping equipment and place in the dramatic
   play area or outdoors. Include items such
   as hiking boots, sweatshirts, raincoats,
   sleeping bags, backpacks, cooking tools,
   and a tent.

2. **Puppets**

   Develop a puppet corner in the dramatic
   play area including various animal puppets that would be seen while camping.

3. **Going Fishing**

   Set up a rocking boat or a large box in the
   classroom or outdoors. Prepare paper fish
   with paper clips attached to them. Include
   a fishing pole made from a wooden dowel
   and a long string with a magnet attached
   to the end.

4. **Going to the Beach**

   In the dramatic play area, set up lawn
   chairs, beach towels, buckets, shovels,
   sunglasses, etc. Weather permitting these
   items could also be placed outdoors.

Arts and Crafts:

1. **Easel Ideas**

   * paint with leaves, sticks, flowers and
     rocks.
   * paint with colors seen in the forest such
     as brown, green, yellow and orange.
   * cut easel paper into the following shapes:
     tent, rabbits, chipmunks, fish.

2. **Camping Collage**

   Collect leaves, pebbles, twigs, pine cones,
   etc. Provide glue and sturdy tagboard.
   Encourage the children to create a collage
   on the tagboard using the materials found
   while camping.

3. Tackle Box

Make two holes approximately three inches apart in the center of the lid of an egg carton. To form the handle, thread a cord through the holes and tie. Paint the box. In the box, place paper clips for hooks and S-shaped styrofoam pieces for worms.

Sensory:

Sensory Table Additions

* leaves
* rocks
* pebbles
* mud and sand
* twigs
* evergreen needles and branches
* water

Large Muscle:

1. Caves

Using large packing boxes or barrels placed horizontally on the playground, allow the children to pretend to be wild animals in caves.

2. "Bear Hunt"

This is a chant. Prepare the children by asking them to listen and watch carefully so that they can echo back each phrase and imitate the motions as they accompany the story. Begin by patting your hands on your thighs to make foot-step sounds.

Let's go on a bear hunt. . .(echo)
We're going to find a bear. . .(echo)
I've got my camera. . .(echo)
Open the door, squeak. . .(echo)
Walk down the walk. . .(echo)
Open the gate, creak. . .(echo)
Walk down the road. . .(echo)
Coming to a wheat field. . .(echo)
Can't go under it. . .(echo)
Can't go over it. . .(echo)
Have to walk through it. . .(echo)
   (stop patting your thighs and rub your
   hands together to make a swishing sound)

Got through the wheat field. . .(echo)
Coming to a bridge. . .(echo)
Can't go under it. . .(echo)
Can't go around it. . .(echo)
Have to walk over it. . .(echo)
   (stop patting your thighs and pound your
   fists on your chest)
Over the bridge. . .(echo)
Coming to a tree. . .(echo)
Can't go under it. . .(echo)
Can't go around it. . .(echo)
We'll have to climb it. . .(echo)
   (stop patting your thighs and place one
   fist on top of the other in a climbing motion)
All the way to the top. . .(echo)
   (look from one side to the other)
Do you see a bear. . .? (echo)
No (shaking head). . .(echo)
We'll have to climb down. . .(echo)
   (place fist under fist to climb down)
Coming to a river. . .(echo)
We can't go under it. . .(echo)
We can't fly over it. . .(echo)
Can't go around it. . .(echo)
We'll have to cross it. . .(echo)
Let's get in the boat. . .(echo)
And row, row, row. . .
   (all sing "Row, Row, Row Your Boat"
   accompanied with rowing motions)
We got across the river. . .(echo)
We're coming to a cave. . .(echo)
We can't go under it. . .(echo)
We can't go over it. . .(echo)
Can't go around it. . .(echo)
We'll have to go in it. . .(echo)
Let's tip-toe
   (use fingertips to pat thighs)
   (whisper)
It's dark inside. . .(echo)
It's very dark inside. . .(echo)
I can see two eyes. . .(echo)
And a big furry body. . .(echo)
And I feel a wet nose. . .(echo)
   (Yell)
It's a BEAR. . . .RUN. . . .(echo)
   (patting hands very quickly)
Run back to the river,
Row the boat across the river,
   (rowing motion)
Run to the tree
Climb up and climb down
   (do climbing motion)
Run to the bridge and cross it
   (pat chest)

67

Run through the wheat field
  (swish hands together)
Run up the road
Open the gate. . . it creaks,
  (open gate)
Run up the walk,
Open the door...it squeaks,
  (open door)
SLAM IT!
  (clap hands together)

Source: *Musical Games, Fingerplays and Rhythmic Activities for Early Childhood.* Marian Wirth, Verna Stassevitch, Rita Shotwell, Patricia Stemmler. Parker Publishing Co. Inc.

Field Trips/Resource People:

1. Department Store

Visit a department store or a sporting goods store where camping tents and other equipment are displayed.

2. Picnic

Pack a picnic lunch or snack and take it to an area campground.

3. Camper Salesperson

Visit a recreational vehicle dealer and tour a large mobile home.

Math:

Camping Scavenger Hunt

Before the children go outdoors, instruct them to find things on your playground that you would see while camping. Sort them and count them when they bring them into the classroom (five twigs, three rocks, etc.).

Social Studies:

1. Pictures

Collect pictures of different campsites. Share them by displaying them in the classroom at the children's eye level.

2. Camping Experiences

At group time ask if any of the children have been camping. Let them tell the rest of the children what they did while they were camping. Ask where they slept, what they ate, where the bathroom was, etc.

Group Time (games, language):

1. What's Missing

Have different pieces of camping equipment available to show the children. Include a canteen, portable stove, sleeping bag, cooking tools, lantern, etc. Discuss each item, and then have the children close their eyes. Take one of the objects away and then have the children guess which object is missing.

2. Camping Safety

Discuss camping safety. Include these points:

* always put out fires before going to sleep.
* swim in safe areas and with a partner.
* when walking, or hiking away from your campsite, always have an adult with you.
* always wear a life jacket in the boat.

3. Pack the Backpack

Bring into the classroom a large backpack. Also have many camping items available such as sweatshirts, flashlights, lanterns, foods, raincoats, etc. The teacher gives the children instructions that they are going to pretend to go on a hike to the beach. What is one thing they will need to bring along? Why? Continue until all of the children have had a chance to contribute.

Cooking:

1. S'Mores

Place a large marshmallow on a square graham cracker. Next place a square of sweet chocolate on top of the marshmallow. After this, place the graham cracker on a baking sheet into a 250-degree oven for about 5 minutes or until the chocolate starts to melt. Remove the s'more and press a second graham cracker square on top of the chocolate. Let cool for a few minutes, and serve while still slightly warm.

2. **Venezuela Breakfast Cocoa**

    1/4 cup water
    3 tablespoons cocoa
    2 tablespoons sugar
    2 cups milk
    1 teaspoon vanilla

    1. Bring the water to a boil in a saucepan.
    2. Stir in the cocoa and sugar until they are blended. Turn the heat very low.
    3. Slowly pour the milk into the saucepan with the cocoa mixture. Stir steadily to keep the mixture from burning. Continue cooking the mixture over low heat for about 2 minutes. Do not let it boil or skin will form on the top.
    4. When the cocoa is hot, remove it from the stove and stir in the vanilla.
    5. Carefully pour the cocoa into the cups. Serve warm.

Source: *Many Hands Cooking.* Terry Touff Cooper and Marilyn Ratner. (New York: Thomas Y. Crowell Company, 1974).

Record:

The following record can be found in preschool educational catalogs.

Camping in the Mountains. Lucille Wood.

Books and Stories:

The following books and stories can be used to complement the theme:

1. **When Insects are Babies.** Gladys Conklin. (New York: Holiday House Pub., 1969).

2. **Spider Silk.** Augusta Goldin. (New York: Thomas Y. Crowell, 1964).

3. **When Peter Was Lost In the Forest.** Hans Peterson. (New York: Coward-McCann Inc., 1970).

4. **Bambi's Fragrant Forest.** Felix Salten. (New York: Golden Press, 1975).

5. **Bailey Goes Camping.** Kevin Henkes. (New York: Greenwillow Books, 1985).

6. **Curious George Goes Hiking.** Margaret Rey and Alan J. Shalleck. (Boston: Houghton Mifflin Company, 1985).

7. **Camping in the Mountains.** Lucille Wood. (Glendale, CA: Bowman, 1971).

Puzzles:

The following puzzles can be found in preschool educational catalogs:

1. **"Leaves"** 5 pieces. Judy/Instructo.

2. **"Tree"** 6 pieces. Judy/Instructo.

3. **"Wild Animals"** (owl, squirrel, ladybug, frog, bird, butterfly) 6 pieces. Judy/Instructo.

4. **"Ladybug"** 5 pieces. Judy/Instructo.

5. **"Owl"** 11 pieces. Judy/Instructo.

6. **"Squirrel"** 11 pieces. Judy/Instructo.

7. **"Raccoon"** 12 pieces. Judy/Instructo.

8. **"Fish"** 6 pieces. Judy/Instructo.

CARS, TRUCKS AND BUSES

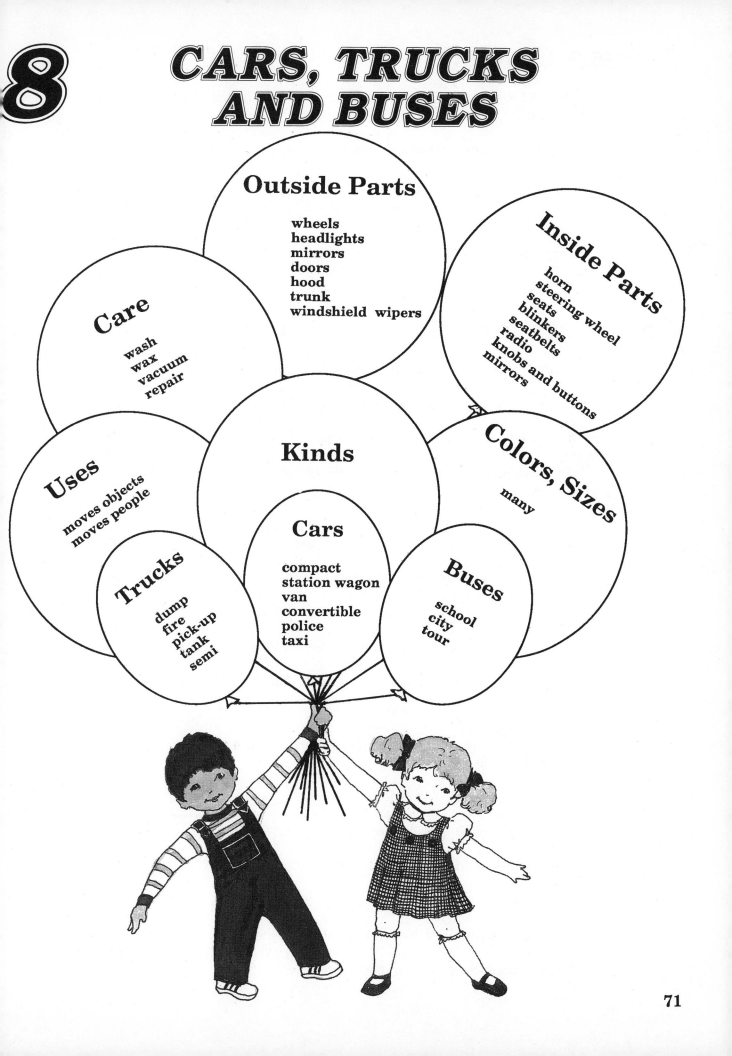

Outside Parts

wheels
headlights
mirrors
doors
hood
trunk
windshield wipers

Inside Parts

horn
steering wheel
seats
blinkers
seatbelts
radio
knobs and buttons
mirrors

Care

wash
wax
vacuum
repair

Uses

moves objects
moves people

Kinds

Colors, Sizes

many

Cars

compact
station wagon
van
convertible
police
taxi

Trucks

dump
fire
pick-up
tank
semi

Buses

school
city
tour

Theme Goals:

Through participating in the experiences provided by this theme, the children may learn:

1. Kinds of cars, trucks and buses.

2. Care of vehicles.

3. Uses of vehicles.

4. Inside and outside parts of vehicles.

5. Colors and sizes of vehicles.

Concepts for the Children to Learn:

1. There are many kinds of cars, trucks and buses.

2. Trucks and buses are usually bigger than cars.

3. Trucks can be used to haul objects.

4. People use cars, trucks and buses to move from place to place.

5. Compact cars are small.

6. A license is needed to drive a car, truck or bus.

7. Cars, trucks and buses need gas to run.

8. Gas can be obtained at a filling station.

9. Vehicles need to be vacuumed, washed, waxed and repaired.

10. Headlights, mirrors and wheels are parts of a car.

Vocabulary:

1. **car**—vehicle used for moving people.

2. **truck**—a wheeled vehicle used to move people and big objects.

3. **bus**—a vehicle that carries many people.

4. **driver**—operates the vehicle.

5. **passenger**—the rider.

6. **fuel**—gas, diesel, etc. used to produce power.

7. **gas**—produces power to move a vehicle.

Bulletin Board

The purpose of the bulletin board is to reinforce color recognition and matching skills, as well as develop one-to-one correspondence concepts. Construct garage shapes out of tagboard. Color each garage a different color and hang on the bulletin board. Hang a push pin in the center of each garage. Next, construct the same number of cars as garages from tagboard. Color each car a different color, to correspond with the colors of the garages. Use a paper punch to make a hole in each car. The children can park each car in its corresponding colored garage.

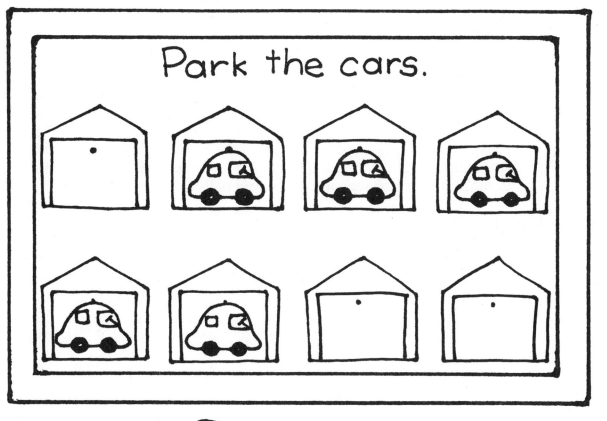

Parent Letter

Dear Parents,

Cars, trucks and buses—these are all transportation vehicles that your child sees on a regular basis. We will be beginning a unit on "Cars, Trucks and Buses" this week. Through participating in the planned experiences, the children will learn that there are many colors, sizes and kinds of cars, trucks and buses. They will also become aware of the occupations associated with the vehicles including taxi drivers, bus drivers and mechanics.

At School This Week

Some of the activities planned for this unit include:

* painting with small cars at the art table.
* looking at many books about trucks, buses and cars.
* setting up a gas station in the dramatic play area.
* a visit with Officer Lewis from the police department, who will show the children his squad car at 10:30 on Thursday.

At Home

You can foster the concepts of this unit at home by taking your child with you the next time you need to buy gas for your car. There are many different types of trucks and cars to observe at the filling station. Also, provide soapy water and a sponge and let your child help you wash the family car. Children enjoy taking part in grown-up activities and this helps to build a sense of responsibility and self-esteem.

Have a good week!

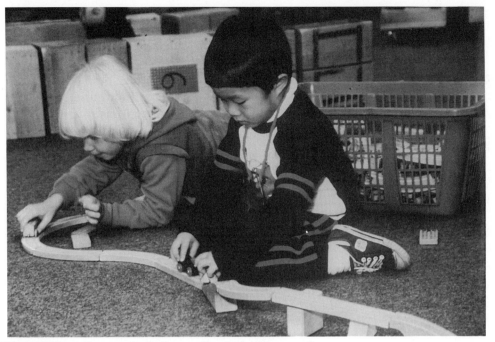

FIGURE 8 Learning the rules of the road.

Fingerplays:

OUR FAMILY CAR

This is our family car
   (make fists as if holding a steering wheel)
The engine purrs like new.
Four wheels and a body,
   (hold up four fingers)
It is painted blue.

Dad and Mom use it for business
   (hold fists as if holding a steering wheel)
Or to drive us to the store.
We take it on vacation
You couldn't ask for more.
   (shake head "no")

In the winter weather
If we should miss the bus,
   (make sad face)
We can still get to our school,
In the family car we trust.
   (hold fists as if holding a steering wheel)

Source: *Everyday Circle Times.* Liz and
Dick Wilmes. (Building Block Publishers,
Illinois, 1983).

WINDSHIELD WIPER

I'm a windshield wiper
   (bend arm at elbow with fingers pointing up)

This is how I go
   (move arm to left and right, pivoting at
   elbow)
Back and forth, back and forth
   (continue back and forth motion)
In the rain and snow.
   (continue back and forth motion)

HERE IS A CAR

Here is a car, shiny and bright.
   (cup one hand and place on other palm)
This is the windshield that lets in the light.
   (hands open, fingertips touching)
Here are wheels that go round and round.
   (two fists)
I sit in the back seat and make not a sound.
   (sit quietly with hands in lap)

THE CAR RIDE

(Left arm, held out bent, is road; right fist
is car.)

"Vroom!" says the engine
   (place car on left shoulder)
As the driver starts the car.
   (shake car)

"Mmmm," says the windows
As the driver takes it far.
   (travel over upper arm)

"Errr," says the tires
As it rounds the final bend,
(turn at elbow, proceed over forearm)

"Ahhh," says the driver
As his trip comes to an end.
(stop car on left flattened palm)

SCHOOL BUS

I go to the bus stop each day
(walk one hand across table)
Where the bus comes to take us away.
(stop, have other hand wait also)
We stand single file
(one behind the other)
And walk down the aisle
(step up imaginary steps onto bus)
When the bus driver talks, we obey.

Science:

1. License Plates

Collect license plates from different states
and different vehicles and place them on a
table for the children to explore.

2. Feely Box

Put transportation toys in a feely box. Include cars, trucks and buses. Individually
let the children feel inside the box and
identify the type of toy.

Dramatic Play:

1. Filling Station

Provide cardboard boxes for cars and hoses
for the gas pumps. Also make available
play money and steering wheels.

2. Bus

Set up a bus situation by lining up chairs
in one or two long rows. Provide a steering
wheel for the driver. A money bucket and
play money can also be provided. If a
steering wheel is unavailable, heavy round
pizza cardboards can be improvised.

3. Taxi

Set up two rows of chairs side by side to
represent a taxi. Use a pizza cardboard, or
other round object, as the steering wheel.
Provide a telephone, dress up clothes for
the passengers and a hat for the driver. A
"TAXI" sign can also be placed by the
chairs to invite play.

4. Fire Truck

Contact the local fire chief and ask to use
old hoses, fire hats and firefighter
clothing.

Arts and Crafts:

1. License Plate Rubbings

Place paper on top of a license plate.
Using the side of a large crayon, rub
across the top of the license plate.

2. Car Painting

Provide several small plastic cars, trucks
and large sheets of white paper. Also have
available low, flat pans of thin tempera
paint. Encourage the children to take the
cars and trucks and roll the wheels in the
paint. They can then transfer the car to
their own paper and make car or truck
tracks on the paper.

3. Designing Cars

Provide the children with large appliance-
sized cardboard boxes. To protect the floor
surface, place a large sheet of plastic
underneath. Provide the children with
paint, markers and collage materials to
decorate the boxes as cars. When the cars
dry, they can be moved into the block
building, dramatic play areas or outdoor
area.

4. Scrapbooks or Collages

Provide magazines for children to cut or
tear out pictures of cars and trucks to
make a collage or small scrapbook.

Sensory:

Sensory Table Additions

* cars and trucks with wet sand
* baby oil and water

Large Muscle:

1. "Fill 'er Up"

The trikes, wagons and scooters can be used outside on the playground. A gas pump can be constructed out of an old cardboard box with an attached hose.

2. Car, Car, Truck

Play this simple variation of "Duck, Duck, Goose" by substituting the words, "Car, Car, Truck".

3. Wash a Car

If possible, wash a compact size car. Provide a hose, sponges, brushes, a bucket and soapy water. If an actual car is not available, children can wash tricycles, bicycles, scooters and wagons.

Field Trips/Resource People:

1. City Bus

Take the children for a ride around town on a city bus. When boarding, allow each child to place his own money in the meter. Observe the length of the bus. While inside, watch how the bus driver operates the bus. Also have a school bus driver visit and tell about the job and the importance of safety on a bus.

2. Taxi Driver

Invite a taxi driver to visit and show the features of the taxi.

3. Patrol Car

Invite a police officer to bring a squad car to the center. The radio, siren and flashing lights can be demonstrated. Let the children sit in the car.

4. Fire Truck

Invite a local firefighter to bring a fire truck to the center. Let the children climb in the truck and observe the parts.

5. Semi-truck Driver

Invite a semi driver to bring his truck. Observe the size, number of wheels and parts of the cab. Let the children sit in the cab.

Math:

1. Cars and Garages

Car garages can be constructed out of empty half-pint milk cartons. Collect and carefully wash the milk cartons. Cut out one side and write a numeral starting with one on each carton. Next, collect a corresponding number of small matchbox cars. Attach a strip of paper with a numeral from one to the appropriate number on each car's top. The children can drive each car into the garage with the corresponding numeral.

2. License Plate Match

Construct two sets of identical license plates. Print a pattern of letters or numerals on each set. Mix them up. Children can try to match the pairs.

3. Car, Truck or Bus Sequencing

Cut out various sized cars, trucks or buses and laminate. Children can sequence them from largest to smallest and vice versa.

4. Sorting

Construct cars, trucks, and buses of different colors and laminate. Children can sort according to color.

Social Studies:

Discussion on Safety

Have a group discussion on safety when riding in a car. Allow children to come up with suggestions. Write them down on a chart and display in classroom during the unit. The addition of pictures or drawings would be helpful for younger children.

Group Time (games, language):

1. Thank You Note

Write a thank you note to a resource person. Allow children to dictate and sign it.

2. Red Light, Green Light

Select one child to pretend to be a traffic light. The traffic light places his back to children lined up at the other end of the room. When the traffic light says "Green Light" or holds up green paper, the other children attempt to creep up on the traffic light. At any time the traffic light can say "Red Light" or hold up a red paper and quickly turn around. Creeping children must freeze. Any child caught moving is sent back to the starting line. Play continues until one child reaches the traffic light. This child becomes the new traffic light.

Cooking:

1. Cracker Wheels

For this recipe each child will need:

4 round crackers
1/2 hot dog
1/2 piece of cheese

Slice hot dogs and place on a cracker. Place cheese over the top. Place in oven at 350 degrees for 3 to 5 minutes or microwave for 30 seconds. Let cool and eat.

2. Greek Honey Twists

3 eggs beaten
2 tablespoons vegetable oil
1/2 teaspoon baking powder
1/4 teaspoon salt
1 3/4 to 2 cups all-purpose flour
vegetable oil
1/4 cup honey
1 tablespoon water
ground cinnamon

Mix eggs, 2 tablespoons oil, baking powder and salt in a large bowl. Gradually stir in enough flour to make a very stiff dough. Knead 5 minutes. Roll half the dough at a time as thin as possible on well-floured surface with a stockinet-covered rolling pin. Cut into wheel shapes. Cover with damp towel to prevent drying.

Heat 2 to 3 inches of oil to 375 degrees. Fry 3 to 5 twists at a time until golden brown, turning once, about 45 seconds on each side. Drain on paper towels. Heat honey and water to boiling; boil 1 minute. Cool slightly. Drizzle over twists; sprinkle with cinnamon. Makes 32 twists.

Source: *Betty Crocker's International Cookbook.* New York: Randon House, 1980.

Books and Stories:

The following books and stories can be used to complement the theme:

1. **I Want to Be a Taxi Driver.** Eugene Baker. (Chicago: Childrens Press, 1969).

2. **The Big Book of Real Trucks.** Elizabeth Cameron. (New York: Grosset and Dunlap, 1970).

3. **ABC of Cars, Trucks and Machines.** Adelaide Holl. (New York: McGraw-Hill, 1970).

4. **Things That Go.** Anne Rockwell. (New York: E. P. Dutton, Inc., 1986).

5. **The Great Big Car and Truck Book.** Richard Scarry. (New York: Western Publishing, 1951).

6. **Cars and Trucks and Things That Go.** Richard Scarry. (New York: Western Publishing, 1974).

7. **When I Ride In a Car.** Dorothy Chlad. (Chicago: Childrens Press, 1983).

8. **Trucks.** Harry McNaught. (New York: Random House, 1976).

9. **Have You Seen Roads?** Joanne Oppenheim. (New York: Young Scott Books, 1969).

10. **The Car Trip.** Helen Oxenbury. (New York: E. P. Dutton, Inc., 1983).

11. **Fill It Up! All About Service Stations.** (New York: Thomas Y. Crowell, 1985).

12. **Big Book of Real Trucks.** George Zaffo. (New York: Grosset and Dunlap, 1976).

13. **The Taxi Book.** Edith T. Kunhardt. (New York: Golden Books, 1985).

14. **Rattle-Rattle Dump Truck.** Darlen Geis. (Los Angeles: Price/Stern/Sloan, 1987).

15. **Josuha James Likes Trucks.** Catherine Petrie. (Chicago: Childrens Press, 1987).

Puzzles:

The following puzzles can be found in preschool educational catalogs:

1. **"Easy Wheels"** 4 pieces. Judy/Instructo.

2. **"Car"** 11 pieces. Judy/Instructo.

3. **"Truck"** 15 pieces. Lauri.

4. **"Transportation Puzzles"** Judy/Instructo.

5. **"Truck"** Judy/Instructo.

6. **"Truck"** Judy/Instructo.

7. **"School Bus"** 12 pieces. Judy/Instructo.

8. **"Diesel Truck"** 11 pieces. Judy/Instructo.

9. **"Transportation"** 20 pieces. Judy/Instructo.

10. **"Great Yellow School Bus"** Floor puzzle. Judy/Instructo.

11. **"Great Orange Dump Truck"** Floor puzzle. Judy/Instructo.

CATS

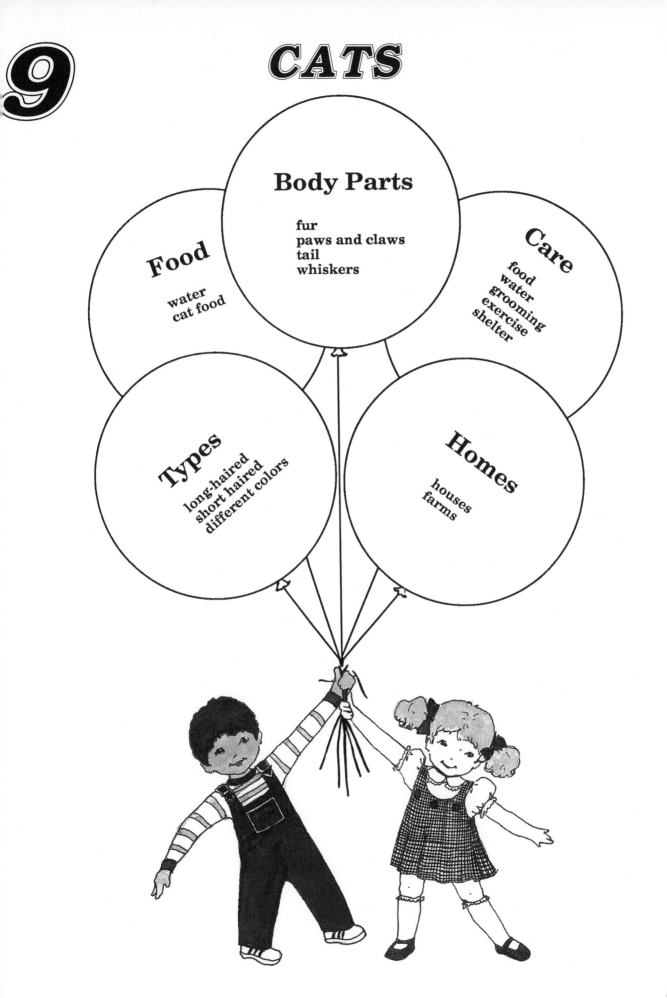

Body Parts

fur
paws and claws
tail
whiskers

Food

water
cat food

Care

food
water
grooming
exercise
shelter

Types

long-haired
short haired
different colors

Homes

houses
farms

Theme Goals:

Through participating in the experiences provided by this theme, the children may learn:

1. Types of cats.

2. Body parts of a cat.

3. Cats need special care.

4. What cats eat, drink and where they live.

Concepts for the Children to Learn:

1. Cats can be black, brown, white, grey or yellow.

2. Cats use their claws for many things.

3. Cats meow and purr to communicate.

4. Cats have legs, eyes, ears, a mouth, nose and tail.

5. Cats have fur on their skin.

6. Cats should be handled carefully and gently.

7. There are many different sizes and types of cats.

8. Cats need food, water, and exercise everyday.

9. Many different people help cats.

10. A kitten is a baby cat.

11. Cats like to play.

Vocabulary:

1. **kitten**—a baby cat.

2. **pet**—an animal kept for pleasure.

3. **paw**—the cat's foot.

4. **veterinarian**—an animal doctor.

5. **leash**—a rope, chain or cord that attaches to a collar.

6. **collar**—a band worn around the cat's neck.

7. **whiskers**—stiff hair growing around the cat's nose, mouth and eyes.

8. **coat**—hair covering the skin.

82

Bulletin Board

The purpose of this bulletin board is to promote visual discrimination and pattern matching skills. Construct cats' bodies and heads out of tagboard, coloring each a different color and fur pattern. Laminate all pieces. Attach cat bodies to the bulletin board. Children then match the heads to the corresponding body.

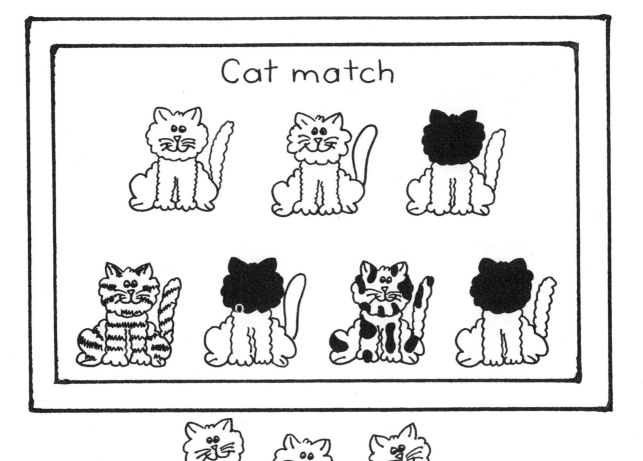

Parent Letter

Dear Parents,

We have many exciting activities planned for this week at school as we begin our study on cats. We will be learning about a cat's body structure, how to care and feed our cats and different types of cats.

At School This Week

Some of the learning experiences planned for the week include:

* taking a field trip to the veterinarian's office.
* making a chart of different types of cats.
* setting up a cat grooming area in dramatic play.

At Home

We will be learning the fingerplay "Two Little Kittens." You may want to try it with your child at home:

Two little kittens found a ball of yarn
   (hold up 2 fingers ... cup hands together to form a ball)
As they were playing near a barn.
   (bring hands together pointed upward for barn)
One little kitten jumped in the hay,
   (hold up 1 finger ... make jumping then wiggling motion)
The other little kitten ran away.
   (make running motion with other hand)

Fingerplays and rhymes help children develop language vocabulary and sequencing skills. The actions that often accompany fingerplays develop fine motor development.

Have a good week!

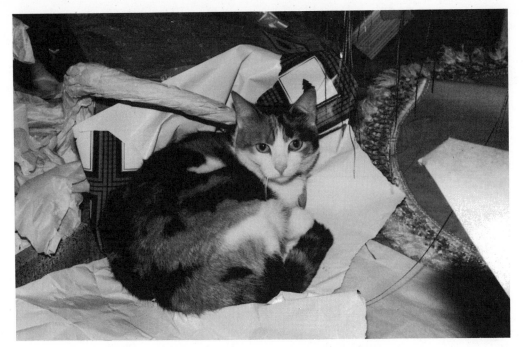

FIGURE 9 Some cats have unique personalities.

Music:

1. "Two Little Kittens"
(Sing to the tune of "Two Little Blackbirds")

Two little kittens sitting on a hill
One named Jack, one named Jill
Run away Jack, run away Jill
Come back Jack, come back Jill
Two little kittens sitting on a hill
One named Jack, one named Jill.

2. "Kitty"
(Sing to the tune of "Bingo")

I have a cat. She's very shy.
But she comes when I call K-I-T-T-Y
K-I-T-T-Y
K-I-T-T-Y
K-I-T-T-Y
and Kitty is her name-o.

Variation: Let children think of other names.

Fingerplays:

MRS. KITTY'S DINNER

Mrs. Kitty, sleek and fat,
  (put thumb up with fingers folded on
  right hand)
With her kittens four.
  (hold up four fingers on right hand)
Went to sleep upon the mat
  (make a fist)
By the kitchen door.

Mrs. Kitty heard a noise.
Up she jumped in glee.
  (thumb up on right hand)
"Kittens, maybe that's a mouse?
  (all 5 fingers on right hand up)
Let's go and see!"

Creeping, creeping, creeping on.
  (slowly sneaking with 5 fingers on floor)
Silently they stole.
But the little mouse had gone
  (mouse is thumb on left hand)
Back into his hole.

A KITTEN

A kitten is fast asleep under the chair.
  (thumb under hands)
And Donald can't find her.
He's looked everywhere.
  (fingers circling eyes to look)
Under the table
  (peek under one hand)
And under the bed
  (peek under other hand)

He looked in the corner, and then Donald said,
"Come Kitty, come Kitty, this milk is for you."
  (curve hands for dish)
And out came kitty calling "mew, mew, mew."

THREE CATS

One little cat and two little cats
went out for a romp one day.
  (hold up 1 finger and then 2 fingers with other hand)
One little cat and two little cats
make how many cats at play?
  (ask how many that makes)
Three little cats had lots of fun
till growing tired away ran _____?
  (take 1 finger away and ask how many ran away)
I really think that he was most unkind
to the _____ little cats that were left behind.
  (how many are left)

KITTEN IS HIDING

A kitten is hiding under a chair,
  (hide one thumb in other hand)
I looked and looked for her everywhere.
  (peer about with hand on forehead)
Under the table and under the bed,
  (pretend to look)
I looked in the corner and then I said,
"Come kitty, come kitty, I have milk for you."
  (cup hands to make dish and extend)
Kitty came running and calling, "Mew, mew."
  (run fingers up arm)

TWO LITTLE KITTENS

Two little kittens found a ball of yarn
  (hold up 2 fingers...cup hands together to form a ball)
As they were playing near a barn.
  (bring hands together pointed upward for barn)

One little kitten jumped in the hay,
  (hold up one finger...make jumping, then wiggling motion)
The other little kitten ran away.
  (make running motion with other hand)

Science:

1. Provide a scale and different cat items (such as cat toys, collar, food dish, etc.) to weigh.

2. During the social studies activity "Share Your Cat," arrange for a cat and a kitten to be in the classroom at the same time. With the help of parents, weigh the cats or kittens and discuss with the children the differences.

3. Set out a magnifying glass to observe different kinds of dry cat food.

4. Talk about a cat who has claws and one that is declawed. Ask various questions such as: "Why do cats have claws? Why are cats declawed? Where do cats go to be declawed? etc."

5. Discuss the various parts of a cat's body and how they can protect the cat. (Examples: fur, whiskers, etc.)

6. Discuss what a cat's body does when it feels danger.

Dramatic Play:

1. **Cat Grooming**

   Provide the children with empty shampoo and conditioner bottles, brushes, combs, ribbons, collars, plastic bathtub, towels, and stuffed animal cats.

2. **Veterinarian's Office**

   Provide various medical supplies such as a stethoscope, bandages and thermometers along with stuffed cats.

3. **Cats!**

Let children pretend they are cats by using cat masks or costumes. Also, you may want to try using yarn balls, boxes to curl up in and empty cat food boxes. Allow the children to act out the story "The Three Little Kitttens" or other cat stories.

4. **Circus or Zoo**

Lions, cheetas, panthers, leopards, and tigers are also cats. Use large boxes for cages.

Arts and Crafts:

1. **Kitty Collage**

Let children find and cut or tear out pictures of cats from greeting cards and magazines. Children can then paste their cats on pieces of construction paper.

2. **Pom Pom Painting**

Set out several different colors of tempera paint. Using pom-pom balls, let children create their own designs on construction paper.

3. **Cat Mask**

Using paper plates or paper bags along with paper scraps, yarn, crayons, scissors and paint, let the children design cat masks.

4. **Paw Prints**

Let children pretend they are cats using their hands and paint to make prints.

Large Muscle:

1. **Bean Bag Toss**

Make a cat shape on plywood with holes of different sizes cut out. The children can try from varying distances to throw bean bags through the holes.

2. **Yarn Balls**

Set up baskets at varying distances from a masking tape line on the floor. Toss yarn balls into the baskets.

3. **Cat Pounce**

Children pretend to be cats and pounce from one line to another.

4. **Climbing Cats**

Bring into the classroom or outside a wooden climber. As cats love to climb; the children can pretend to be cats and climb on the climber.

5. **Cat Movements**

Write down all the words that describe how cats move. Allow the children to demonstrate the movements. Also use music in the background.

Field Trips/Resource People:

1. **Pet Store**

Take a field trip to a pet store. Ask the manager how to care for cats. Observe the different types of cats, cages, collars, leashes and food.

2. **Veterinarian's Office**

Take a field trip to a veterinarian's office or animal hospital. Compare the similarities and differences to a doctor's office.

3. **Variety Store**

Visit a variety store and observe pet accessories.

4. **Resource People**

Invite resource people. Suggestions include:

* cat groomer
* humane society representative

* pet store owner
* veterinarian
* parents to bring in pet cats

Math:

1. Matching Game

Have the children match the number of cats on a card to the correct numeral. (Cat stickers work well.)

2. How Many Paper Clips

Make several different sizes of cats out of tagboard. Children measure each cat with the paper clips.

3. Whisker Count

Make several cat faces with one numeral on each face. Children attach the correct number of whiskers (pipe cleaners, felt, paper strips, etc.) according to the numeral on the cat.

Social Studies:

1. Chart

Make a chart with the children of different types of cats.

2. Displays

Display different pictures of cats around the room.

3. Share Your Cat

Invite the children and the parents to bring in a pet cat on specified days. (Have your camera ready! Take pictures and display them on a bulletin board.)

4. Cat Safety

Discuss cat safety with the class. Items that may be discussed include why cats use their claws, what to do if you find a stray cat, the uses of collars and leashes.

Group Time (games, language):

1. Copy Cats

Have one child be the cat and clap a rhythm for the group. The other children listen and then be the copy cats. They clap the same rhythm as the cat did. Another child now becomes the cat and creates a rhythm for the copy cats to imitate.

2. Nice Kitty

One child is chosen to be the kitty. The rest of the children sit in a circle. As the kitty goes to each child in the circle he pets the kitty and says nice kitty, but the kitty makes no reply. Finally the kitty meows in response to one child. That child must run around the outside of the circle as the kitty chases him. If the child returns to his original place before the kitty can catch him the child becomes the new kitty.

3. Listen Carefully

The children should sit in a circle. One child is selected to be the mother cat. After mother cat has left the room, choose several other children to be kittens. All of the children cover their mouths with both hands and the kittens start saying meow, meow, meow. When the mother cat returns she should listen carefully to find all of her kittens. When she has found them all, another child should be chosen mother cat and the game can continue.

4. Farmer in the Dell

The children can play "Farmer in the Dell."

Cooking:

1. Cheese Cat

English muffins
cheese slices

Allow the children to cut out a cat face on
their own slice of cheese. Put the cheese
on top of the English muffin and bake
long enough to melt the cheese.

2. Cat Face

1/2 peach (head)
almonds (ears)
red hots (eyes)
raisin (nose)
stick pretzels (whiskers)

Create a cat face using the ideas above or
a variety of other items.

Records:

The following records can be found in preschool educational catalogs:

1. **I Like Cats.** Marion Crume.

2. **Be a Frog, a Bird or a Tree.** Rachel Carr. "Stretch like a Cat"

3. **Singing, Swinging.** Sharon, Lois and Bram. "The Cat Came Back"

4. **Birds, Beast, Bugs and Little Fishes.** Pete Seeger. "My Little Kitty"

Books and Stories:

The following books and stories can be used to complement the theme:

1. **Our Cat Flossie.** Ruth Brown. (New York: E. P. Dutton, 1986).

2. **Karen and the Little Lost Kitten.** Peter Seymour. (Los Angeles: Inter-
visual Communications, Inc., 1982).

3. **Kittens, Kittens, Kittens.** Edith Kunhardt. (New York: Golden Books, 1987).

4. **One Little Kitten.** Tana Hoban. (New York: Scholastic, 1979).

5. **Two Little Kittens Are Born.** Betty Schilling. (New York: Scholastic,
1980).

6. **The Curious Little Kitten.** Linda Hayward. (New York: Golden Press,
1982).

7. **Cats.** F. Henrie. (New York: Franklin Watts, Inc., 1980).

8. **I Love Cats.** Catherine Matthias. (Chicago: Childrens Press, 1987).

9. **Hi Cat!** Ezra Jack Keats. (New York: Macmillan, 1970).

10. **Oh No Cat.** Janice May Udry. (New York: Coward, McCann and
Geognegan, 1976).

11. **The Cat in the Hat.** Dr. Seuss. (New York: Harper and Row, 1973).

12. **Angus and The Cat.** Marjorie Flack. (New York: Doubleday, 1971).

13. **Momo's Kitten.** Mitsu and Taro Yashima. (New York: Viking Press, 1961).

14. **How Kittens Grow.** Millicent Selsam. (New York: Four Winds Press, 1975).

Puzzles:

The following puzzles can be found in preschool educational catalogs:

1. **"Kitten"** 5 pieces. Judy/Instructo.

2. **"Cat and Kittens"** 13 pieces. Judy/Instructo.

3. **"Animal Mothers and Babies Puzzle Set"** 13 pieces. Lakeshore.

4. **"Kitten"** (Beginner's Mini Puzzle Set) 4 pieces. Lakeshore.

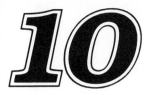

10 CHRISTMAS

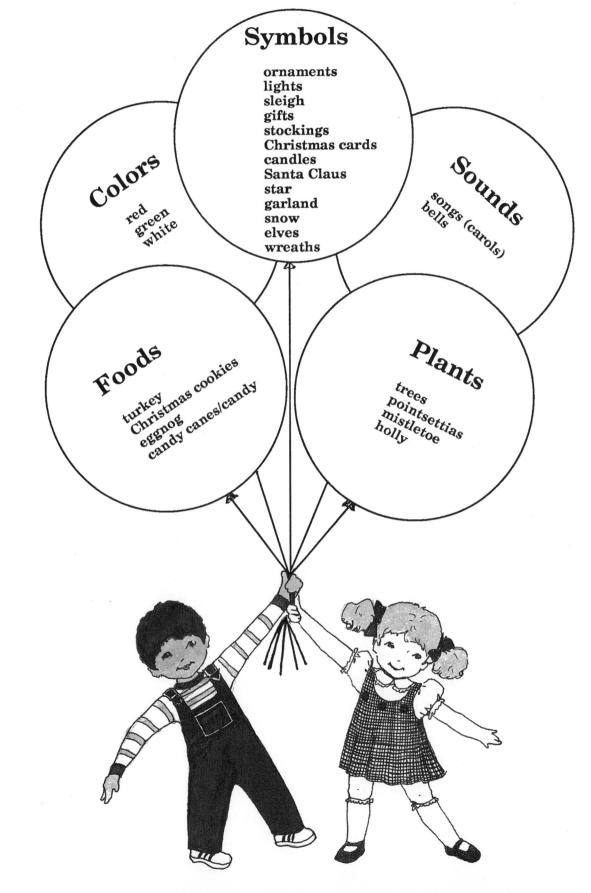

Symbols

ornaments
lights
sleigh
gifts
stockings
Christmas cards
candles
Santa Claus
star
garland
snow
elves
wreaths

Colors

red
green
white

Sounds

songs (carols)
bells

Foods

turkey
Christmas cookies
eggnog
candy canes/candy

Plants

trees
pointsettias
mistletoe
holly

Theme Goals:

Through the experiences provided by this theme, the children may learn:

1. Christmas colors.
2. Christmas foods.
3. Christmas plants.
4. Symbols of Christmas.
5. Sounds heard at Christmas.

Concepts for the Children to Learn:

1. Red, green and white are Christmas colors.
2. Turkey, Christmas cookies and candy are Christmas foods.
3. Santa Claus, reindeer, stockings, and Christmas trees are symbols of Christmas.
4. Decorating Christmas trees is a Christmas activity.
5. Christmas ornaments and garland are hung on Christmas trees.
6. There are special Christmas songs.
7. Bells and Christmas carols are sounds heard at Christmas.
8. Pointsettias, pine trees and mistletoe are Christmas plants.
9. Many people spend Christmas with their families and friends.
10. At Christmas time some people hang special stockings that are filled with candy and small gifts.

Vocabulary:

1. **Santa Claus**—a jolly man that wears a red suit and symbolizes Christmas.
2. **pine tree**—a tree decorated for the Christmas holidays.
3. **wreath**—a decoration made from evergreen branches.
4. **elf**—Santa's helper.
5. **star**—a treetop decoration.
6. **stocking**—a large Christmas sock.
7. **reindeer**—an animal used to pull Santa's sleigh.
8. **present**—a gift.
9. **ornament**—decoration for the home or tree.
10. **carol**—a Christmas song.
11. **pinata**—brightly colored paper mache figure that is filled with candy and gifts.

Bulletin Board

The purpose of this bulletin board is to foster positive self-concept, as well as name recognition. Construct a stocking out of tagboard for each child in your class. Print the name across the top and punch a hole in the top with a paper punch. Hang a Christmas poster or teacher-made poster in the center of the bulletin board. Next, attach push pins to the bulletin board, allowing enough room for each stocking to hang on a pin. The children can hang their own stocking on the bulletin board as they arrive each day.

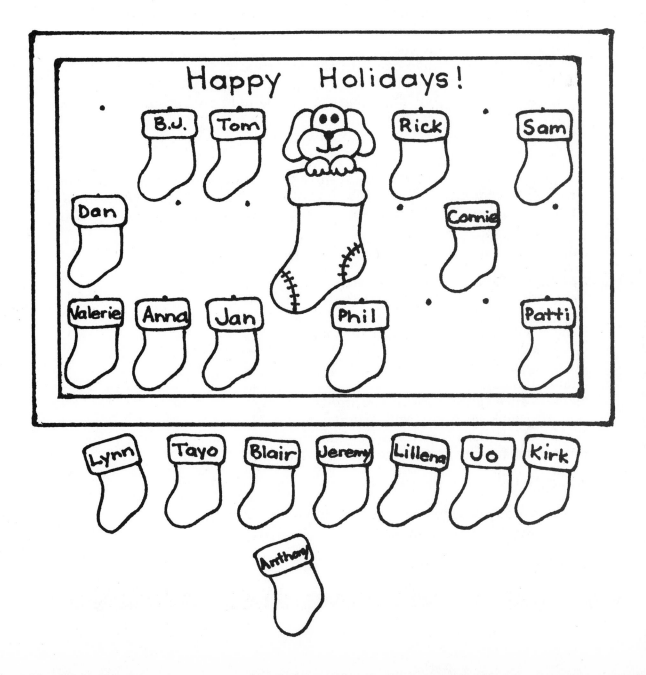

Parent Letter

Dear Parents,

The Christmas season is approaching. All we need to do is drive through the downtown area to see decorations and busy shoppers everywhere. Songs of Christmas are heard, and Santa is in the thoughts and sentences of every child. This week at school we will be participating in many Christmas activities. The children will learn the colors, plants, and symbols that are associated with the Christmas season.

At School This Week

A few of the Christmas learning experiences planned for the week include:

* creating ornaments to decorate the classroom Christmas tree.
* painting with pine boughs at the easel.
* making Christmas cookies.
* designing Christmas cards in the art area.
* practicing songs for our Holiday program. Keep your eyes open for a special invitation! The program will be held on December 19th at 3:30. Mark your calendar.

At Home

Music and singing are wonderful ways to communicate our feelings and we often have many feelings this time of year! When singing Christmas carols, encourage traditional songs as well as this new song:

I'm a Little Pine Tree
(Sing to the tune of "I'm a Little Teapot")

I'm a little pine tree tall and straight
Here are my branches for you to decorate
 (extend arms)
First we'll put the shiny star on top.
 (touch head)
Just be careful the balls don't drop
 (clap hands)
Now be sure to plug in all the lights
So I will look very gay and bright.
Then put all the presents under me.
I'm all set for Christmas, as you can see!

Reminder

Our last day of school will be December 23. We will begin school again on January 3 of the new year.

Happy holidays to you and yours!

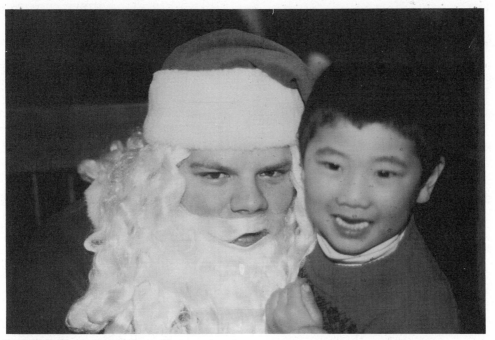

FIGURE 10 Visiting Santa is an exciting time for children.

Music:

1. **"Rudolph the Red-Nosed Reindeer"** (traditional)

2. **"Jingle Bells"** (traditional)

3. **"The Twelve Days of Christmas"** (traditional)

4. **"We Wish You a Merry Christmas"** (traditional)

5. **"Peppermint Stick Song"**

Oh I took a lick of my
peppermint stick
And I thought it tasted yummy.
Oh it used to hang on my
Christmas tree,
But I like it better in my tummy.

6. **"S-A-N-T-A"**
(Sing to the tune of "B-I-N-G-O")

There was a man on Christmas Day
And Santa was his name-o.
S-A-N-T-A
S-A-N-T-A
S-A-N-T-A
And Santa was his name-o.

7. **"Up on the House Top"** (traditional)

8. **"Santa Claus is Coming to Town"** (traditional)

9. **"Circle Christmas Verse"**

Two, four, six, eight.
Santa Claus don't be late;
Here's my stocking, I can't wait!
Two, four, six, eight.

10. **"Christmas Chant"**

With a "hey" and a "Hi" and a "ho-ho-ho,"
Somebody tickled old Santa Claus' toe.
Get up ol' Santa, there's work to be done,
The children must have their holiday fun.
With a "hey" and a "hi" and a "ho-ho-ho,"
Santa Claus, Santa Claus,
GO-GO-GO!

11. **"Santa's in His Shop"**
(Sing to the tune of "The Farmer in the Dell")

Santa's in his shop
Santa's in his shop
What a scene for Christmas
Santa's in his shop.

95

Other verses:

Santa takes a drum
The drum takes a doll
The doll takes a train
The train takes a ball
The ball takes a top
They're all in the shop
The top stays in the shop

Pictures could be constructed for use during the singing of each toy.

Fingerplays:

SANTA'S WORKSHOP

Here is Santa's workshop.
  (form peak with both hands)
Here is Santa Claus.
  (hold up thumb)
Here are Santa's little elves
  (wiggle fingers)
Putting toys upon the shelves.

HERE IS THE CHIMNEY

Here is the Chimney.
  (make fist and tuck in thumb)
Here is the top.
  (cover with hand)
Open it up quick
  (lift hand up)
And out Santa will pop.
  (pop out thumb)

FIVE LITTLE CHRISTMAS COOKIES

(hold up five fingers, take one away as
directed by poem)

Five little Christmas cookies on a plate by
the door,
One was eaten and then there were four.

Four little Christmas cookies, gazing up at
me
One was eaten and then there were three.

Three little Christmas cookies, enough for
me and you
One was eaten and then there were two.

Two little Christmas cookies sitting in the
sun
One was eaten and then there was one.

One little Christmas cookie, better grab it
fast
As you can see the others surely didn't
last.

PRESENTS

See all the presents by the Christmas tree?
  (hand shades eyes)
Some for you,
  (point)
And some for me—
  (point)

Long ones,
  (extend arms)
Tall ones,
  (measure hand up from floor)
Short ones, too.
  (hand to floor—low)
And here is a round one
  (circle with arms)
Wrapped in blue.

Isn't it fun to look and see
  (hand shade eyes)
All of the presents by the Christmas tree?
  (arms open wide)

Science:

1. Making Candles

Candles can be made for Christmas gifts.
This experience provides an opportunity
for the children to see how a substance
can change from solid to liquid and back
to a solid form. The children can place
pieces of paraffin in a tin can that is bent
at the top, forming a spout. A red or green
crayon piece can be used to add color.

The bottom of the tin cans should be
placed in a pan of water and heated on the
stove until the paraffin is melted. Mean-
while, the children can prepare small
paper cups.

In the bottom of each paper cup mold place a wick. Wicks can be made by tying a piece of string to a paper clip and a pencil. Then lay the pencil horizontally across the cup allowing the string to hang vertically into the cup. When the wax is melted, the teacher should carefully pour the wax into the cup. After the wax hardens, the candles can be used as decorations or presents. This activity should be restricted to four- and five-year-old children. Constant supervision of this activity is required for safety.

2. **Add to the Science Area:**

   * pine needles and branches with magnifying glasses
   * pine cones with a balance scale
   * red, green and white materials representing different textures

3. **Bells**

   Collect bells of various shapes and sizes. Listen for differences in sounds in relationship to the sizes of the bells.

4. **Feely Box**

   A feely box containing Christmas items such as bows, cookie cutters, wrapping paper, non-breakable ornaments, stockings, bells, candles, etc. can be placed on the science table.

Dramatic Play:

Gift Wrapping

Collect and place in the dramatic play area empty boxes, scraps of wrapping paper, comic paper, wallpaper books and scraps. Scissors, tape, bows and ribbon should also be provided.

Arts and Crafts:

1. **Christmas Chains**

   Cut sheets of red, green and white construction paper into strips. Demonstrate

how to form the links. The links can be pasted, taped or stapled, depending upon the developmental level of the children.

2. **Cookie Cutter Painting**

   Provide Christmas cookie cutters, paper and shallow pans containing red and green paint. The children can apply the paint to the paper using the cookie cutters as printing tools.

3. **Rudolph**

   Begin the activity by encouraging the children to trace their shoe. This will be used for Rudolph's face. Then the children should trace both of their hands which will be used as the reindeer's antlers. Finally, cut out a red circle to be used as the reindeer's nose. Have the children paste all the pieces together on a sheet of paper and add facial features.

4. **Designing Wrapping Paper**

   The children can design their own wrapping paper using newsprint, ink stampers, felt-tip colored markers, tempera paint, etc. Glitter can also be glued onto the paper.

5. **Creating Christmas Cards**

   Paper, felt-tip colored markers and crayons should be available at the art table. Christmas stencils can also be provided.

6. **Pine Branch Painting**

   Collect short pine boughs to use as painting tools. The tools can be placed at the easel or used with a shallow pan of tempera paint at tables.

7. **Candy Cane Marble Painting**

   Cut red construction paper into candy cane shapes. Marble paint with white tempera paint.

8. **Seasonal Stencils**

   Spread glue inside a seasonal stencil. Apply glitter over the glued area.

9. Glittery Pine Cones

Paint pine cones with tempera paint, sprinkle with glitter and allow the paint to dry. The glittery pine cones can be used for classroom decoration, presents or taken home.

10. Paper Wreaths

Purchase green muffin tin liners. To make the paper wreaths, cut out a large ring from light tagboard or construction paper for each child in the class. The children can glue the green muffin tin liners to the ring, adding small pieces of red yarn, crayons or felt-tip marker symbols to represent berries if desired.

11. Playdough Cookies

Using red, green and white playdough and Christmas cookie cutters, the children can make playdough cookies.

Favorite Playdough

Combine and boil until dissolved:
2 cups water
1/2 cup salt
food coloring or tempera

Mix while very hot:
2 tablespoons salad oil
2 tablespoons alum
2 cups flour

Knead approximately five minutes until smooth. Store in an airtight covered container.

Sensory:

1. Add to the Sensory Table:

* pine branches, needles and cones
* scented red and green playdough
* icicles or snow (if possible) with thermometers
* water for a sink and float activity add different Christmas objects such as bells, plastic stars, and cookie cutters

* Add scents such as peppermint and ginger to water

2. Holiday Cubes

Prepare ice cube trays using water colored with red and green food coloring. Freeze. Place in the sensory table.

Field Trip/Resource People:

1. Christmas Tree Farm

Plan a trip to a Christmas tree farm so the children can cut down a Christmas tree. Check your state's licensing requirements regarding the use of fresh Christmas trees and decorations in the center or classroom.

2. Caroling

Plan to go Christmas caroling at a local nursing home or even for another group of children. After caroling, Christmas cookies could be shared.

Math:

1. Christmas Card Sort

Place a variety of Christmas cards on a table in the math area. During self-selected or self-initiated periods the children can sort by color, pictures, size, etc.

2. Christmas Card Puzzles

Collect two sets of identical Christmas cards. Cut the covers off the cards. Cut one of each of the identical sets of cards into puzzle pieces. The matching card can be used as a form for the children to match the pieces on.

Group Time (games, language):

1. Find the Christmas Bell

For this activity the children should be standing in a circle. One child is given a bell. Then the child should hide, while the remainder of the children cover their eyes. After the child has hidden, he begins to ring the bell, signaling the remainder of the children to listen for the sound and identify where the bell is hidden. Turns should be taken, allowing each child an opportunity to hide and ring the bell.

2. **"Guess What's Inside"**

Wrap a familiar object inside of a box. Let the children shake, feel and try to identify the object. After this, open the box and show the children the object. This activity works well in small groups as well as large groups.

Cooking:

1. Candy Canes

Prepare the basic sugar dough recipe for cookie cutters. Divide the recipe in half. Add red food coloring to one half of the dough. Show the children how to roll a piece of red dough in a strip about 3 inches long by 1/2 inch wide. Repeat this process using the white dough. Then twist the two strips together, shaping into a

candy cane. Bake the cookies in a 350-degree oven for 7 to 10 minutes.

2. Basic Sugar Dough for Cookie Cutters

1/2 cup butter
1 cup sugar
1 egg
1/2 teaspoon salt
2 teaspoons baking powder
2 cups flour
1/2 teaspoon vanilla

Cut into desired shapes. Place on lightly greased baking sheets. Bake 8 minutes at 400 degrees. This recipe makes approximately 3 to 4 dozen cookies.

3. Eggnog

4 eggs
2 teaspoons vanilla
4 tablespoons honey
4 cups milk

Beat all of the ingredients together until light and foamy. Pour into glasses or cups and shake a little nutmeg on the top of the eggnog. This adds color and flavor. The recipe makes one quart.

GIFTS FOR PARENTS

Wax Paper Placemats
wax paper that is
   heavily waxed
crayon shavings
paper designs
dish towel
scissors

Use at least one of the
   following:
yarn
fabric
lace
dried leaves

Cut the wax paper into
   12 inch by 20 inch
   sheets (2 per mat).

Place crayon shavings between the wax paper. Then decorate with other items. Place towel on wax paper and press with warm iron until crayon melts. Fringe the edges.

Popsicle Stick Picture
   Frames
popsicle sticks (10 per
   frame)
glue
picture

Make a background of
   sticks and glue picture

in place. Add additional sticks around the edges, front and back for the frame and for support. For a free standing frame add more popsicle sticks to both the front and the back at the bottom.

Refrigerator Magnets
small magnets
glue
any type of decoration
   (paper cut outs,
   plaster of paris molds,
   yarn, styrofoam
   pieces, buttons, etc.)

Glue the decorations to the magnet.

Service Certificate
paper
crayons
pencils
lace
ribbon

Have the children write and decorate a certificate that states some service they will do for their parents. (Example: This certificate is good for washing the dishes; sweeping the floor; picking up my toys; etc.)

Ornaments
plaster of paris
any mold
glitter
yarn
straw

Pour the plaster of paris into the mold. Decorate with glitter and let dry. If so desired, place a straw into the mold and string with yarn or thread.

Refrigerator Clothespin
clothespins
glue
sequins/glitter/beads
small magnet

Let the children put glue on one side of the clothespin. Sprinkle this area with glitter, sequins or beads. Then assist the child in gluing the magnet to the other side.

Patchwork Flowerpot
precut fabric squares
glue

tins (for glue)
flower pots

Let the children soak the fabric squares one at a time in the glue. Press onto the pot in a patchwork design. Let dry overnight.

Snapshot Magnet
snapshot
plastic lid
scissors (preferably pinking shears)
glue
magnet

Using the lid, trace around the back of the picture. Cut the picture out and glue into the lid. Glue the magnet to the underside of the lid.

Holiday Pin
outline of a heart, wreath etc. cut out of tagboard
glue
sequins, beads, buttons, yarn
purchased backing for a pin

Let the children decorate the cardboard figure with glue and other decorating items. Glue onto purchased backing for a pin.

Flowers with Vase
styrofoam egg carton
pipe cleaner
scissors
glass jar or bottle
liquid starch
colored tissue paper (cut into squares)
glue yarn
paintbrush

Cut individual sections from egg carton and

punch a hole in the bottom of each. Insert a pipe cleaner through the hole as a stem. Use the scissors to cut the petals.

For the vase: Using the paintbrush, cover a portion of the jar with liquid starch. Apply the tissue paper squares until the jar is covered. Add another coat of liquid starch. Dip the yarn into the glue and wrap it around the jar. Insert the flower for a decoration.

Pine Cone Ornament
pine cones
paint
paintbrush
glue
glitter
yarn

Paint the pine cones. Then roll the pine cones in the glue and then into a dish filled with glitter. Tie a loop of yarn for hanging.

Paper Weights
glass furniture glides
crepe paper
crayons
glue
plaster of paris
felt piece
scissors

Children decorate a picture and then cut it to fit the glide. Place the picture face down into the recessed part of the glide. Pour plaster of paris over the top of the picture and let it dry. Glue a felt piece over the plaster.

Rock Paper Weight
large rocks
paint

Let the children paint a
design on a rock they
have chosen and give
to their parents as a
present.

Soap Balls
1 cup Ivory Snow
detergent
1/8 cup of water
food coloring
colored nylon netting
ribbon

Add the food coloring to
the water and then
add the Ivory Snow
detergent. Shape the
mixture into balls or
any shape. Wrap in
colored netting and tie
with ribbon.

Closet Clove Scenter
orange
cloves
netting
ribbon

Have the children push
the pointed ends of
the cloves into an
orange. Cover the
orange completely.
Wrap netting around
the orange and tie it
with the ribbon. These
make good closet or
dresser drawer
scenters.

Handprint Wreath
colored construction
paper
scissors
glue
pencil
cardboard/tagboard circle

Let the children trace
their hand and cut it

out. Glue the palm of
the hand to the card-
board circle. Using a
pencil roll the finger-
tips of the hand until
curly.

Bird's Nest
1 can sweetened con-
densed milk
2 teaspoons vanilla
3 to 4 cups powdered
milk
1 cup confectioners sugar
yellow food coloring

Mix all the ingredients
together and add food
coloring to tint the
mixture to a yellow
brown color. Give each
child a portion and let
him mold a bird's
nest. Chill for 2 hours.
If so desired, green
tinted coconut may be
added for grass and
put in the nest. Add
small jelly beans for
bird's eggs.

Flower Pots
plaster of paris
1/2 pint milk containers
straws (3 to 4 for each
container)
scissors
construction paper
paint
paintbrush
stapler

Cut the cartons in half
and use the bottom
half. Pour 1 to 3 in-
ches of plaster into
the containers. Stick 3
or 4 straws into the
plaster and let
harden. After plaster
has hardened, remove
the plaster very
carefully from the
milk carton. Let the
children paint the

plaster pot and make
flowers from construc-
tion paper and staple
the flowers to the
straws.

Cookie Jar
coffee can with lid or
oatmeal box
construction paper
crayons or felt-tip
markers
glue
scissors

Cover the can with con-
struction paper and
glue to seal. Let the
children decorate their
cans with crayons or
felt-tip markers. For
an added gift, make
cookies in the
classroom to send
home in the jars.

Felt Printing
felt
glue
wood block
tempera paint
scissors

Let the children cut the
felt pieces into any
shape. Glue the shape
onto the wood block.
Dip into a shallow
pan of tempera paint.
Print on newspaper to
test.

Napkin Holder
paper plates
scissors
yarn
paper punch
crayons
clear shellac

Cut one paper plate in
half. Place the inside
together and punch
holes through the
lower half only. Use

yarn to lace the plates together. Punch a small hole at the top for hanging. Decorate with crayons or felt-tip markers. Coat with shellac. May be used as a potholder, napkin or card holder.

Clay Figures
4 cups flour
1 1/2 cup water
1 cup salt
paint
paintbrush

Combine flour, water and salt. Knead for 5 to 10 minutes. Roll and cut dough into figures. (Cookie cutters work well.) Make a hole at the top of the figure. Bake in a 250-degree oven for 2 hours or until hard. When cool, paint to decorate.

Key Holder
8 popsicle sticks
construction paper or a cutout from a greeting card
self-adhesive picture hanger
yarn

Glue five sticks together edge to edge. Cut a 1

3/4 inch piece of stick and glue it across the 5 sticks. Glue 2 sticks across the top parallel to the 5 sticks. Turn the sticks over. Cut paper or a greeting card to fit between the crossed sticks. Place on the self-adhesive hanger and tie yarn to the top for hanging.

Planter Trivets
7 popsicle sticks
felt
glue

Glue four popsicle sticks into a square, the top two overlapping the bottom ones. Fill in the open space with the remaining three and glue into place.

Pencil Holder
empty soup cans
construction paper or contact paper
crayons or felt-tip markers
glue
scissors

Cover the can with construction or contact paper. Decorate with crayons or markers and use as a pencil holder.

Plaster Hand Prints
plaster of paris
1 inch deep square container
paint
paintbrush

Pour plaster of paris into the container. Have the child place his hand in the plaster to make a mold. Let the mold dry and remove it from the container. Let the child paint the mold and give as a gift with the following poem:

My Hands

Sometimes you get discouraged
Because I am so small
And always have my fingerprints
on furniture and walls
But everyday I'm growing up
and soon I'll be so tall
that all those little handprints
will be hard for you to recall
So here's a little handprint
just for you to see
Exactly how my fingers looked
When I was little me.

Books and Stories:

The following books and stories can be used to complement the theme:

1. **The Cowboy's Christmas.** Joan Walsh Anglud. (New York: A. Margaret K. McElderly Book, 1972).

2. **Father Christmas.** Raymond Briggs. (New York: Coward, McCann and Goeghegan, Inc., 1973).

3. **The Biggest Christmas Tree on Earth.** Fernando Krahn. (Boston: Little, Brown and Company, 1978).

4. **Christmas Is a Time of Giving.** Joan Walsh Anglud. (New York: Harcourt, Brace and World, 1961).

5. **Where's Prancer?** Syd Hoff. (New York: Harper, 1960).

6. **The Christmas Piñata.** Jack Kent. (New York: Parents Magazine Press, 1975).

7. **The Night After Christmas.** James Stevenson. (New York: Greenwillow Books, 1981).

8. **Keeping Christmas.** William F. Strucker. (Maryland: Stemmer House Publications, 1981).

9. **Twelve Days of Christmas.** Brian Wildsmith. (New York: Franklin Watts, Inc., 1972).

10. **Clifford's Christmas.** Norman Bridwell. (New York: Scholastic Inc., 1984).

11. **The Berenstain Bears' Christmas Tree.** Stan and Jan Berenstain. (New York: Random House, 1980).

12. **The Christmas Sled.** Carol North. (New York: Golden Books, 1984).

13. **Santa's Hat.** Claire Schumacher. (New York: Prentice Hall Books, 1987).

14. **The Father Christmas Letter.** J.R. Tolkien. (Boston: Houghton Mifflin, 1976).

15. **That's Not Santa.** Leonard Kessler. (New York: Scholastic Book Services, 1981).

16. **Santa Makes a Change.** Sol Chanelles. (New York: Parents Magazine Press, 1970).

17. **Nicholas Who Wanted to be Santa Claus.** James C. Crimmins. (New York: J.B. Lippincott Company, 1962).

18. **Arthur's Christmas Cookies.** Lillian Hoban. (New York: Harper and Row, 1972).

19. **The Little Drummer.** Ezra Jack Keats. (New York: Macmillan Company, 1968).

20. **The Twelve Days of Christmas.** Cathie Shuttleworth (ill.) (New York: Derrydale Books, 1987).

21. **How the Grinch Stole Christmas.** Dr. Seuss. (New York: Random House, 1957).

22. **The Christmas Snowman.** Diane Sherman. (Chicago: Rand McNally & Co., 1977).

23. **Blue Bug's Christmas.** Virginia Poulet. (Chicago: Childrens Press, 1987).

24. **A Christmas Card for Mr. McFizz.** Obren Bokich. (Chicago: Childrens Press, 1987).

Puzzles:

The following puzzles can be found in preschool educational catalogs:

1. **"Christmas Tree"** 15 pieces. Judy/Instructo.

2. **"Santa Claus"** 17 pieces. Judy/Instructo.

3. **"Santa's Elves"** 14 pieces. Puzzle People.

4. **"Santa and Mrs. Claus"** 17 pieces. Puzzle People.

CIRCUS

11

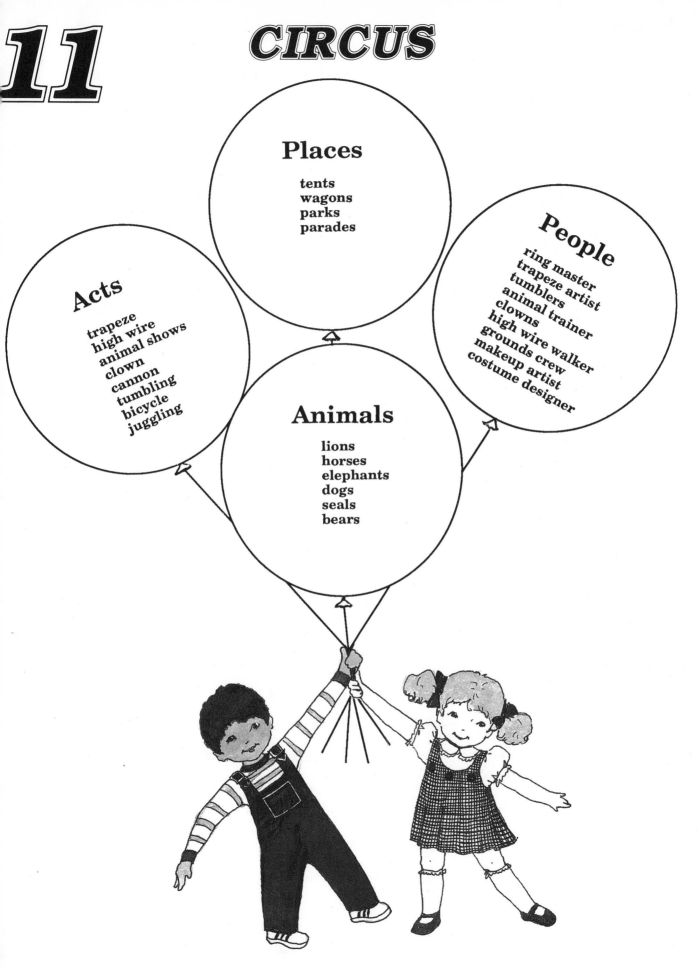

Places
tents
wagons
parks
parades

People
ring master
trapeze artist
tumblers
animal trainer
clowns
high wire walker
grounds crew
makeup artist
costume designer

Acts
trapeze
high wire
animal shows
clown
cannon
tumbling
bicycle
juggling

Animals
lions
horses
elephants
dogs
seals
bears

Theme Goals:

Through participating in the experiences provided by this theme, the children may learn:

1. Different circus acts.

2. People who work for a circus.

3. Animals that perform in a circus.

4. Places to watch a circus.

Concepts for the Children to Learn:

1. The circus is fun.

2. Many adults and children enjoy the circus.

3. The circus can be performed under a big tent.

4. An animal trainer teaches animals tricks.

5. Circus shows have colorful clowns.

6. Clowns wear makeup.

7. Music is played at the circus.

8. People and animals do special tricks in the circus.

9. Many people work at the circus.

Vocabulary:

1. **circus**—traveling show with people and animals.

2. **circus parade**—a march of people and animals at the beginning of the performance.

3. **clowns**—people who wear makeup and dress in silly clothes.

4. **trapeze**—short bar used for swinging.

5. **ring master**—person in charge of the circus performance.

6. **makeup**—colored face paint.

7. **stilts**—long sticks a performer stands on to be taller.

Bulletin Board

The purpose of this bulletin board is to develop color recognition and matching skills. Construct eight clown faces with collars out of tagboard. Color each collar a different color using felt-tip markers. Hang these pieces on the bulletin board. Next, construct eight hat pieces out of tagboard. Color each one a different color, to correspond with the colors of the clowns' collars. Punch holes in the hats, and use push pins to hold the hats above the appropriate clown. The children can match the colored hats to the clown wearing the same colored collar.

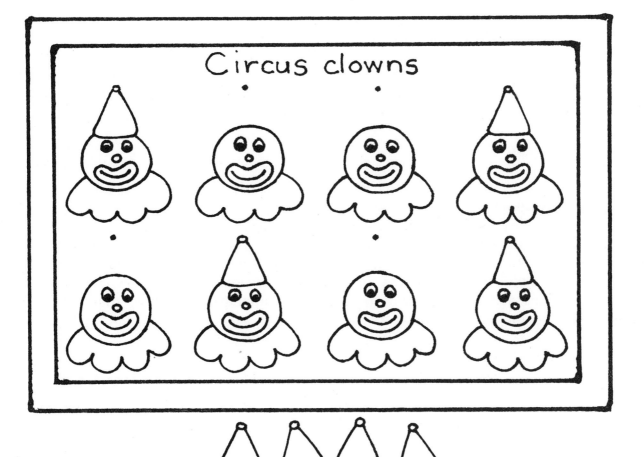

Parent Letter

Dear Parents,

This week at school we are starting a unit that is fun for everyone—the circus! It will be a very exciting week! Developing an awareness of special people and animals enhances an appreciation of others. It also stimulates children's curiousity to learn more about other people and jobs people have. The children will be learning about the many acts and performances people and animals do at the circus.

At School This Week

Some of the many fun and exciting things we will be doing this week include:

* listening to the story *Harriet Goes to the Circus* by Betsy and Guilio Maestro.
* dressing up in clown suits and applying makeup in the dramatic play area.
* acting out a small circus of our own.
* making clown face puppets.

We will have a very special visitor come to our room on Friday—a clown! He will show us how he applies his makeup and will perform for us. You are invited to join us for the fun at 3:00 p.m. to share in this activity.

At Home

It has been said that the circus is perhaps the world's oldest form of entertainment. Pictures of circus acts drawn over 3,000 years ago have been discovered on walls of caves. Most children enjoy clowns and dressing up as clowns. Prepare clown makeup with your child by adding a few drops of food coloring to cold cream. Have your child use his fingers or a clean paintbrush to paint his face. This activity will help develop an awareness of colors, as well as realize that appearances can change but the person remains the same!

Have a great week!

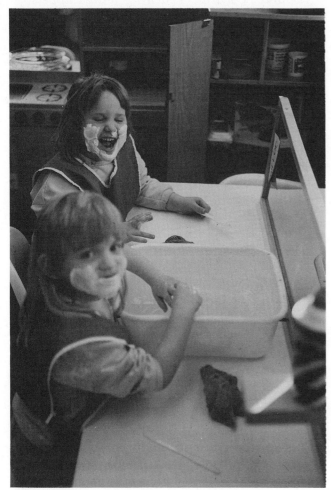

FIGURE 11 Clowning around.

Music:

1. "Circus"
(Sing to the tune of "Did You Ever See a Lassie")

Let's pretend that we are clowns, are clowns, are clowns.
Let's pretend that we are clowns.
We'll have so much fun.
We'll put on our makeup and make people laugh hard.
Let's pretend that we are clowns.
We'll have so much fun.

Let's pretend that we are elephants, are elephants, are elephants.
Let's pretend that we are elephants.
We'll have so much fun.
We'll sway back and forth and stand on just two legs.
Let's pretend that we are elephants.
We'll have so much fun.

Let's pretend that we are on a trapeze, a trapeze, a trapeze.
Let's pretend that we are on a trapeze.
We'll have so much fun.
We'll swing high and swoop low and make people shout "oh!"
Let's pretend that we are on a trapeze.
We'll have so much fun!

2. "The Ring Master"
(Sing to tune of "The Farmer and the Dell")

The ring master has a circus.
The ring master has a circus.
Hi-ho the clowns are here.
The ring master has a circus.

The ring master takes a clown.
The ring master takes a clown.
Hi-ho the clowns are here.
The ring master takes a clown.

The clown takes an elephant...

Use clowns, elephants, lions, tigers, tightrope walker, trapeze artist, acrobat, etc.

Fingerplays:

GOING TO THE CIRCUS

Going to the circus to have a lot of fun.
  (hold closed fist, and raise fingers to indicate number)
The animals parading one by one.
Now they are walking 2 by 2,
A great big lion and a caribou.
Now they are walking 3 by 3,
The elephants and the chimpanzee.
Now they are walking 4 by 4,
A striped tiger and a big old bear.
Now they are walking 5 by 5,
It makes us laugh when they arrive.

ELEPHANTS

Elephants walk like this and like that.
  (sway body back and forth)
They're terribly big; they're terribly fat.
  (spread arms wide in a circular motion)
They have no hands, they have no toes,

109

And goodness gracious, what a NOSE!
(put arms together and sway for
elephant nose)

Source: *Creative Teaching with Puppets.*
Barbara Rountree and others. (The Learning Line, Inc.: Alabama, 1981).

FIVE LITTLE CLOWNS

Five little clowns running through the
door.
(hold up one hand, put down one finger
at each verse)
One fell down and then there were four.
Four little clowns in an apple tree.
One fell out and then there were three.
Three little clowns stirring up some stew.
One fell in and then there were two.
Two little clowns having lots of fun.
One ran away and then there was one.
One little clown left sitting in the sun.
He went home and then there were none!

CIRCUS CLOWN

I'd like to be a circus clown
And make a funny face,
(make a funny face)
And have all the people laugh at me
As I jump around the place.
(act silly and jump around)

THE CIRCUS IS COMING

The circus is coming hurray, hurray!
(clap hands)
The clowns are silly; see them play.
(make a face)
The animals parade one by one
(walk fingers on lap)
While clowns juggle balls for fun.
(pretend to juggle)
The lion growls; the tigers roar,
(paw in the air)
While the elephant walks on all fours.
(swing arms like an elephant trunk)
The circus is coming hurray, hurray!
(clap hands)

Science:

1. Circus Balloons

Cut several pieces of tagboard into circles.
If desired, cover the balloons with
transparent contact or lamination paper.
On each table have three cups of colored
water—red, yellow and blue—with a brush
in each cup. The child can mix all or any
two colors and see which colors they can
create for their circus balloons.

2. Shape the Clown

Cut several large outlines of clowns' heads
from tagboard or construction paper and
many eyes, hats, ears, noses, ruffles and
bowties. Make a large die with an ear,
nose, hat, eye, ruffle and bowtie. (One on
each of the six sides.) The children can
take turns rolling the die to construct
their clown face. If a child rolls a die with
the shape they already have, they must
wait for their next turn.

Source: *Teacher-made Games.* (Parent-Child Early Education: Missouri, 1980).

3. Seal and Ball Color/Word Match

Cut several seals out of different colored
tagboard. Out of the same colors cut
several balls. Write the correct color on
each ball. The children match each ball
with the word on it to the correct seal.

4. Sizzle Fun

Pour 1 inch of vinegar in a soda or catsup
bottle. Put 2 teaspoons of baking soda inside
a balloon. Quickly slip the open end of the
balloon over the soda bottle. Watch the
balloon fill with gas created by the interaction of the vinegar with the baking
soda.

5. Texture Clown

Construct a large clown from tagboard. Use different textured materials to create the clown's features. Make two sets. Place the extra set in a box or a bag. The children may pick a piece of textured material from the bag and match it to the identical textured piece used as a clown feature.

6. Make Peanut Butter

Take the shells off of fresh peanuts. Blend peanuts in a blender until smooth. Add 1 1/2 to 2 tablespoons of oil per cup of peanuts and blend well. Add 1/2 teaspoon salt per cup if desired. Spread on bread or crackers and eat for snack.

Dramatic Play:

1. Clown Makeup

Prepare clown makeup be mixing 1 part facial cream with 1 drop food coloring. Place clown makeup by a large mirror in the dramatic play area. The children apply makeup to their faces. Clown suits can also be provided if available.

2. Circus

Set up a circus in your classroom. Make a circle out of masking tape on the floor. The children can take turns performing in the ring. The addition of hoola-hoops, animal and clown costumes, tickets, and chairs would extend the children's play in this area.

3. Animal Trainers

Each child can bring in their favorite stuffed animals on an assigned day. The children can pretend to be animal trainers for the circus. They may select to act out different animal performances.

Arts and Crafts:

1. Clown Stencils

Cut several clown figures out of tagboard. Place felt-tip markers, crayons, pencils and stencils on the art table. The children can trace the stencils.

2. Easel Ideas

* clown face shaped paper
* circus tent shaped paper

3. Circus Wagons

Collect old cardboard boxes and square food containers. The children can make circus wagons by decorating the boxes. When each child is through making their train, all of the boxes can be placed together for a circus train.

4. Clown Face Masks

Provide paper plates and felt-tip markers to make paper plate clown masks. Glue the plate to a tongue depressor. The children can use the masks as puppets.

5. Playdough Animals

Prepare playdough by combining:

2 cups flour
1 cup salt
1 cup hot water
2 tablespoons oil
4 teaspoons cream of tartar
food coloring

Mix the ingredients. Then knead the mixture until smooth. This dough may be kept in a plastic bag or covered container. If the dough becomes sticky, add additional flour.

6. Peanut Shell Collages

Provide peanut shells, glue and paper for the children to create collages with.

Sensory:

Provide rubber or plastic animal figurines for the children to play with in water.

Large Muscle:

1. Tightrope Walker

Place a balance beam and a stick for the children to hold perpendicular to their bodies.

2. Dancing Elephants

Provide each child a scarf and play music. The children can pretend to be dancing elephants.

3. Bean Bag Toss

Make a large clown or other circus person or animal bean bag toss out of thick cardboard. Cut the eyes, nose and mouth holes all large enough for the bean bags to go through. For older children, assign each hole a certain number of points and maintain a score chart.

4. Can Stilts

Provide large tin cans and thick string or twine for the children to make can stilts. Once completed, the children stand on the cans and walk around the room.

5. Tightrope Transition

As a transition, place a ten-foot line of masking tape on the floor. The children can pretend to tight rope walk over to the next activity.

6. Monkey, Monkey, Clown

Play Duck, Duck, Goose but change the words to Monkey, Monkey, Clown.

Field Trips/Resource People:

1. Clown Makeup

Invite a clown to demonstrate putting on makeup. Then have the clown put on a small skit and talk about the circus.

2. The Circus

If possible, go to a circus or circus parade in your area.

Math:

1. Clown Hat Match

Make sets of matching colored hats. On one set print a numeral. On the matching hats print an identical number of dots. The children match the dots to the numbers.

2. Circus Sorting

Find several pictures of symbols that represent a circus. Also include other pictures. Place all pictures in a pile. The children can sort pictures into two piles. One pile will represent circus objects.

3. Growing Chart

Make a giraffe growing chart. If desired, another animal can be substituted. Record each child's height on the chart at various times during the year.

Social Studies:

1. Circus Life

Read *You Think It's Fun to be a Clown!* by David A. Adler. When finished, discuss the lives of circus people.

2. Body Parts

Make a large clown out of tagboard. Make corresponding matching body parts such as arms, legs, ears, shoes, hands, and fingers. The children can match the parts.

Group Time (games, language):

1. Making a Clown

Give each child a paper and one crayon. Have children draw as you recite this fingerplay:

Draw a circle round and big,
Add a few hairs as a wig.
Make a circle for a nose,
Now a smile, broad and wide.
Put an ear on either side.
Add some eyes, but not a frown.
Now you have your very own clown.

This activity should only be used with older children when it is developmentally appropriate.

Source: *The Everything Book For Teacher's of Young Children.* Valerie Indenbaum and Marcia Shapiro. (Partner Press: Michigan, 1985).

2. Circus Pictures

Place pictures of clowns and circus things around the room at the children's eye level. Introduce the pictures at group time and discuss each picture.

3. Who Took My Nose?

Prepare red circles from construction paper. Seat the children in a circle. Give each child a red circle to tape on their nose. Then, have everyone close their eyes. Tap one child. This child should get up and go to another child and take his nose.

When the child returns to his place the teacher claps her hands and all the children open their eyes. The children then try to identify the child who took the nose.

4. Clown Lotto

Adhere clown face stickers, or draw simple clown faces, on several 2 inch × 2 inch pieces of tagboard. Also prepare lotto boards using the same stickers or drawings. To play, turn all cards face down. Children take turns choosing a card from the table and seeing if it matches a picture on their game boards.

Cooking:

1. Clown Snack

Place a pear in the middle of a plate. Sprinkle grated cheese on the pear for hair. Add raisin eyes, a cherry nose and a raisin mouth. Finally, make a ruffle collar from a lettuce leaf.

2. Cheese Popcorn

1/4 cup butter
1/4 cup dry cheddar cheese
3 cups popped popcorn

Melt butter and grate cheese. Mix together and pour over popcorn. Stir until well coated. Salt to taste if desired.

Source: *Super Snacks.* Jean Warren. (Alderwood Manor, WA: Warren Publishing House, 1982).

BUBBLE SOLUTIONS

BUBBLE SOLUTION #1

1 cup of water
2 tablespoons liquid
    detergent
1 tablespoon glycerine
1/2 teaspoon sugar

BUBBLE SOLUTION #2

2/3 cup liquid dish
    detergent
1 gallon of water
1 tablespoon glycerine
    (optional)

Allow solution to sit in
    an open container for
at least a day before use.

BUBBLE SOLUTION #3

3 cups water
2 cups Joy liquid
    detergent
1/2 cup Karo syrup

Records:

The following records can be found in preschool educational catalogs:

1. **Pretend.** Hap Palmer.

2. **Animals and Circus.** Lucille Wood.

3. **"Circus Parade"** on the record **Rhythm Time.** Lucille and Tanner Wood.

Books and Stories:

The following books and stories can be used to complement the theme:

1. **The Circus Baby.** Petersham, Maud and Miska. (New York: Macmillan Company, 1950).

2. **Circus.** Bea Shenk De Reghiers. (New York: Viking Press, 1966).

3. **Let's Go to the Circus.** Tony Palazzo. (New York: Doubleday and Company, 1961).

4. **Harold's Circus.** Crockett Johnson. (New York: Scholastic, 1959).

5. **Pantomine Trip to the Circus.** Esther Nelson. (New York: Sterling Publishing Co., 1975).

6. **The Circus—Bigger, Better than Ever.** Herb Clement. (New York: A.S. Burns and Co., 1974).

7. **Joey the Clown.** D.B. Kabaleusky. (Japan: Gakken Co., 1971).

8. **Harriet Goes to the Circus.** Betsy and Guilio Maestro. (New York: Crown Publishers Inc., 1977).

9. **Circus Numbers.** Rodney Peppe. (New York: Delacorte Press, 1969).

10. **The Big Show.** Felix Sutton. (New York: Doubleday and Company, 1971).

11. **Come to the Circus.** Charles P. Fox. (Chicago: Reilly and Lee Co., 1960).

12. **Born on the Circus.** Fred Powledge. (New York: Harcourt, Brace and Jovanovich, 1976).

13. **Circus Work.** Mark Taylor. (Boston: Allyn and Bacon Inc., 1978).

14. **You Think It's Fun to be a Clown!** David A. Adler. (New York: Doubleday and Company, 1980).

15. **Bear Circus.** William Pene Du Bois. (New York: Viking Press, 1971).

16. **Carousel.** D. Crews. (New York: Greenwillow Books, 1982).

Puzzles:

The following puzzles can be found in preschool educational catalogs:

1. **"Clown Face"** Puzzle People.

2. **"Elephant/Balloon Colors"** Puzzle People.

3. **"Seal Balancing Ball"** 7 pieces. Judy/Instructo.

4. **"Cycling Clown"** 8 pieces. Judy/Instructo.

5. **"Circus Elephant"** 10 pieces. Judy/Instructo.

6. **"Clown Face"** 15 pieces. Judy/Instructo.

7. **"Merry-Go-Round"** 18 pieces. Judy/Instructo.

8. **"Pudgy Clown"** 14 pieces. Puzzle People.

9. **"Balloon Man"** 15 pieces. Lauri.

12

CLOTHING

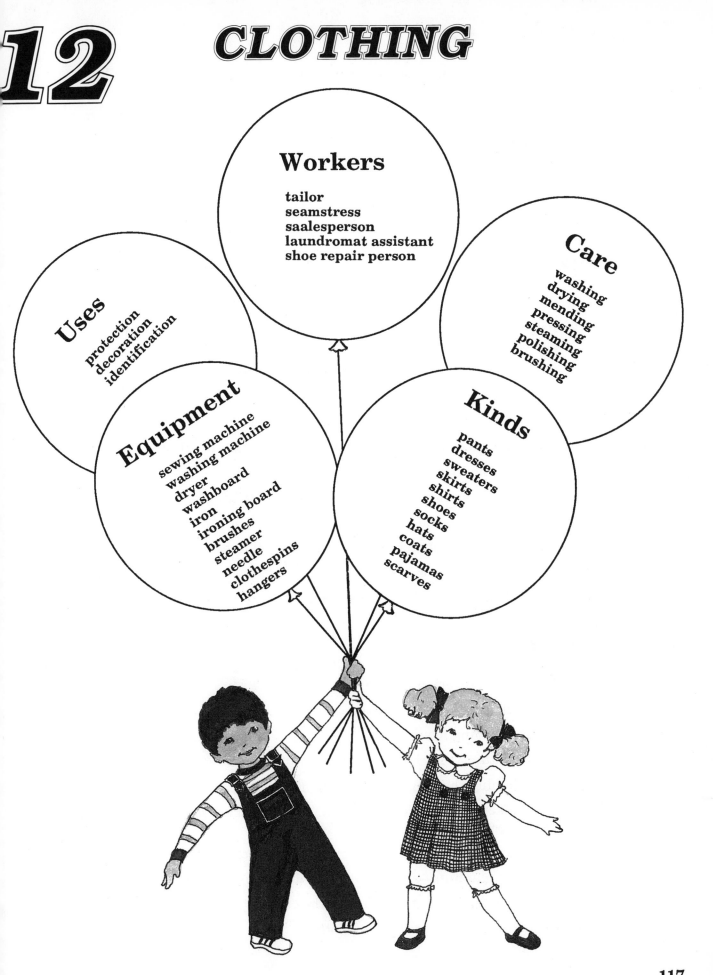

Workers

tailor
seamstress
saalesperson
laundromat assistant
shoe repair person

Care

washing
drying
mending
pressing
steaming
polishing
brushing

Uses

protection
decoration
identification

Equipment

sewing machine
washing machine
dryer
washboard
iron
ironing board
brushes
steamer
needle
clothespins
hangers

Kinds

pants
dresses
sweaters
skirts
shirts
shoes
socks
hats
coats
pajamas
scarves

Theme Goals:

Through participating in the experiences provided by this theme, the children may learn:

1. Types of clothing.
2. Clothing workers.
3. Uses of clothing.
4. Care of clothing.
5. Equipment used with clothing.

Concepts for the Children to Learn:

1. Clothing is a covering for our body.
2. Pants, dresses, shirts and sweaters are some of the clothing we wear on our bodies.
3. Shoes, socks and boots are clothing for our feet.
4. Gloves and mittens are coverings for our hands.
5. Hats and scarves are coverings for our head.
6. Protection, decoration and identification are uses for clothing.
7. There are many colors and sizes of clothing.
8. A tailor and a seamstress make and mend clothing.
9. Clothing needs to be cleaned.
10. Clothespins and hangers are used to hang clothes.
11. Clothes identify workers.
12. Needles, brushes and irons are needed to care for clothing.

Vocabulary:

1. **clothing**—a covering for the body.
2. **shirt**—clothing that covers the chest and sometimes arms.
3. **shoes**—clothing for our feet.
4. **skirt**—clothing that hangs from the waist.
5. **hat**—clothing that covers our head.
6. **coat/jacket**—a piece of clothing that is often used for warmth and is worn over other clothing.
7. **clothespin**—a clip used to hang clothes on a clothesline or a hanger.
8. **washing machine**—an appliance used to clean clothes.
9. **dryer**—an appliance that dries clothes.
10. **laundromat**—a place to clean clothes.

Bulletin Board

The purpose of this bulletin board is to develop visual perception and discrimination skills. A "Sort the Clothes" bulletin board can be an addition to the clothing unit. Construct shorts and shirt pieces out of tagboard. The number used will be dependent upon the size of the bulletin board and the age of the children. Draw a pattern on a pair of shorts and the same pattern on one of the shirts. Continue, drawing a different pattern for each shorts and shirt set. Hang the shorts on the bulletin board, and hang a push pin on top of the shorts, so the children can hang the corresponding patterned shirt on top of the shorts.

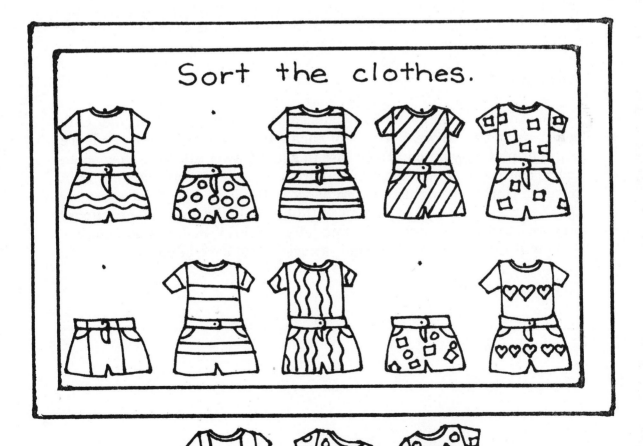

Parent Letter

Dear Parents,

This week we will be beginning a unit on clothing. Through participating in this unit, the children will learn about many different kinds of clothing. They will also become aware of the care of clothing and purposes of clothing.

At School This Week

Some of the learning experiences planned for the week include:

* sorting clothes hangers by color.
* going to a laundromat in the dramatic play area.
* making newspaper skirts at the art table.
* washing doll clothes in the sensory table.

We will also be taking a walk to the Corner Laundromat on Tuesday afternoon. We will be looking at the big laundry carts, washers and dryers, and folding tables. If you would like to join us, please contact me. We will be leaving the center at 3:00 p.m.

At Home

You can foster the concepts introduced in this unit by letting your child select what he will wear to school each day. To promote independence, begin by placing your child's clothes in a low drawer allowing easy access to the clothes. To make mornings more enjoyable, encourage your child to select clothes at night that can be worn the next day. Find a location to place the clothes. Also, if your child has doll clothes, fill the kitchen sink or a tub with soapy water, and let your child wash the doll clothes. This will help your child become aware of the care of clothes.

Have a fun week!

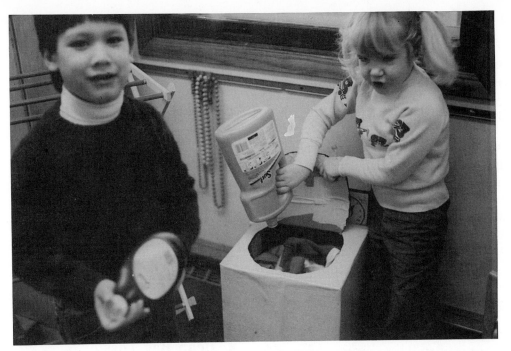

FIGURE 12 Clothes need to be "washed" in order the get them clean.

Fingerplay:

DRESS FOR THE WEATHER

If you go without your coat
  (put on coat)
When the wind is damp and chill,
  (hug self)
You'll end up in bed, my friend,
  (shake finger)
Feverish, sneezing and ill.
  (look sick, sneeze)
Wear your boots through snow and mud
  (put on boots)
And during a thunderstorm.
Also wear a waterproof coat and hat
  (put on coat and hat)
To keep yourself dry and warm.

Source: *Finger Frolics.* Cromwell, Hibner and Faitel. (Michigan: Partner Press, 1983).

Science:

Fabric Sink and Float

Provide various kinds of clothing and fabric on the science table along with a large tub of water. The children can test the different types of clothing to see which will sink and which will float. Some clothing articles will sink while other clothing articles float until they become saturated with water. After a test has been made, the clothes can be hung to dry.

Dramatic Play:

1. **Clothing Store**

   Place dress-up clothing on hangers and a rack. A cash register, play money, bags and small shopping carts can also be provided to extend the play.

2. **Party Clothes**

   Provide dressy clothes, jewelry, shoes, hats and purses.

3. **Uniforms**

   Collect occupational clothing and hats, such as police officer shirts and hats, a firefighter's hat, nurse and doctor lab coats, and artist smocks. High school athletic uniforms can also be provided. After use, store this box so the uniforms are available upon request for other units.

4. Hanging Clothes

String a low clothesline in the classroom or outdoors. Provide clothespins and doll clothes for the children to hang up.

5. Laundromat

Collect two large appliance-sized boxes. Cut a hole in the top of one to represent a washing machine, and cut a front door in the other to represent a dryer. A laundry basket, empty soap box and play clothing may be welcomed additions to extend the play.

Arts and Crafts:

1. Dress the Paper Doll

Prepare clothing to fit paper dolls out of construction paper scraps. For younger children, the dolls can be pre-cut. Older children may be able to cut their own dolls if the lines are traced on paper and a simple pattern is provided.

2. Newspaper Skirts

Depending upon the developmental level of the children, newspaper skirts can be constructed in the classroom. Begin by stapling about ten sheets of newspaper across at the top. Draw a bold line about two inches from the staples. Then instruct the children to vertically cut from the bottom edge of the paper, all the way up to the bold line creating strips. String pieces can be attached by stapling to the top of both sides to enable the skirt to be tied in the back.

3. Easel Ideas

* feature clothes-shaped easel paper
* paint using tools created by attaching small sponges to a clothespin

Sensory:

1. Washing Clothes

Fill the sensory table with soapy water and let the children wash doll clothing.

After being washed, the clothes can be hung on a low clothesline.

2. Add to the Sensory Table:

* clothespins

Large Muscle:

1. Clothespin Drop

Collect clothespins and a series of jars with mouth openings of varying widths. The children can stand near the jar and drop the clothespins into it. To ensure success, the younger children should be guided to try the jar with the largest opening.

2. Bean Bag Toss

Bean bags can be tossed into empty laundry baskets.

3. Clothes Race

Fill bags with large-sized clothing items. Give a bag to each child. Signal the children to begin dressing up with the clothing. The object is to see how quickly they can put all of the clothes items in the bag over their own clothing.

Field Trips/Resource People:

1. Clothing Store

Visit a children's clothing store. Look at the different colors, sizes and types of clothing.

2. Tailor/Seamstress

Invite a seamstress to visit your classroom to show the children how they make, mend and repair clothing. The seamstress can demonstrate tools and share some of the clothing articles they have made.

3. Laundromat

Take a walk to a local laundromat. Observe the facility. Point out the sizes of the different kinds of washing machines and dryers. Explain the use of the laundry carts and folding tables.

Math:

1. Clothes Seriation

Provide a basketful of clothes for the children to line up from largest to smallest. Include hats, sweatshirts, shoes and pants. Use clothing items whose sizes are easily distinguishable.

2. Line 'em Up

Print numerals on clothespins. The children can attach the clothespins on a low clothesline and sequence them in numerical order.

3. Hanger Sort

Colored hangers can be sorted into laundry baskets or on a clothesline by color.

4. Sock Match

Collect many different pairs of socks. Combine in a laundry basket. The children can find the matching pairs and fold them.

Social Studies:

1. Weather Clothing

Bring in examples of clothing worn in each of the four seasons. Provide four laundry baskets. Label each basket with a picture representing either a sunny hot day, a rainy day, a cold day and a fall or spring day. Then encourage the children to sort the clothing according to the weather label on the basket.

2. Who Wears It?

At group time, hold up clothing items and ask the children who would wear it. Include baby clothes, sports uniforms and occupational clothing, ladies clothes, men's clothes, etc.

Group Time:

Look Closely

While the children are sitting on the floor in a circle, call out the clothes items that one child is wearing. For example, say, "I see someone who is wearing a red shirt and pants." The children can look around the circle and say the name of the child who is wearing those items.

Cooking:

1. Graham Crackers

Wear chef uniforms, and make your own graham crackers for snack.

1/2 cup margarine
2/3 cup brown sugar
1/2 cup water
2 3/4 cups graham flour
1/2 teaspoon salt
1/2 teaspoon baking powder
1/8 teaspoon cinnamon

Beat margarine and sugar till smooth and creamy. Add the remainder of the ingredients and mix well. Let the mixture sit for 30 to 45 minutes. Sprinkle flour on a board or table top. Roll out dough to 1/8 inch thick. Cut the dough into squares, logs or whatever. Place on an oiled cookie sheet. Bake at 350 degrees for twenty minutes until lightly brown. This recipe should produce a sufficient quantity for eight children.

2. Irish Gingerbread

1 or 2 teaspoons butter
2 cups flour
1 1/2 teaspoon baking soda
1 teaspoon cinnamon
1 teaspoon ground ginger
3/4 teaspoon salt
1 egg
2 egg yolks
1 cup molasses
1/2 cup soft butter
1/2 cup sugar
1/2 cup quick-cooking oatmeal
1 cup hot water

Preheat the oven to 350 degrees. Grease the bottom of the baking pan with 1 or 2 teaspoons of butter. Measure the flour, baking soda, cinnamon, ginger and salt and sift them together onto a piece of waxed paper. In a mixing bowl, combine the butter with the sugar by stirring them with the mixing spoon until they are blended. Add the egg and egg yolks. With the mixing spoon, beat the mixture until it is fluffy. Stir in the molasses.

Add the sifted dry ingredients, the oatmeal, and the hot water one fourth at a time to the egg and molasses mixture, stirring after each addition. Pour the mixture into the greased pan. Bake 50 to 55 minutes. Test with a toothpick. Make gingerbread people with cookie cutters. Decorate: make clothes for the gingerbread people using coconut, nuts, raisins, etc.

Source: *Many Hands Cooking.* Terry Touff Cooper and Marilyn Ratner. (New York: Thomas Y. Crowell Co., 1974).

3. Pita or Pocket Bread

1 package of yeast
1/4 cup of lukewarm water
3 cups of flour
   (white, whole wheat or any combination)
2 teaspoons of salt

Dissolve the yeast in the water and add the flour and salt. Stir into a rough sticky ball. Knead on a floured board or table until smooth, adding more flour, if necessary. Divide the dough into 6 balls and knead each ball until smooth and round. Flatten each ball with a rolling pin until 1/4 inch thick and about 4 to 5 inches in diameter.

Cover the dough with a clean towel and let it rise for 45 minutes. Arrange the rounds upside down on baking sheets. Bake in a 500-degree oven for 10 to 15 minutes or until brown and puffed in the center. The breads will be hard when they are removed from the oven, but will soften and flatten as they cool. When cooled, split or cut the bread carefully and fill with any combination of sandwich filling.

DRAMATIC PLAY CLOTHES

The following list contains names of clothing articles to save for use in the dramatic play area:

aprons	socks	coats
boots	purses	ear muffs
pajamas	jewelry—rings	raincoats
shirts	bracelets	snow pants
dresses	necklaces	shorts
skirts	clip-on earrings	sweatsuits
hats	shoes	suspenders
gloves/mittens	slippers	billfolds
scarves	robes	ties
leotards	slacks	belts
swimsuits	sweaters	

Record:

The following record can be found in preschool educational catalogs:

Learning Basic Skills Through Music by Hap Palmer. "What Are You Wearing?"

Books and Stories:

The following books and stories can be used to complement the theme:

1. **New Shoes!** Dorothy Corey. (Niles, IL: Albert Whitman & Co., 1985).

2. **Max's New Suit.** Rosemary Wells. (New York: Dial Press, 1979).

3. **Elizabeth Jane Gets Dressed.** Anne Tyrrell. (Woodbury, NY: Barron's, 1987).

4. **Not So Fast, Songololo.** Niki Daly. (New York: Atheneum, 1986).

5. **Hiram's Red Shirt.** Mable Watts. (New York: Golden Press, 1981).

6. **Shoes.** Elizabeth Winthrop. (New York: Harper and Row, 1986).

7. **The Red Jacket Mix-up.** Ari Hill. (New York: Golden Press, 1986).

8. **Dots, Spots, Speckles and Stripes.** Tara Hoban. (New York: Greenwillow Books, 1987).

9. **I Can Be a Textile Worker.** Christine Maloney Fitz-Gerald. (Chicago: Childrens Press, 1987).

10. **What Was It Before It Was a Sweater?** Roseva Shreckhise. (Chicago: Childrens Press, 1985).

11. **The Patchwork Quilt.** Valerie Flournoy. (New York: Dial Press, 1985).

12. **I Can Get Dressed.** Nicole Rubel. (New York: Macmillan, 1984).

13. **Socks for Supper.** Jack Kent. (New York: Parents Magazine Press, 1978).

14. **Katy No-Pocket.** Emmy Payne. (Boston, MA: Houghton Mifflin Company, 1972).

Puzzles:

The following puzzles can be found in preschool educational catalogs:

1. **"Dressable Dolls"** Puzzle People.

2. **"Rain"** Judy/Instructo.

3. **"Occupational Hats"** Puzzle People.

4. **"Shoes, Occupations"** Judy/Instructo.

5. **"Boy/Girl Doll with Clothes"** Puzzle People.

6. **"Dressing Puzzles"** 7 pieces. Puzzle People.

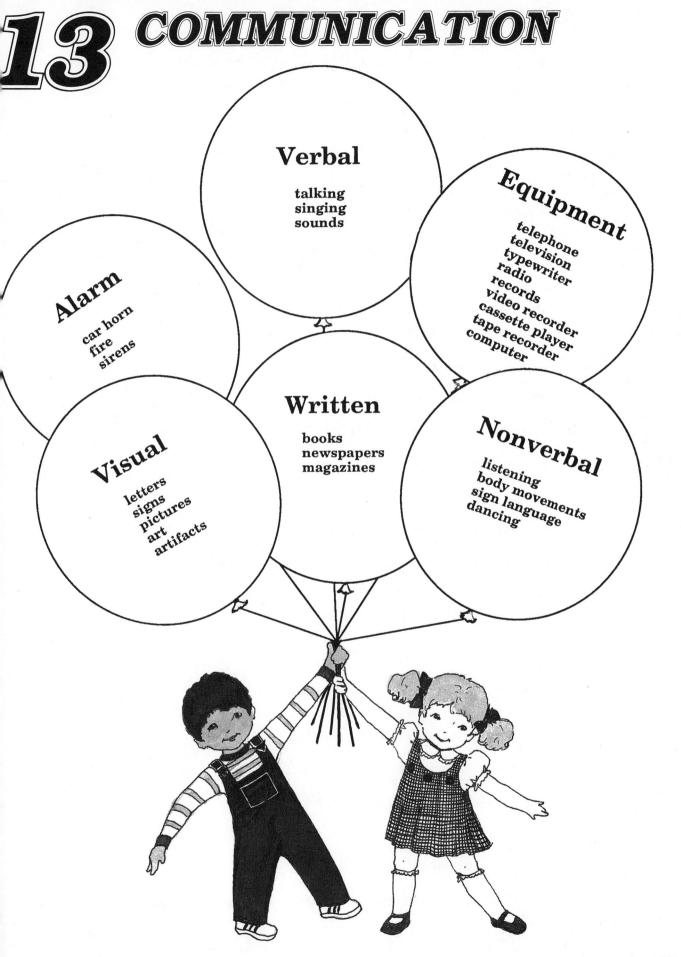

Verbal

talking
singing
sounds

Equipment

telephone
television
typewriter
radio
records
video recorder
cassette player
tape recorder
computer

Alarm

car horn
fire
sirens

Written

books
newspapers
magazines

Nonverbal

listening
body movements
sign language
dancing

Visual

letters
signs
pictures
art
artifacts

Theme Goals:

Through participating in the experiences provided by this theme, the children may learn:

1. Visual communication skills.

2. Nonverbal communication skills.

3. Verbal communication skills.

4. Communication equipment.

Concepts for the Children to Learn:

1. Talking is a form of communication.

2. Listening is a way to communicate.

3. Our hands can communicate.

4. Our faces can communicate.

5. Sign language is a way of communication.

6. The telephone is a communication tool.

7. Letters are a way of communicating.

8. Machines can transmit messages.

9. Typewriters, televisions, radios and computers are equipment for communicating.

10. Signs are a way of communicating.

11. Books are a form of communication.

Vocabulary:

1. **communication**—sharing information.

2. **typewriter**—a machine that prints letters.

3. **newspaper**—words printed on paper.

4. **sign language**—making symbols with our hands to communicate.

5. **Braille**—a system of printing for blind people.

6. **alphabet**—letter symbols that are used to write a language.

7. **signs**—symbols.

Bulletin Board

The purpose of this bulletin board is to assist older children in learning their home telephone number. Construct a telephone and receiver for each child. See the illustration. Affix each child's telephone number to the telephone. Laminate this card. For younger children, receivers can be attached to the telephones but left off the hook. The children can hang up their receiver when they arrive at school. Older children can match their receiver to their number and correct themselves by the color match. Later, white receivers for each child could be used to see if they know their telephone number. Telephones can be prepared for dialing by fastening the rotary dial with a brass fastener. Then the children can practice calling home by dialing their own number.

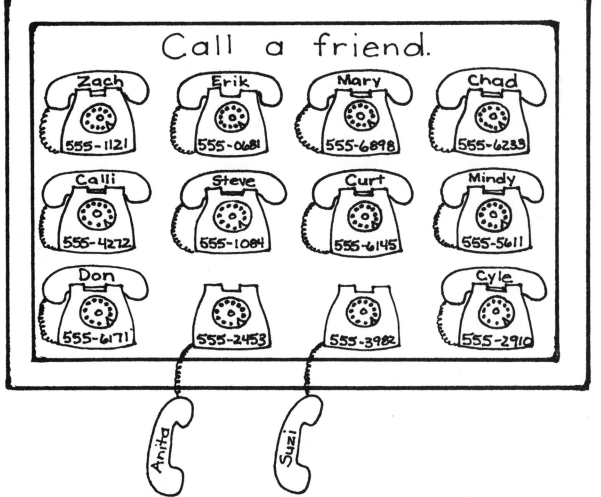

Parent Letter

Dear Parents,

This week at school we will be talking about communication or how we get our ideas across to others. Through this unit the children will become aware of the different ways we communicate: through our voices, letters, using hands and our bodies. They will also become familiar with machines that are used to communicate such as the television, radio, computer, typewriter and telephone.

At School This Week

Some of the learning experiences planned for this week include:

* a sign language demonstration.
* a phone booth in the dramatic play area.
* a typewriter in the writing center.
* songs and books about communication.

At Home

It is important for children to know their telephone number for safety reasons. Help your children learn your home telephone number. (This is also something we will be practicing at school.) To make practicing more fun, construct a toy telephone with your child. Two paper cups or empty tin cans and a long piece of rope, string or yarn are needed to make a telephone. Thread the string through the two cups and tie knots on the ends. Have two people hold the cups and pull the string taut. Take turns talking and listening. The sound vibrations travel through the string—and you won't hear a busy signal!

Have a nice week!

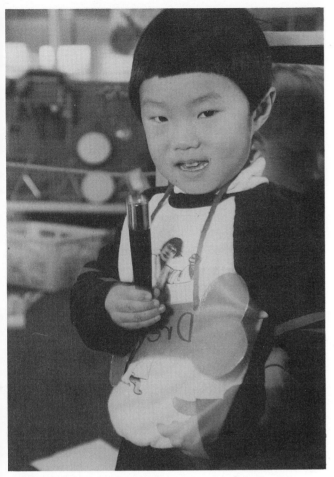

FIGURE 13 Microphones are just one way of communicating.

Music:

1. **Call a Friend**
   (Sing to the tune of "Row, Row, Row Your Boat")

   Call, call, call a friend.
   Friend, I'm calling you.
   Hi, hello, how are you.
   Very good, thank you!

2. **A Letter, A Letter**
   (Sing to the tune of "A Tisket, A Tasket")

   A letter, a letter, I can make a letter.
   I take my arms and take my legs and I
   can make a _____.

   Encourage the children to make letters of
   the alphabet with their body parts.

   Source: *Musical Games, Fingerplays and
   Rhythmic Activities for Early Childhood.*
   Wirth, Stassevitch, Shotwell and Stemmler.

3. **Twinkle, Twinkle Traffic Light**
   (Sing to the tune of "Twinkle, Twinkle
   Little Star")

   Twinkle, twinkle traffic light
   Standing on the corner bright.
   Green means go, we all know
   Yellow means wait, even if you're late.
   Red means STOP!
     (pause)
   Twinkle, twinkle traffic light
   Standing on the corner bright.

4. **I'm a Little Carrier**
   (Sing to the tune of "I'm a Little Teapot")

   I'm a little mail carrier, short and stout.
   Here is my hat, and here is my pouch.
     (point to head, point to side)
   I walk around from house to house,
   Delivering mail from my pouch.
     (pretend to take things out of a bag)

Fingerplays:

BODY TALK

When I smile, I tell you I'm happy.
  (pointers at the corner of mouth)
When I frown I tell you that I'm sad
  (pointers pull down corners of mouth)
When I raise my shoulders and tilt my
head I tell you "I don't know"
  (raise shoulders, tilt head, raise hands,
  shake head)

HELPFUL FRIENDS

Mail carriers carry a full pack
Of cards and letters on their backs.
  (hold both hands over one shoulder)
Step, step, step! Now ring, ring ring!
  (step in place and pretend to ring bell)
What glad surprises do they bring?

MY HANDS

My hands can talk
In a special way.
These are some things
They help me to say.
"Hello"
  (wave)

"Come Here"
  (beckon towards self)
"It's A–OK"
  (form circle with thumb and pointer)
"Now Stop"
  (hand out–palm up)
"Look"
  (hands shading eyes)
"Listen"
  (cup hand behind ear)
Or "It's far, far away"
  (point out into the distance)
And "Glad to meet you, how are you to-day."
  (shake neighbor,s hand)

Science:

1. Telephones

Place telephones, real or toy, in the classroom to encourage the children to talk to each other. Also, make your own telephones by using two large empty orange juice concentrate cans, removing one end for the removal of content. After washing the cans, connect with a long string. The children can pull the string taut. Then they can take turns talking and listening to each other.

2. Sound Shakers

Using identical small orange juice cans, pudding cups or empty film containers, fill pairs of the containers with different objects. Included may be sand, coins, rocks, rice, salt, etc. Replace the lids. Make sure to secure the lids with glue or heavy tape to avoid spilling. To make the containers self-correcting, place numbers or like colors on the bottoms of the matching containers.

3. Feely Box

Prepare a feely box which includes such things as tape cassette, pen, pencil, block letters, an envelope and anything else that is related to communication. The children can place their hand in the box and identify objects using their sense of touch.

4. Training Telephones

Contact your local telephone company to borrow training telephones. Place the telephone on the science table along with a chart listing the children's telephone numbers. The children can sort, match and classify the wires.

5. Vibrations

Encourage the children to gently place their hand on the side of the piano, guitar, record player, radio, television, etc. in order to feel the vibrations. Then have the children feel their own throats vibrate as they speak. A tuning fork can also be a teaching aid when talking about vibrations.

6. Telephone Parts

Dismantle an old telephone and put it on the science table for the children to discover and explore the parts.

Dramatic Play:

1. Post Office

In the dramatic play area place a mailbox, envelopes, old cards, paper, pens, old stampers, ink pads, hats and mailbags. During self-selected or self-initiated play periods, the children can play post office.

2. Telephone Booth

Make a telephone booth from a large refrigerator-sized cardboard box. Inside, place a toy phone. Place in the dramatic play area.

3. Television

Obtain a discarded television console to use for puppetry or storytelling experiences. Remove the back and set, allowing just the wooden frame. If desired, make curtains.

4. Radio Station

Place an old microphone, or one made from a styrofoam ball and cardboard with records in the dramatic play area.

5. Puppet Show

Place a puppet stand and a variety of puppets in the dramatic play area for the children to use during the self-selected or self-directed play period.

Arts and Crafts:

1. Record Player Art

Place a piece of round paper or a paper plate with a hole punched in the center on a record player turn table. Turn the record player on. The children can use crayons or markers to draw softly on the paper while the record player is spinning.

2. Easel Idea

Cut easel paper in the shape of a book, record, radio or other piece of communication equipment.

3. Traffic Lights

Provide red, yellow and green circles, glue and construction paper for the children to create a traffic light.

4. Stationery

Provide the children with various stencils or stamps to make their own stationery. It can be used for a gift for a parent or a special person. Children could then dictate a letter to a relative or friend.

Large Muscle:

Charades

Invite children one at a time to come to the front of the group. Then whisper something in the child's ear, like "You're very happy." The child then uses his hands, face, feet, arms, etc. to communicate this feeling to the other children. The group of children then identifies the demonstrated feeling.

Field Trips/Resource People:

1. Post Office

Visit a local post office. Encourage the children to observe how the mail is sorted.

2. Phone Company

Visit a local phone company.

3. Radio Station

Visit a local disc jockey at the radio station.

4. Television Station

If available, visit a local television station. Observe the cameras, microphones and other communication devices.

5. Sign Language Demonstration

Invite someone to demonstrate sign language.

Math:

Phone Numbers

Make a list of the children's names and telephone numbers. Place the list by a toy, trainer, or unhooked telephone.

Social Studies:

Thank You

Let the children dictate a group thank you letter to one of your resource visitors or field trip representatives. Before mailing the letter, provide writing tools for children to sign their names.

Group time (games, language):

1. Telephone

Play the game telephone by having the children sit in a circle. Begin by whispering a short phrase into a child's ear. That child whispers your message to the next child. Continue until the message gets to the last child. The last child repeats the message out loud. It is fun to see how much it has changed. (This game is most successful with older children.)

2. What's Missing?

Place items that are related to communication on a tray. Include a stamp, a telephone, a record, a pocket radio, etc. The children can examine the objects for a few minutes. After this they should close their eyes while you remove an object. Take away one object. Then let the children look at the tray and identify which object is missing.

3. Household Objects Sound Like...

Make a tape of different sounds around the house. Include a radio, television, alarm clock, telephone, vacuum cleaner, flushing toilet, door bells, egg timer, etc. Play the tape for the children, letting them identify the individual sounds.

Cooking:

Edible Envelope

Spread peanut butter on a graham cracker. Add raisins to represent an address and a stamp.

FINGERPAINT RECIPES

Liquid Starch Method

liquid starch (put in
   squeeze bottles)
dry tempera paint in
   shakers

Put about 1 tablespoon of liquid starch on the surface to be painted. Let the child shake the paint onto the starch. Mix and blend the paint. Note: If this paint becomes too thick, simply sprinkle a few drops of water onto the painting.

Soap Flake Method

Mix in a small bowl:
soap flakes
a small amount of water

Beat until stiff with an eggbeater. Use white soap on dark paper, or add to the soap and use it on light-colored paper. This gives a slight three-dimensional effect.

Wheat Flour Paste

3 parts water
1 part wheat paste flour
coloring

Stir flour into water. Add coloring. (Wallpaper paste can be bought at low cost in wallpaper stores or department stores.)

Uncooked Laundry Starch

A mixture of 1 cup laundry/liquid starch, 1 cup cold water and 3 cups soap flakes will provide a quick fingerpaint.

Flour and Salt I
1 cup flour
1 1/2 cups salt
3/4 cup water
coloring

Combine flour and salt. Add water. This has a grainy quality, unlike the other fingerpaints, providing a different sensory experience. Some children enjoy the different touch sensation when 1 1/2 cup salt is added to the other recipes.

Flour and Salt II

2 cups flour
2 teaspoons salt
3 cups cold water
2 cups hot water
coloring

Add salt to flour, then pour in cold water gradually and beat mixture with egg beater until it is smooth. Add hot water and boil until it becomes clear. Beat until smooth, then mix in coloring. Use 1/4 cup food coloring to 8 to 9 ounces of paint for strong colors.

Instantized Flour Uncooked Method

1 pint water (2 cups)
1 1/2 cups instantized flour (the kind used to thicken gravy)

Put the water in the bowl and stir the flour into the water. Add color. Regular flour may be lumpy.

Cooked Starch Method

1 cup laundry starch dissolved in a small amount of cold water
5 cups boiling water added slowly to dissolve starch
1 tablespoon glycerine (optional)

Cook the mixture until it is thick and glossy. Add 1 cup mild soap flakes. Add color in separate containers. Cool before using.

Cornstarch Method

Gradually add 2 quarts water to 1 cup cornstarch. Cook until clear and add 1/2 cup soap flakes. A few drops of glycerine or oil of wintergreen may be added.

Flour Method

Mix 1 cup flour and 1 cup cold water. Add 3 cups boiling water and bring all to a boil, stirring constantly. Add 1 tablespoon alum and coloring. Paintings from this recipe dry flat and do not need to be ironed.

TIPS

1. Be sure you have running water and towels nearby or provide a large basin of water where children can rinse off.

2. Fingerpaint on smooth table, oil cloth, or cafeteria tray. Some children prefer to start fingerpainting with shaving cream on a sheet of oil cloth.

3. Food coloring or powdered paint may be added to mixture before using, or allow child to choose the colors he wants sprinkled on top of paint.

4. Sometimes reluctant children are more easily attracted to paint table if the fingerpaints are already colored.

Records:

The following records can be found in preschool educational catalogs:

1. **Jambo Songs and Chants.** Ella Jenkins.

2. **Community Helpers.** (Bowmar/Noble Publishers, Inc.)

3. **Creative Movement and Rhythmic Exploration.** Hap Palmer.

4. **Listening Skills for Pre-readers.** (Classroom Materials, Inc.: New York).

5. **You'll Sing a Song and I'll Sing a Song.** Ella Jenkins.

Books and Stories:

The following books and stories can be used to complement the theme:

1. **I Can Sign My ABC's.** Susan Gibbons Chaplin. (Washington, DC: Gallaudet University Press, 1986).

2. **Hand Talk; An ABC of Fingerspelling and Sign Language.** Remy Charlip. (New York: Parent's Magazine Press, 1974).

3. **My First Book of Sign.** Pamela Baker. (Washington, DC: Gallaudet University Press, 1986).

4. **The Telephone Book.** Maida Silverman. (New York: Golden, 1985).

5. **Jambo Means Hello.** Muriel Feelings. (New York: The Dial Press, 1974).

6. **Listen Rabbit.** Aileen Fisher. (New York: Thomas Y. Crowell Company, 1964).

7. **I Read Signs.** Tom Funk. (New York: Holiday House, 1962).

8. **I Read Symbols.** Tara Hoban. (New York: Greenwillow, 1983).

9. **Listening for Sounds.** Adelaide Hall. (New York: The Bobbs Merrill Company, 1970).

10. **How We Communicate.** Bobbie Kalman. (New York: Crabtree Publishing Company, 1986).

11. **Listen Children Listen.** Myra Cohn Livingston. (New York: Harcourt, Brace Jovanovich, Inc., 1972).

12. **Marcel Marceou Alphabet Book.** George Mendoza. (New York: Doubleday and Company, 1970).

13. **Red Light Says Stop.** Barbara Rinkoff. (New York: Lothrop, Lee and Shepard Company, 1974).

14. **Early Words.** Richard Scarry. (New York: Random House, 1976).

15. **A Button in Her Ear.** Ada B. Litchfield. (Chicago: Albert Whitman and Company, 1976).

16. **Gobble, Growl, Grunt.** Peter Spier. (New York: Doubleday and Company, 1971).

17. **Noisy.** S. Hughes. (New York: Lothrop, Lee and Shepard Company, 1985).

Puzzles:

The following puzzles can be found in preschool educational catalogs:

1. **"Alphabet Dog"** 26 pieces. Judy/Instructo.

2. **"Telephone Line Person"** 11 pieces. Judy/Instructo.

3. **"T.V. Reporter"** 18 pieces. Judy/Instructo.

4. **"Mail Carrier"** 11 pieces. Judy/Instructo.

14 CONSTRUCTION TOOLS

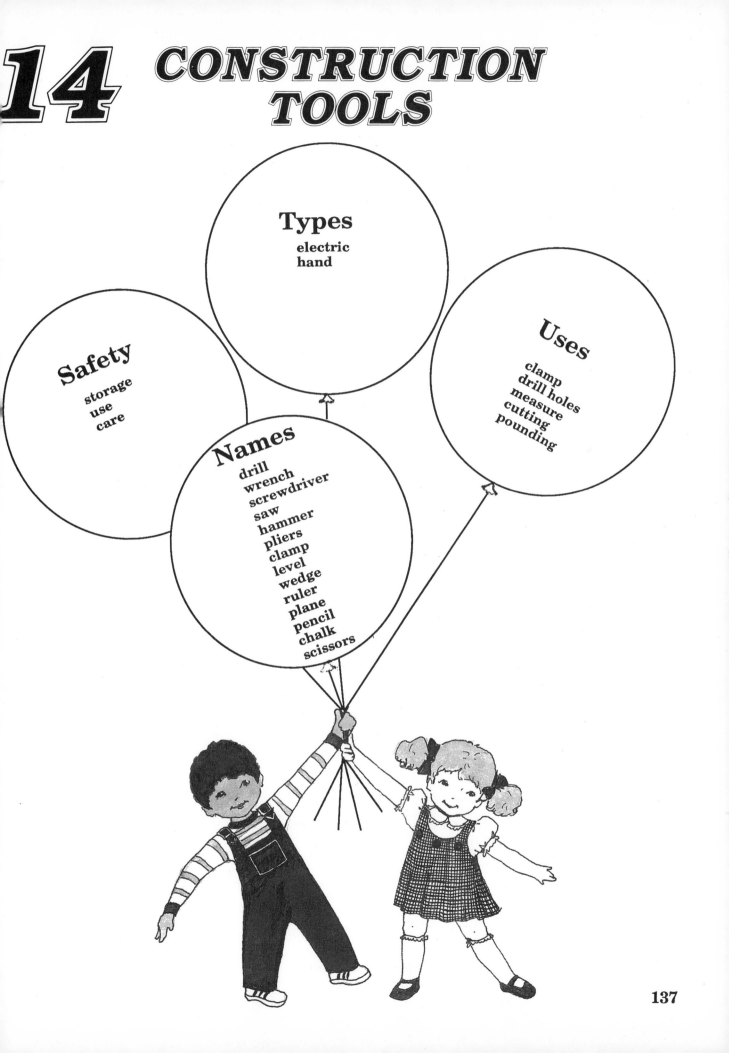

Types
electric
hand

Safety
storage
use
care

Uses
clamp
drill holes
measure
cutting
pounding

Names
drill
wrench
screwdriver
saw
hammer
pliers
clamp
level
wedge
ruler
plane
pencil
chalk
scissors

Theme Goals:

Through participating in the experiences provided by this theme, the children may learn:

1. Types of tools.
2. Names of common tools.
3. Functions of tools.
4. Tool safety.

Concepts for the Children to Learn:

1. Tools can be electric or hand powered.
2. Tools are helpful when building.
3. Pliers, tweezers and clamps hold things.
4. Drills, nails, and screws make holes.
5. Planes, saws, and scissors cut materials.
6. Hammers and screwdrivers are used to put in and remove nails and screws.
7. Rulers are used for measuring.
8. To be safe, tools need to be handled with care.
9. Goggles should be worn to protect our eyes when using tools.
10. After use, tools need to be put away.

Vocabulary:

1. **tool**—an object to help us.
2. **drill**—a tool that cuts holes.
3. **wrench**—a tool that holds things.
4. **screwdriver**—a tool that turns screws.
5. **saw**—a cutting tool with sharp edges.
6. **hammer**—a tool used to insert or remove objects such as nails.
7. **pliers**—a tool used for holding.
8. **clamp**—a tool used to join or hold things.
9. **ruler**—a measuring tool.
10. **wedge**—a tool used for splitting.
11. **plane**—a tool used for shaving wood.

Bulletin Board

The purpose of this bulletin board is to develop awareness of types of tools, as well as foster visual discrimination skills. A shadow tool match bulletin board can be constructed by drawing about six or seven tool pieces on tagboard. See the illustration. These pieces can be colored and cut out. Next, trace the pieces on black construction paper to make shadows of each piece. These shadow pieces can be attached to the bulletin board. Magnet pieces can be applied to both the shadows and the colored tool pieces, or a push pin can be placed above the shadow and a hole can be punched in the colored tool piece. The children can match the colored tool piece to its corresponding shaped shadow.

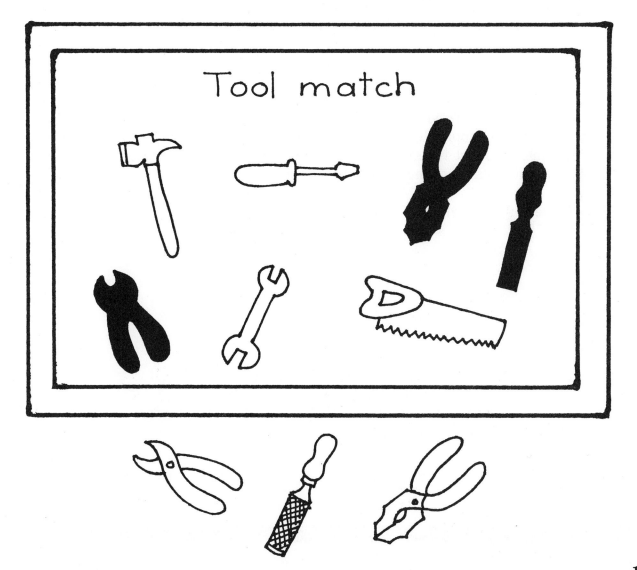

Parent Letter

Dear Parents,

The unit for this week will focus on construction tools. This unit will help your child become more aware of many kinds of tools, their purposes, and tool safety. During the week, the children will have opportunities to use many hand tools at the woodworking bench.

At School This Week

Some of the activities the children will participate in this week include:

* painting with screwdrivers and wrenches.
* exploring wood shavings in the sensory table.
* setting up a mechanic's shop where the children can pretend to fix cars.
* a visit on Wednesday from Mr. Smith, a local shoe repairer. Mr. Smith will show us the tools he uses to repair shoes.

At Home

To develop memory skills recall with your child all of the tools we use in our homes—from cooking and cleaning tools to gardening tools. Count the number of tools that are in each room of your house. Which room contains the most tools? This will promote the mathematical concepts of rational counting and vocabulary of most and least.

Have a nice week!

Music:

"This Is the Way"
(Sing to the tune of "Mulberry Bush")

This is the way we saw our wood,
saw our wood, saw our wood.
This is the way we saw our wood,
so early in the morning.

Other verses: pound our nails
drill a hole
use a screwdriver

Fingerplays:

CARPENTER'S HAMMER

The carpenter's hammer goes rap, rap, tap
  (make hammer motion)
And his saw goes see, saw, see.
  (make saw motions)
He planes and measures and hammers and
saws
  (act out each one)
While he builds a house for me.
  (draw house with index fingers)

JOHNNY'S HAMMER

Johnny works with one hammer, one hammer, one hammer.
Johnny works with one hammer, then he works with two.

Say the same words adding one hammer each time. Children are to pretend to hammer using various body parts.

Verse 1: 1 hand hitting leg.
Verse 2: 2 hands hitting legs.
Verse 3: use motions for verses 1 and 2, plus tap one foot.
Verse 4: verses 1, 2, and 3 plus tap other foot.
Verse 5: verses 1 to 4, plus nod head. At the end of verse 5 say, "Then he goes to sleep," and place both hands by side of head.

You can also change the name used in the fingerplay to include names of children in your classroom.

THE COBBLER

Cobbler, cobbler mend my shoe.
  (point to shoe)
Get it done by half past two.
  (hold up two fingers)
Half past two is much too late.
Get it done by half past eight.
  (hold up eight fingers)

Science:

1. **Exploring Levels**

   Place levels and wood scraps on a table for the children to explore while being closely supervised.

2. **Hammers**

   Collect a variety of hammers, various-sized nails and wood scraps or styrofoam. Allow the children to practice pounding using the different tools and materials.

3. **The Wide World of Rulers**

   Set up a display with different types and sizes of rulers. Include the reel type. Paper and pencils can also be added to create interest.

Dramatic Play:

1. **The Carpenter**

   Place a carpentry box with scissors, rulers and masking tape in the woodworking area. Also, provide large cardboard boxes and paint, if desired.

2. **Shoemaker Store**

   Set up a shoemaker's store. Provide the children with shoes, toy hammers, smocks, cash registers and play money. The children can act out mending, buying and selling shoes.

Arts and Crafts:

1. **Rulers**

   Set rulers and paper on the table. The children can then experiment creating lines and geometric shapes.

2. Tool Print

Pour a small amount of thick-colored tempera paint in a flat pan. Also, provide the children with miniature tools such as wrenches, screwdrivers and paper. The children then can place the tools in the paint pan, remove them and print on paper.

Sensory:

1. Scented Playdough

Prepare playdough and add a few drops of extract such as peppermint, anise, or almond. Also collect a variety of scissors, and place in the art area with the playdough.

2. Wood Shavings

Place wood shavings in the sensory table along with scoops and pails.

Large Muscle:

The Workbench

In the woodworking area place various tools, wood and goggles for the children to use. It is **very** important to discuss the safety and limits used when at the workbench prior to this activity. An extra adult is helpful to supervise this area.

Field Trips/Resource People:

1. Shoe Repair Store

Visit a shoe repair store. Observe a shoe being repaired.

2. Wood Worker

Invite a parent or other person into the classroom who enjoys woodworking as a hobby.

Math:

1. Use of Rulers

Discuss how rulers are used. Provide children with rulers so that they may measure various objects in the classroom. Allow them to compare the lengths. Also, measure each child and construct a chart including each child's height.

2. Weighing Tools

Place scales and a variety of tools on the math table. Let the children explore weighing the tools.

Social Studies:

1. Tool Safety

Discuss the safe use of tools. Allow the children to help decide what classroom rules are necessary for using tools. Make a chart containing these rules to display in the woodworking area.

2. Helper Chart

Design a helper chart for the children to assist with clean-up and care of the classroom tools. Each day select new children to assist, assuring that everyone gets a turn. To participate the children can be responsible for cleaning the dirty tools and putting them away.

Group Time (games, language):

1. Tool of the Day

Each day of this unit, introduce a "tool of the day." Explain how each tool is used and who uses it. If possible, leave the tool out for children to use on the wood working bench.

2. Thank You Letter

Using a pencil as a tool, let the children dictate a thank-you note to any resource person or field trip site coordinator that has contributed to the program.

Cooking:

"Hands On" Cookies

3 cups brown sugar
3 cups margarine or butter
6 cups oatmeal
1 tablespoon baking soda
3 cups flour

Place all of the ingredients in a bowl. Let the children use clean child-size wooden hammers to mash and knead. Form into small balls and place on ungreased cookie sheet. Butter the bottom of a glass. Dip the bottom of the glass into a saucer with sugar. Use the glass to flatten the balls. Bake in an oven preheated to 350 degrees for 10 to 12 minutes. Makes 15 dozen.

SCIENCE MATERIALS AND EQUIPMENT

Teachers need to continuously provide science materials for the classroom. Materials that can be collected include:

acorns and other nuts
aluminum foil
ball bearings
balloons
binoculars
bird nests
bones
bowls and cups
cocoon
corks
discorded clock
dishpans
drinking straws
drums
egg cartons
eyedroppers and basters
eggbeaters
fabric scraps
filter paper
flashlight
flowers
gears
insect nests
insects
jacks
kaleidoscope

locks and keys
magnets—varying
    strengths, sizes
marbles
magnifying glasses—good
    lenses
microscope
measuring cups and
    spoons
milk cartons
mirrors—all sizes
moths
musical instruments
newspapers
nails, screws, bolts
paper bags
paper of various types
plants
paper rolls and spools
plastic bags
plastic containers with
    lids—many sizes
plastic tubing
pots, pans, trays, muffin
    tins
prisms

pulleys
rocks
rubber tubing
ruler
safety goggles—child size
scales
scissors—assorted sizes
screen wire
sieves, sifters and funnels
seeds
sand paper
spatulas
sponges
stones
string
styrofoam
tape
thermometers
tongs and tweezers
tuning forks
tools—hammer, pliers
waxed paper
weeds
wood and other building
    materials
wheels

Books and Stories:

The following books and stories can be used to complement the theme:

1. **The Tool Box.** Anne and Harlow Rockwell. (New York: Macmillan Company, 1972).

2. **Fix-It.** David McPhail. (New York: Dutton, 1984).

3. **Tool Book.** Gail Gibbons. (New York: Holiday House, 1982).

4. **In Christina's Tool Box.** Dianne Homan. (Chapel Hills, NC: Lollipop Power, 1981).

5. **Mr. Bell's Fixit Shop.** Ronne Peltzman. (New York: Golden Press, 1981).

6. **What Was It Before It Was a Chair?** Roseva Screckhise. (Chicago: Childrens Press, 1985).

7. **Betsy's Fixing Day.** Gunilla Wolde. (New York: Random House, 1978).

Puzzles:

The following puzzles can be found in preschool educational catalogs:

1. **"Carpenter"** Judy/Instructo.

2. **"Car Mechanic"** Judy/Instructo.

3. **"Construction Worker"** Judy/Instructo.

15 CREATIVE MOVEMENT

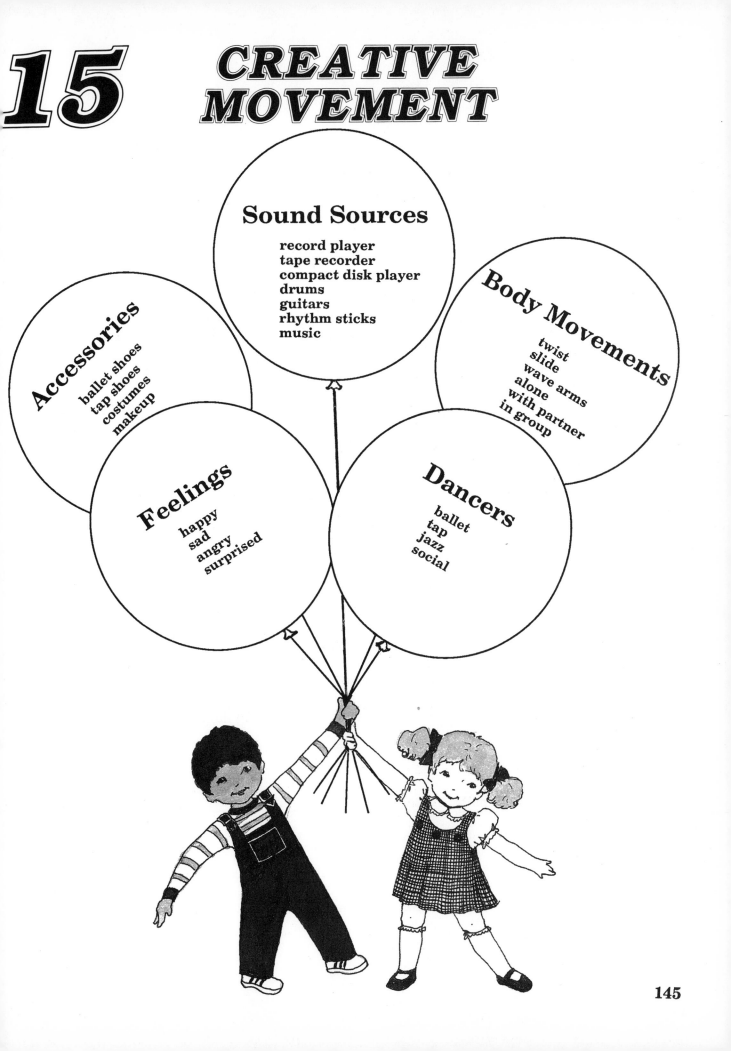

Sound Sources

record player
tape recorder
compact disk player
drums
guitars
rhythm sticks
music

Body Movements

twist
slide
wave arms
alone
with partner
in group

Accessories

ballet shoes
tap shoes
costumes
makeup

Feelings

happy
sad
angry
surprised

Dancers

ballet
tap
jazz
social

Theme Goals:

Through participating in the experiences provided by this theme, the children may learn:

1. Creative movement accessories.

2. Creative movement sound sources.

3. Body movements used in creative movement.

4. Expression of feelings through creative movement.

5. Types of dancers.

Concepts for the Children to Learn:

1. People can dance to music.

2. The record player, tape recorder and compact disk player are all sound sources used for dance.

3. Dancing and moving can be done alone, with a partner, or in a group.

4. Our bodies can move in many different ways.

5. Ballet, tap, jazz and social are some types of dances.

6. Happy, sad, angry and surprised are feelings that can be expressed through dance.

7. Some dancers wear special costumes and makeup.

8. Ballet and tap dancers wear special shoes.

9. Our bodies can move to the sound of drums, guitars and rhythm sticks.

10. We can twist, slide and wave our arms during dance.

Vocabulary:

1. **dance**—a pattern of body movements.

2. **movement**—change in body position.

3. **ballet**—movement that usually tells a story.

4. **music**—sounds made by instruments or voices.

Bulletin Board

The purpose of this bulletin board is to develop one-to-one correspondence skills and the ability to match a set to the matching written numeral. Construct tank tops, each of a different color from a sheet of tagboard. See the illustration. Print a numeral that would be developmentally appropriate for the group of children on each tank top. Draw a corresponding number of black dots below each numeral. Construct a tutu ruffle from white tagboard for each top. Place colored dots on each ruffle. Trace ruffles onto black construction paper. Laminate all pieces. Staple tank tops and shadow ruffles to bulletin board. The children can match the ruffles with dots to the corresponding tank top, using holes in white ruffles and push pins in shadow ruffles.

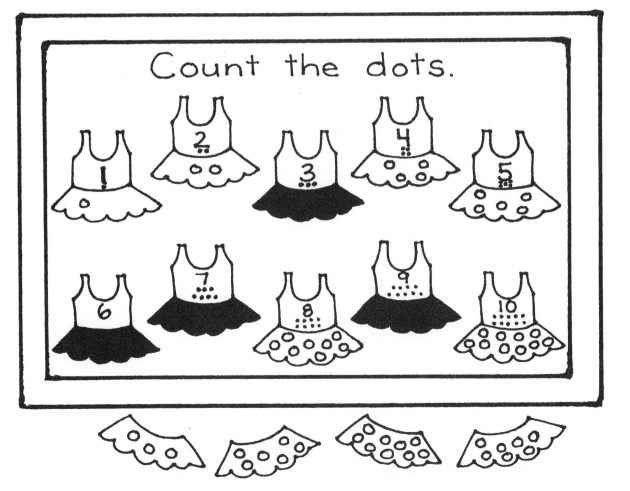

Parent Letter

Dear Parents,

Children love to dance, and they are constantly on the move. So this week at school we will be enjoying a unit on creative movement. Throughout the week the children will discover the different ways our bodies move, and also learn about various forms of dance. Some of the activities for the week include:

* singing songs and moving to music.
* dancing in the dance studio that will be set up in the dramatic play area.
* watching other people move.
* participating in an aerobics class.

Field Trip This Week

On Thursday, at 2:30 p.m. we will be taking a bus to a dance studio. At the studio, we will observe dancers and learn a few steps from a dance instructor. To assist with the trip, we need several parents to accompany us. Please call the school if you are available.

At Home

As your child develops, he will show increased control and interest in perfecting and improving motor skills. To foster the development of large muscle skills, balance and body coordination, provide opportunities each day for vigorous play. Give suggestions such as "How fast can you hop?", "How far can you hop on one foot?" etc. Also ask your child to walk on a curved line, a straight line or a balance beam.

Have a good week!

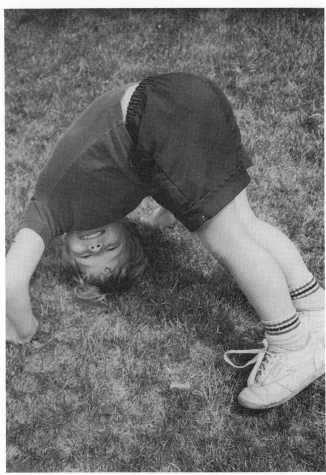

FIGURE 15 Exercise can be creative.

Fingerplays:

The following circle games are from *Finger Frolics: Fingerplays for Young Children* by Cromwell, Hibner and Faitel. (Partner Press: 1983).

HOP AND TWIRL

Make a circle and we'll go around.
First walk on tiptoe so we don't make a sound.
Tip, toe, around we go.
Then hop on our left foot, and then on our right.
Then hop together. What a funny sight!
Now stop hopping and twirl around
Now we're ready to settle down.

A CIRCLE

Around in a circle we will go.
Little tiny baby steps, make us go very slow.

And then we'll take some great giant steps,
As big as they can be.
Then in our circle we'll stand quietly.

STAND IN A CIRCLE

Stand in a circle and clap your hands.
Clap, clap, clap, clap.
Now put your hands over your head.
Slap, slap, slap, slap.
Now hands at your sides and turn around.
Then in our circle we'll all sit down.

ONE TO TEN CIRCLE

Let's make a circle and around we go,
Not too fast and not too slow.
One, two, three, four, five,—six, seven, eight, nine, ten
Let's face the other way and go around again,
One, two, three, four, five—six, seven, eight, nine, ten.

PARTNER GAME

Pick a partner, take a hand.
Then in a circle partners stand.
Take two steps forward,
And two steps back.
Then bow to your partner
And clap, clap, clap.
Wrap your elbows
And around you go.
Not too fast and not too slow.
Change elbows.
Go around again.
Then stand in a circle
And count to ten.

Science:

1. **Magnet Dancers**

On a piece of tagboard, draw pictures of three-inch dancers. Stickers or pictures from magazines can also be used. Cut the dancers out and attach paper clips to the back side. Use a small box and a magnet to make these dancers move. Hold the dancers up on one side of the box and move the dancer up by holding and moving a magnet on the other side of the box.

2. Kaleidoscopes

On the science table, put a number of kaleidoscopes. The tiny figures inside appear to be dancing.

3. Dancing Shoes

Place various types of dancing shoes at the science table. Let the children compare the shape, size, color and texture of the shoes. The children may also enjoy trying the shoes on for size and dancing in them.

Dramatic Play:

1. Dance Studio

Add to the dramatic play area tap shoes, tutus, ballet shoes, tights and leotards, and either a record player with records or tape player with tapes.

2. Fitness Gym

Add to the dramatic play area a small mat, head bands, wrist bands, sweat shirts, sweat pants, leotards and music.

Arts and Crafts:

1. Stencils

The teacher can construct stencils from tagboard. Shapes such as shoes, ballerinas, circles, etc. can be made and added to the art table for use during self-selected activity periods.

2. Musical Painting

Provide a tape recorder with head phones and a tape of children's music or classical music at the easel. The children can listen and move their brushes to the music if desired.

Large Muscle:

1. Streamer/Music Activity

In the music area provide streamers. Play a variety of music, allowing the children, if desired, to move to the different rhythms.

2. Do As I Say

Provide the children verbal clues for moving. For example, say, "Move like you are sad," "Show me that you are tired," "You just received a special present," or "Show me how you feel."

3. Animal Movement

Ask a child to act out the way a certain animal moves. Examples include: frog, spider, caterpillar, butterfly, etc.

4. Balance

Add a balance beam or balance strip to the indoor or outdoor environment.

5. Roly-Poly

The children can stretch their bodies out on the floor. When touched by a teacher, the child rolls into a tight ball.

6. Dancing Cloud

Using an inflated white balloon or ball, let the children stand in a circle and bounce or hit it to each other.

7. Obstacle Course

Set up an obstacle course indoors or outdoors depending on the weather. Let the children move their bodies in many different ways. They can run or crawl through the course. Older children may enjoy hopping or skipping.

Field Trips/Resource People:

1. Field Trips

* dance studio
* health club
* gymnasium

2. Resource People

* a dancer or dance instructor
* gymnast
* aerobics instructor

Math:

1. Matching Leotards to Hangers

Using plastic hangers, prepare a numeral on each of the hangers. Provide the children with a box of leotards. Have a printed numeral on each. Encourage the children to match the numbered leotard with the identically numbered hanger.

2. Following Steps

Using tagboard, cut out some left feet and right feet. Write the numerals from one to ten on the feet and arrange them in numerical order. Place the footprints on the floor, securing them with masking tape. Encourage the children to begin the walk on the numeral one and continue in the correct sequence.

3. Ballet Puzzle

Purchase a large poster of a ballet dancer. Laminate the poster or cover it with clear contact paper. Cut the poster into several large shapes. Place the puzzle in the manipulative area. During self-selected play periods, the children can reconstruct the puzzle.

Social Studies:

Social Dancing

Let each child choose a partner. Encourage the children to hold hands. Play music as a background, so the partners can move together.

Group Time (games, language):

1. Balloon Bounce

Blow up balloons for the children to use at group time. Play music and have children bounce the balloons up in the air. Let the balloons float to the ground when the music ends. Supervision is required for this activity. Broken balloons should be immediately removed from the environment.

3. Toy Movements

Form a circle and move like different toys. Try to include as many actual toys as you can, so that the children can observe each toy moving, and then can more easily pretend to be that toy.
* jack in the box
* wind-up dolls
* roll like a ball
* skates

4. Rag Doll

Repeat the following poem as the child creates a dance with a rag doll.

If I were a rag doll
And I belonged to you,
Whenever I would try to dance,
This is what I'd do.

Cooking:

1. Orange Buttermilk Smoothie

1 quart buttermilk
3 cups orange juice
1/2 teaspoon cinnamon
1/4 cup honey

Blend in a blender until the mixture is smooth. Enjoy!

2. Indian Flat Bread

2 cups all purpose flour
1/4 cup unflavored yogurt
1 egg, slightly beaten
1 1/2 teaspoons baking powder
1 teaspoon sugar
1/4 teaspoon salt
1/4 teaspoon baking soda
1/2 cup milk
vegetable oil
poppy seeds

Mix all ingredients except milk, vegetable oil and poppy seeds. Stir in enough milk to make a soft dough. Turn dough onto lightly-floured surface. Knead until smooth, about 5 minutes. Place in greased

151

bowl; turn greased side up. Cover and let rest in warm place 3 hours.

Divide dough into 6 or 8 equal parts. Flatten each part on lightly-floured surface, rolling it into 6 inch x 4 inch leaf shape about 1/4 inch thick. Brush with vegetable oil; sprinkle with poppy seeds.

Place 2 cookie sheets in oven; heat oven to 450 degrees. Remove hot cookie sheets from oven; place breads on cookie sheets. Bake until firm, 6 to 8 minutes. Makes 6 to 8 breads.

Source: *Betty Crocker's International Cookbook*. (New York: Random House, 1980).

MOVEMENT ACTIVITIES

Listen to the Drum

Accessory: drum
fast
slow
heavy
soft
big
small

Choose a Partner

Make a big shape
go over
go under
go through
go around

To Become Aware of Time

Run very fast
Walk very slowly
Jump all over the floor quickly
Sit down on the floor slowly
Slowly grow up as tall as you can
Slowly curl up on the floor as small as possible

To Become Aware of Space

Lift your leg up in front of you
Lift it up backwards, sideways
Lift your leg and step forward, backwards, sideways and around and around

Reach up to the ceiling
Stretch to touch the walls
Punch down to the floor

To Become Aware of Weight

To feel the difference between heavy and light, the child should experiment with his own body force.
Punch down to the floor hard
Lift your arms up slowly and gently
Stomp on the floor
Walk on tip-toe
Kick out one leg as hard as you can
Very smoothly and lightly slide one foot along the floor

Moving Shapes

1. Try to move about like something huge and heavy: elephant, tug boat, bulldozer.
2. Try to move like something small and heavy: a fat frog, a heavy top.
3. Try moving like something big and light: a beach ball, a parachute, a cloud.
4. Try moving like something small and light: a feather, a snowflake, a flea, a butterfly.

Put Yourself Inside Something

(bottle, box, barrel)
You're *outside* of something—now get into it
You're *inside* of something—now get out of it
You're *underneath* something
You're *on top of* something
You're *beside* or *next to* something
You're *surrounded* by it

Pantomine

1. You're going to get a present. What is the shape of the box? How big is the box? Feel it. Hold it. Unwrap it. Take it out. Put it back in.
2. Think about an occupation. How does the worker act?
3. Show me that it is cold, hot.
4. You are two years old (sixteen, eighty, etc.)
5. Show me: It's very early in the morning, late in the afternoon.
6. Show me: What is the weather like?
7. Pretend you are driving, typing, raking leaves.
8. Take a partner. Pretend you're playing ball.

Records:

The following records can be found in preschool educational catalogs:

1. **Dance, Sing, and Listen.** Esther Nelson and Bruce Haack.

2. **Creative Movement and Rhythmic Exploration.** Hap Palmer.

3. **Songs, Rhythms and Chants for the Dance.** Ella Jenkins.

4. **Music for Creative Movement.** (Kimbo Records).

5. **Simple Folk Dances.** (Kimbo Records).

Books and Stories:

The following books and stories can be used to complement the theme:

1. **Twelve Dancing Princesses.** The Grimm Brothers. (New York: Charles Scribner and Sons, 1966).

2. **The Dancing Camel.** Betsy Byars. (New York: Viking Press, 1965).

3. **Shake My Sillies Out.** Raffi. (New York: Crown Publishers, Inc., 1987).

4. **I Danced in My Red Pajamas.** Edith Thacher Hurd. (New York: Harper and Row, 1982).

5. **Singing and Dancing Games for the Very Young.** Esther L. Nelson. (New York: Sterling Publishing Company, Inc., 1977).

6. **The Dancing School.** Eleanor Schick. (New York: Harper and Row, 1966).

7. **Kiki Dances.** Charlotte Steiner. (New York: Doubleday, 1949).

8. **My Body: How it Works.** Jane Werner Watson. (New York: Western Publishing Company, 1972).

Puzzles:

The following puzzles can be found in preschool educational catalogs:

1. **"Playground & Kid's Puzzle"** Lauri.

2. **"Kids"** 18 pieces. Lauri.

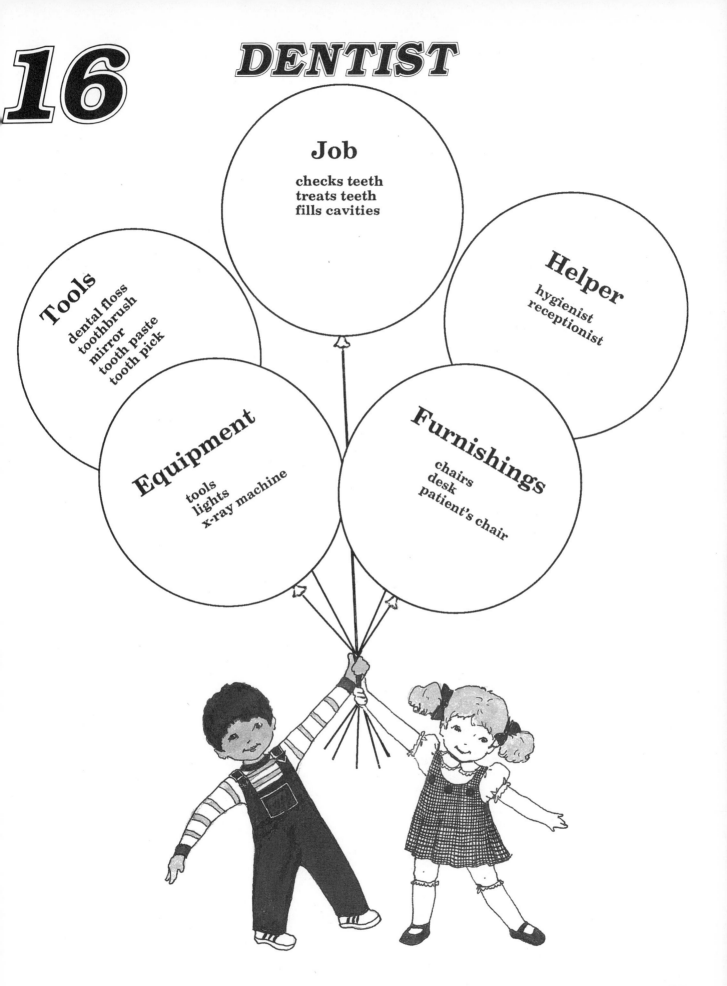

16 **DENTIST**

Job
checks teeth
treats teeth
fills cavities

Helper
hygienist
receptionist

Tools
dental floss
toothbrush
mirror
tooth paste
tooth pick

Equipment
tools
lights
x-ray machine

Furnishings
chairs
desk
patient's chair

Theme Goals:

Through participating in the experiences provided by this theme, the children may learn:

1. How the dentist helps us.

2. Dentist's tools.

3. The name of the dentist's assistant.

4. Proper tooth care.

5. Dental equipment.

6. Dental office furnishings.

Concepts for the Children to Learn:

1. The dentist helps keep our teeth healthy.

2. Teeth are used to chew food.

3. Teeth should be brushed after each meal.

4. A hygienist helps the dentist.

5. A dentist removes decay from our teeth.

6. Pictures of our teeth are called x-rays.

7. A toothbrush and paste are used to clean teeth.

8. Dental floss helps clean between teeth.

9. The dentist's office has special machines.

Vocabulary:

1. **toothbrush**—a brush to clean teeth.

2. **toothpaste**—a paste to clean our teeth.

3. **dentist**—a person who helps keep our teeth healthy.

4. **teeth**—used to chew food.

5. **hygienist**—the dentist's assistant.

6. **cavity**—tooth decay.

7. **toothpick**—a stick-like tool used for removing food parts between our teeth.

8. **dental floss**—a string used to clean between the teeth.

Bulletin Board

The purpose of this bulletin board is to develop a positive self-concept and assist in name recognition. Prepare an attendance bulletin board by constructing a toothbrush out of tagboard for each student and teacher. See the illustration. Color the toothbrushes and print the children's names on them! Laminate. Punch holes in each toothbrush. Observe who brushed by observing who hung their toothbrush on a push pin on the bulletin board.

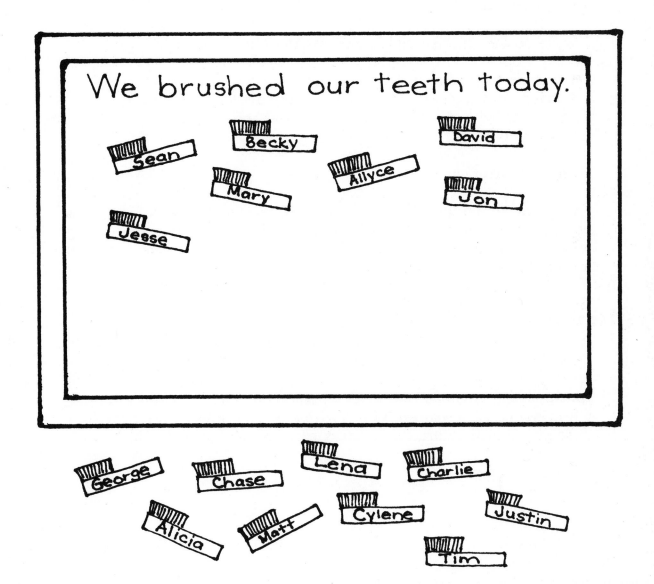

Parent Letter

Dear Parents,

This week we are continuing our study of community helpers with a unit on the dentist. The dentist is an important helper for us because our teeth are very important. Children are very aware of their teeth at this age. Many of the older five year olds will soon begin losing their baby teeth. Through the experiences provided in this unit the children may learn that the dentist is a person who helps us to keep our teeth healthy. They will also spend some time learning about the importance of tooth care.

At School This Week

Some of the experiences planned for the week include:

* making toothpaste.
* string painting with dental floss at the art table.
* painting with discarded toothbrushes at the easel.
* exploring tools that a dentist uses.

Special Visitor

On Tuesday, January 13, we will meet Mrs. Jones, the dental hygienist at Dr. Milivitz's dental clinic. Mrs. Jones will discuss proper toothbrushing and will pass out toothbrush kits. You are invited to join our class at 10:00 a.m. for her visit.

At Home

Good habits start young! Dental cavities are one of the most prevalent diseases among children. It has been estimated that 98 percent of school-aged children have at least one cavity. You and your child can spend some time each day brushing your teeth together. Sometimes a child will more effectively brush if someone else is with him. It is important for children to realize that they are the primary caretakers of their teeth!

Have a good week!

Music:

1. "Brushing Teeth"
(Sing to the tune of "Mulberry Bush")

This is the way we brush our teeth,
brush our teeth, brush our teeth.
This is the way we brush our teeth,
so early in the morning.

2. "Clean Teeth"
(Sing to the tune of "Row, Row, Row Your Boat")

Brush, brush, brush your teeth
Brush them everyday.
We put some toothpaste on our brush
To help stop tooth decay.

Fingerplays:

MY TOOTHBRUSH

I have a little toothbrush.
   (use pointer finger)
I hold it very tight.
   (make hand into fist)
I brush my teeth each morning,
and then again at night.
   (use pointer finger and pretend to brush)

MY FRIEND THE TOOTHBRUSH

My toothbrush is a tool.
I use it everyday.
I brush and brush and brush and brush
to keep the cavities away.
   (pretend to brush teeth)

Science:

1. Tools

Place some safe dental products on the sensory table. Include a mirror, dental floss, toothbrush, toothpaste, etc. A dentist may even lend you a model of a set of teeth.

2. Acid on Our Teeth

Show the children how acid weakens the enamel of your teeth. Place a hard-boiled egg into a bowl of vinegar for 24 hours. Observe how the egg shell becomes soft as it decalcifies. The same principle applies to our teeth if the acid is not removed by brushing. (This activity is only appropriate with older children.)

3. Making Toothpaste

In individual plastic bags, place 4 teaspoons of baking soda, 1 teaspoon salt and 1 teaspoon water. Add a drop of food flavoring extract such as peppermint, mint or orange. The children can mix their own toothpaste.

4. Sugar on Our Teeth

Sugar found in sweet food can cause cavities on tooth enamel if it is not removed by rinsing or brushing. To demonstrate the effect of brushing, submerge white eggshells, which are made of enamel, into a clear glass of cola for 24 hours. Observe the discoloration of the eggshell. Apply toothpaste to toothbrush. Brush the eggshell removing the stain. Ask the children, "What caused the stain?"

Arts and Crafts:

1. Easel Ideas

* paint with discarded toothbrushes
* paint on tooth-shaped easel paper

2. Toothbrushes and Splatter Screen

Provide construction paper, splatter screens and discarded toothbrushes. The children can splatter paint onto the paper using the toothbrush as a painting tool.

3. Dental Floss Painting

Provide thin tempera paint, paper and dental floss. The child can spoon a small amount of paint onto their paper and can hold on to one end of the dental floss while moving the free end through the paint to make a design.

Sensory:

Additions to the Sensory Table

* toothbrushes and water
* peppermint extract added to water

Large Muscle:

1. Drop the Toothbrush

Set a large plastic open mouth bottle on the floor. Encourage the children to try to drop the toothbrushes into the mouth of the bottle.

2. Sugar, Sugar, Toothbrush

Play like Duck, Duck, Goose. The toothbrush tries to catch the "sugar" before it gets around the circle to where the "toothbrush" was sitting. Game can continue until interest diminishes.

Field Trips/Resource People:

1. The Dentist

Visit the dentist's office. Observe the furnishings and equipment.

2. The Hygienist

Invite a dental hygienist to visit the classroom. Ask the hygienist to discuss

tooth care and demonstrate proper brushing techniques. After the discussion, provide each child with a disclosing tablet to check their brushing habits.

Group Time (games, language):

Pass the Toothpaste

Play music and pass a tube of toothpaste around the circle. When the music stops, the person who is holding the toothpaste stands up and claps their hands three times (or some similar action). Repeat the game.

Cooking:

1. Happy Teeth Snacks

* apple wedges
* orange slices
* asparagus
* cheese chunks
* milk
* cucumber slices
* cauliflower pieces

2. Smiling Apples

apples, cored and sliced
peanut butter
mini-marshmallows, raisins or peanuts

Spread peanut butter on one side of each apple slice. Place 3 to 4 mini-marshmallows, raisins or peanuts on the peanut butter of one apple slice. Top with another apple slice, peanut butter side down.

Records:

The following records can be found in preschool educational catalogs:

1. **Let's Go to the Dentist.** Captain Kangaroo. Columbia Records.

2. **Health and Safety.** "Brush Away." Hap Palmer.

3. **Singable Songs for the Very Young.** "Brush Your Teeth" Raffi. Kimbo Educational.

Books and Stories:

The following books and stories can be used to complement the theme:

1. **My Dentist.** Harlow Rockwell. (New York: Greenwillow Books, 1975).

2. **Our Tooth Story—A Tale of Twenty Teeth.** E. and Leonard Kessler. (New York: Dodd, Mead and Company, 1972).

3. **Albert's Toothache.** Barbara Williams. (New York: E.P. Dutton, 1974).

4. **Alligator's Toothache.** Diane deGroat. (New York: Crown Publishers, 1977).

5. **Teeth.** Michael Ricketts. (London: MacDonald and Company, 1971).

6. **How Many Teeth.** Paul Showers. (New York: Thomas Y. Crowell Company, 1962).

7. **I Want to Be a Dentist.** Carla Greene. (Chicago: Childrens Press, 1960).

8. **Bugs Bunny Goes to the Dentist.** Seymour Reit. (New York: Western Publishing Company, 1978).

9. **A Visit to the Dentist.** Bernard Garn. (New York: Grosset and Dunlap, 1960).

10. **Michael and the Dentist.** Bernard Wolf. (New York: Four Winds Press, 1980).

11. **Tom Visits the Dentist.** Nigel Snell. (London: H. Hamilton Publishers, 1979).

12. **The Tooth Book.** Theo LeSeig. (New York: Beginner Books, 1981).

Puzzles:

The following puzzles can be found in preschool educational catalogs:

1. **"Dentist"** Judy/Instructo. White.

2. **"Dentist"** Judy/Instructo. Black.

3. **"Brushing Teeth"** A See-Quees sequence puzzle.

17 DOCTORS AND NURSES

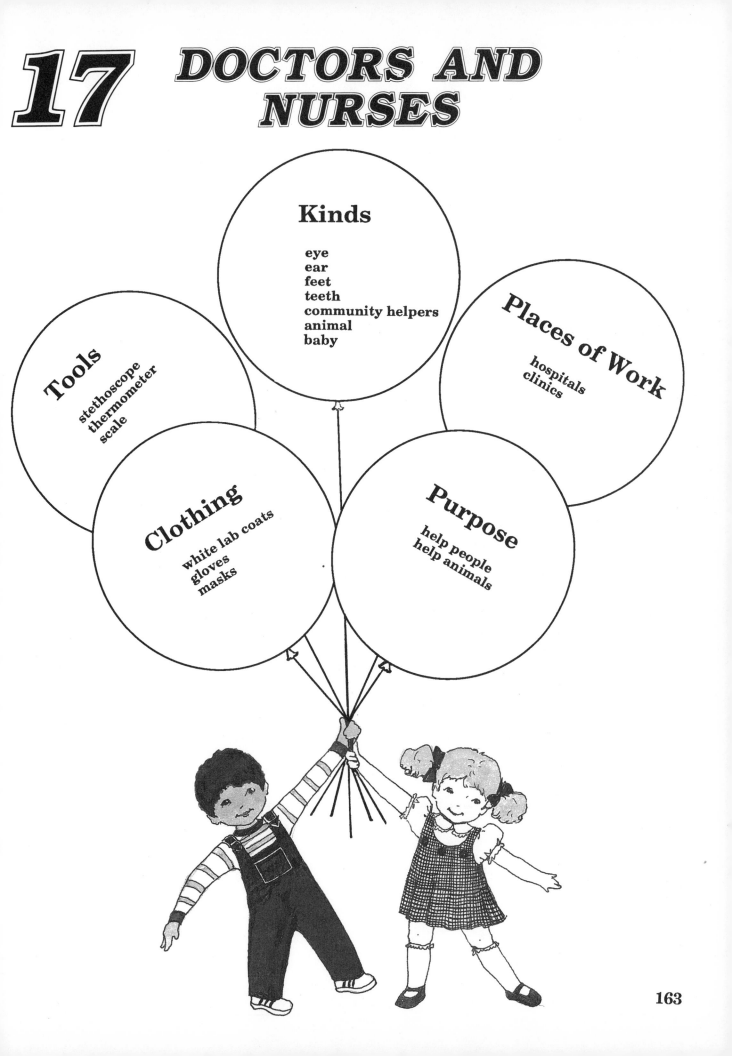

Kinds

eye
ear
feet
teeth
community helpers
animal
baby

Places of Work

hospitals
clinics

Tools

stethoscope
thermometer
scale

Clothing

white lab coats
gloves
masks

Purpose

help people
help animals

Theme Goals:

Through participating in the experiences provided in this theme, the children may learn:

1. Kinds of doctors and nurses.

2. Places doctors and nurses work.

3. Tools used by doctors and nurses.

4. Clothing worn by doctors and nurses.

5. How doctors and nurses help people.

Concepts for the Children to Learn:

1. Doctors and nurses are community helpers.

2. Doctors and nurses help to keep people and animals healthy.

3. Doctors and nurses work in hospitals and clinics.

4. Lab coats, gloves and masks are clothing doctors and nurses may wear.

5. Special doctors and nurses care for our eyes, ears, feet and teeth.

6. A stethoscope is a tool used to check heartbeats and breathing.

7. Thermometers are used to check body temperature.

Vocabulary:

1. **doctor**—a person who helps keep our bodies healthy.

2. **nurse**—assists the doctor.

3. **stethoscope**—a tool used for checking heartbeat and breathing.

4. **thermometer**—tool for checking body temperature.

5. **patient**—a person who goes to see a doctor.

6. **pediatrician**—a children's doctor.

7. **veterinarian**—an animal doctor.

8. **ophthalmologist**—eye doctor.

Bulletin Board

The purpose of this bulletin board is to develop skills in identifying written numerals and matching sets to numerals. Construct bandages out of manilla tagboard as illustrated. Laminate. Collect small boxes and cover with white paper if necessary. The number will be dependent upon the developmental age of children. Plastic bandage boxes or 16-count crayon boxes may be used. On each box place a numeral. Affix the box to a bulletin board by stapling. The children can place the proper number of bandages in each box.

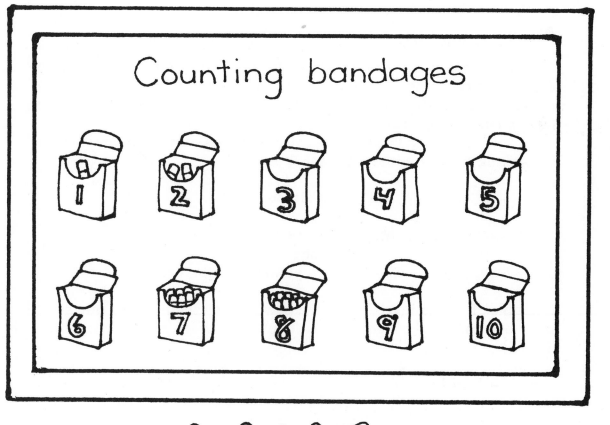

Parent Letter

Dear Parents,

I hope everyone in your family is happy and healthy this week! Speaking of healthy, we are starting a unit on doctors and nurses this week. The children will be learning about the different types of doctors and nurses and how they help people. They also will be introduced to some of the tools used by doctors and nurses.

At School This Week

A few of the learning experiences planned for the week include:

* listening to the story *Tommy Goes to the Doctor*.
* taking our temperatures with forehead strips and recording them on a chart in the science area.
* dressing up as doctors and nurses in the dramatic play area.
* experimenting with syringes (no needles!) and water in the sensory table.

At Home

There are many ways to integrate this unit into your home. To begin, discuss the role of your family doctor. Talk about your child's visit to a physician. This will help to alleviate anxiety and fears your child may have about the procedures and setting.

Let your child help you prepare this nutritious snack at home. We will be making it for Wednesday's snack as well.

Peanut Butter Balls

1/2 cup peanut butter
1/2 cup honey
3/4 to 1 cup powdered milk

Combine all of the ingredients in a bowl. Shape the mixture into small balls and roll in chopped nuts, coconut or graham cracker crumbs, if desired.

Have a healthy week!

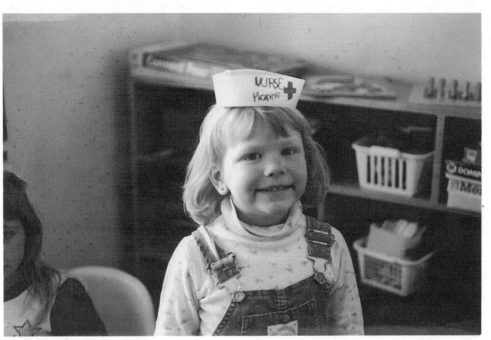

FIGURE 17 Being a nurse is an important profession in our society.

Music:

1. The Doctor in the Clinic
(Sing to the tune of "Farmer in the Dell")

The Doctor in the clinic.
The doctor in the clinic.
Hi-ho the derry-o,
The doctor in the clinic.

The doctor takes a nurse...
The nurse takes a patient...
The patient gets help...
The patient gets better...

2. "To The Hospital"
(Sing to the tune: "Frere Jacques")

To the hospital, to the hospital,
We will go, we will go.
We will see the doctors,
And we'll see the nurses,
Dressed in white, dressed in white.

Fingerplays:

MISS POLLY'S DOLLY

Miss Polly had a dolly that was sick, sick, sick
   (cradle arms and look sad)

She called for the doctor to come quick,
quick, quick.
   (clap hands three times)
The doctor came with his coat and his hat.
   (point to your shirt and head)
And rapped on the door with a rap, rap, rap.
   (pretend to knock three times)
He looked at the dolly and he shook his head
   (shake head)
And he said, "Miss Polly, put her straight
to bed."
   (shake finger)
Then he wrote on a paper for some pills,
pills, pills.
   (hold left hand out flat, pretend to write
   with right hand)
I'll be back in the morning with my bill,
bill, bill.
   (hold left hand out flat, wave it up and
   down as if waiting to be handed cash)

Note: The doctor may be male or female.
Substitute pronouns.

DOCTOR DAY

My father said,
"It's doctor day,"
Then he and I
We're on our way
To see our friend

167

The doctor who
Would check me out
As doctors do.
She had more things
Than I can tell
To help her keep
The people well.
She checked me up
And all the while
She wore a big
And friendly smile.
So now I hope
That someday you
May go to see
The doctor too!

Source: *Everyday Circle Times*. Liz and
Dick Wilmes. (Building Blocks Publishing:
Illinois, 1983).

Science:

1. Thermometer

Place a variety of unbreakable thermometers on the science table. Include a candy, meat and an outdoor thermometer. Also include a strip thermometer that can be safety used on children's foreheads.

2. Casts

Ask personnel at a local hospital to save clean, discarded casts. Place the casts on the science table, allowing the children to observe the materials, try them on for size as well as feel their weight.

3. Stethoscope

Place a stethoscope on the science table for the children to experiment with. After each child uses it, wipe the ear plugs with alcohol to prevent the transmission of disease.

4. Doctors' Tools

In a feely box place several tools that a doctor uses. Include a thermometer, gauze, stethoscope, rubber hammer, and a tongue depressor.

5. Making Toothpaste

Mix four teaspoons baking soda, one teaspoon salt, and one teaspoon peppermint flavoring. Then add just enough water to form a thick paste.

Dramatic Play:

1. Doctors and Nurses

Make a prop box for a doctor and nurse. Include a white coat, plastic gloves, a thermometer, gauze, tape, masks, eye droppers, tweezers, tongue depressors, eye chart, cots, blankets, pencil and paper, empty and washed medicine bottles, a stethoscope, a scale and syringes without needles. A first-aid kit including gauze and tape, bandages, butterflies, a sling, and ace bandages can be placed in this box. Place the prop boxes in the dramatic play area.

2. Animal Clinic

Place stuffed animals with the doctor tools in the dramatic play area.

3. Eye Doctor Clinic

Ask a local eye doctor for discontinued eye glass frames. Place the frames with a wall chart in the dramatic play area.

Arts and Crafts:

1. Cotton Swab Painting

Place cotton swabs, cottonballs and tempera paint on a table in the art area. The cotton swabs and balls can be used as painting tools.

2. Body Tracing

Trace the children's bodies by having them lie down on a large piece of paper. The body shape can be decorated at school by the child with crayons and felt-tip markers. The shapes could also be taken home and decorated with parental assistance.

3. Eye Dropper Painting

Provide eye droppers, thin tempera paint and absorbent paper. Designs can be made by using the eye dropper as a painting tool. Another method is to prepare water colored with food coloring in muffin tins. Using heavy paper towels with construction paper underneath for protection, the children will enjoy creating designs with the colored water.

Field Trips/Resource People:

1. Doctor's Office

Visit a doctor's office.

2. Classroom Visitor

Invite a nurse or doctor to visit the classroom. Encourage them to talk briefly about their jobs. They can also share some of their tools with the children.

3. The Hospital

Visit a local hospital.

Math:

1. Weight and Height Chart

Prepare a height and weight chart out of tagboard. Record each child's height and weight on this chart. Repeat periodically throughout the year to note bodily changes.

2. Tongue Depressor Dominoes

Make a set of dominoes by writing on tongue depressors. Divide each tongue depressor in half with a felt-tip marker. On each half place a different number of dots. Consider the children's developmental level in determining the number of dots to be included. Demonstrate to interested children how to play dominoes.

3. Bandage Lotto

Construct a bandage lotto game using various sizes and shapes of bandages. Place it on a table for use during self-selected activity time.

Social Studies:

Pictures

Display various health-related pictures in the room at the children's eye level, including doctors and nurses.

Group Time (games, language):

1. Doctor, Doctor, Nurse

Play Duck, Duck, Goose inserting the words Doctor, Doctor, Nurse.

2. What's Missing?

Place a variety of doctors' and nurses' tools on a large tray. Tell the children to close their eyes. Remove one item from the tray. Then have the children open their eyes and guess which item has been removed. Continue playing the game using all of the items as well as providing an opportunity for each child.

Cooking:

1. Mighty Mixture

Mix any of the following:
A variety of dried fruit (apples, apricots, pineapple, raisins)
A variety of seeds (pumpkin, sunflower)
A variety of nuts (almond, walnuts, pecans)

2. Vegetable Juice

Prepare individual servings of vegetable juice in a blender by adding 1/2 cup of cut up vegetables and 1/4 cup water. Salt to taste. Vegetables that can be used include: celery, carrots, beets, tomatoes, cucumbers, and zucchini.

Books and Stories:

The following books and stories can be used to complement the theme:

1. **Your Friend the Doctor.** The Staff of American Medical Association. (Chicago: Reilly and Lee Books, 1969.)

2. **My Doctor.** Harlow Rockwell. (New York: Macmillan Publishing Co., 1973.)

3. **Too Many Lollipops.** Robert Quakenbush. (New York: Parents Press Magazine, 1975.)

4. **Tommy Goes to the Doctor.** Gunilla Wolde. (Boston: Houghton Mifflin Company, 1979.)

5. **What It's Like to Be a Doctor.** Arthur Shay. (Chicago: Reilly and Lee Books, 1971.)

6. **Curious George Goes to the Hospital.** H.A. Rey. (Boston: Houghton Mifflin Company, 1966.)

7. **Doctor Rabbit.** Jan Wahl. (New York: Delacorte Press, 1970.)

8. **Jenny's in the Hospital.** Seymour Reit. (Racine, WI: Western Publishing Company, Inc., 1984.)

9. **My Daddy is a Nurse.** Mark Wandro. (Reading, MA: Addison-Wesley, 1981.)

10. **Going to the Doctor.** Fred Rogers. (New York: G.P. Putnam's Sons, 1986.)

11. **I Can Be an Animal Doctor.** Kathryn Wentzel Lumley. (Chicago: Childrens Press, 1985).

Puzzles:

The following puzzles can be found in preschool educational catalogs:

1. "**Female Nurse**" 11 pieces. Judy/Instructo.

2. "**Female Doctor**" 16 pieces. Judy/Instructo.

3. "**Male Nurse**" 14 pieces. Judy/Instructo.

4. "**Male Doctor**" 11 pieces. Judy/Instructo.

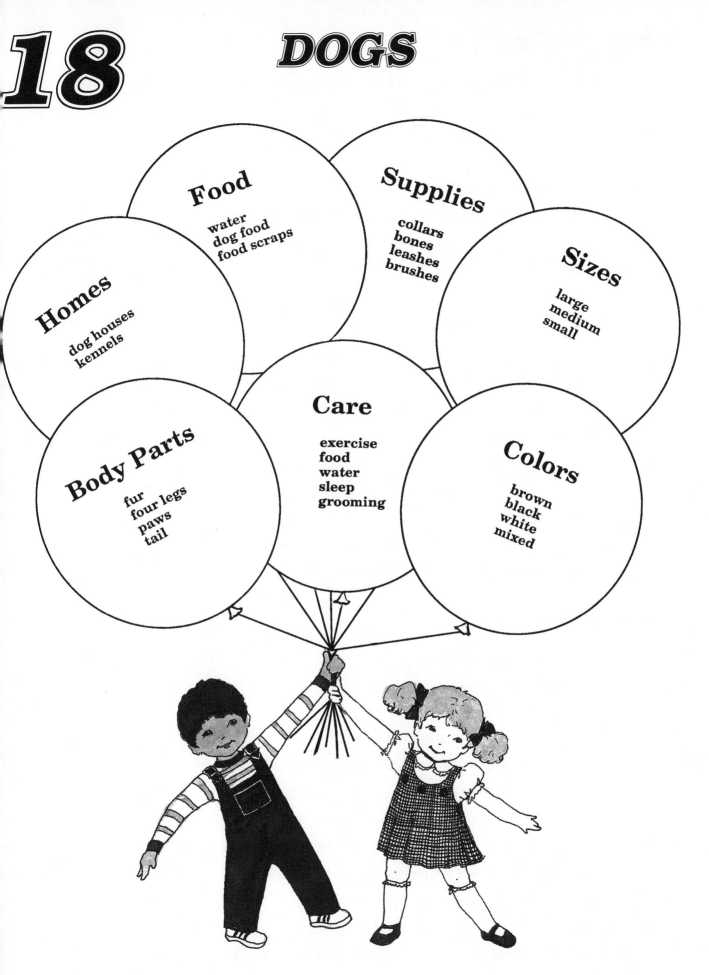

18 DOGS

Food
water
dog food
food scraps

Supplies
collars
bones
leashes
brushes

Sizes
large
medium
small

Homes
dog houses
kennels

Care
exercise
food
water
sleep
grooming

Colors
brown
black
white
mixed

Body Parts
fur
four legs
paws
tail

Theme Goals:

Through participating in the experiences provided by this theme, the children may learn:

1. Dog's body parts.

2. Types of dogs.

3. Dogs need special care.

4. Dogs can be trained to do special tasks and tricks.

Concepts for the Children to Learn:

1. There are many different sizes of dogs.

2. Dogs have a keen sense of smell and hearing.

3. Dogs growl and bark to communicate.

4. Dogs may bark at strangers to protect their owners and their space.

5. Dogs have legs, eyes, ears, a mouth, nose and tail.

6. Dogs have fur on their skin.

7. Dogs enjoy being handled carefully and gently.

8. Some dogs help people.

9. There are many different colors, sizes and kinds of dogs.

10. Dogs need food, water and exercise every day.

11. Dogs can be taught to do tricks.

Vocabulary:

1. **puppy**—a baby dog.

2. **pet**—an animal kept for pleasure.

3. **paw**—the dog's foot.

4. **veterinarian**—an animal doctor.

5. **guide dog**—a dog trained to help blind people.

6. **leash**—a rope, chain or cord that attaches to a collar.

7. **collar**—a band worn around the dog's neck.

8. **obediance school**—a school where dogs are taught to obey.

9. **whiskers**—stiff hair growing around the dog's nose, mouth and eyes.

10. **bone**—an object a dog uses to chew on.

11. **coat**—hair or fur covering the skin.

12. **doghouse**—a place for dogs to sleep and keep warm.

Bulletin Board

The purpose of this bulletin board is to develop color recognition and matching skills. Prepare the bulletin board by cutting dog shapes out of tagboard or construction paper. Use rubber cement to attach a different colored paper collar to each dog's neck. Also cut out dog dishes from colored construction paper. Attach the pieces to the bulletin board as illustrated. Use lengths of yarn or string for children to match the color of each dog's collar to the corresponding dog dish.

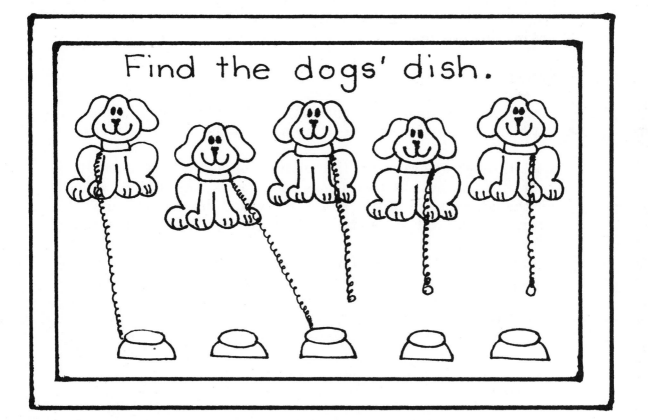

Parent Letter

Dear Parents,

This week at school we will be starting a unit on a favorite subject of children of all ages—dogs! We will be learning about their basic physical features such as coat and body. We will also learn about caring for a dog, the roles of dogs in people's lives, dog training, as well as things families need to consider when choosing a dog. This unit is designed so that the children will develop an awareness of and respect dogs as pets.

At School This Week

Some of the learning experiences planned for the week include:

* creating paw prints at the art table (dipping paw-shaped sponges into paint and applying it to paper).
* sorting various sized dog biscuits.
* listening to the children's stories about their own dogs.
* setting up a "pet store" in the dramatic play area, complete with stuffed animals and many dog accessories.
* baking dog biscuits!

At Home

To foster parent-child interaction and reinforce at home some of the concepts we are working on at school, try some of the following ideas:

* Look through magazines to find pictures of dogs and puppies. Help your child tear out pictures of dogs and puppies. This activity is good for the development of fine motor and visual discrimination skills. An interesting collage can be made by gluing these pictures onto a piece of paper.
* If you don't have access to a dog, visit a pet shop to observe the puppies. At the same time note all of the dog supplies available.

Have a good week!!

Music:

1. "Bingo"

There was a farmer had a dog
And Bingo was his name-o.
B-I-N-G-O
B-I-N-G-O
B-I-N-G-O
And Bingo was his name-o.

2. "Six Little Dogs"
(Sing to the tune of "Six Little Ducks")

Six little dogs that I once knew,
fat ones, skinny ones, fair ones too.
But the one little dog with the brown
curly fur,
He led the others with a grr, grr, grr.
Grr, grr, grr
Grr, grr, grr
He led the others with a grr, grr, GRR!

Fingerplays:

FRISKY'S DOGHOUSE

This is Frisky's doghouse;
   (pointer fingers touch to make a roof)
This is Frisky's bed;
   (motion of smoothing)
Here is Frisky's pan of milk;
   (cup hands)
So that he can be fed.

Frisky has a collar
   (point to neck with fingers)
With his name upon it, too;
Take a stick and throw it,
   (notion of throwing)
He'll bring it back to you.
   (clap once)

FIVE LITTLE PUPPIES

Five little puppies were playing in the
sun.
   (hold up hands, fingers extended)

This one saw a rabbit, and he began to run.
   (bend down first finger)
This one saw a butterfly, and he began to race.
   (bend down second finger)
This one saw a pussy cat, and he began to chase.
   (bend down third finger)
This one tried to catch his tail, and he went round and round.
   (bend down fourth finger)
This one was so quiet, he never made a sound.
   (bend down thumb.)

FIVE LITTLE PUPPIES

Five little puppies jumping on the bed,
   (hold up five fingers)
One fell off and bumped his head,
   (hold up one finger—tap head)
Mama called the doctor and the doctor said,
"No more puppies jumping on the bed."
   (shake index finger)

Science:

1. Additions to the science table or area may include:

   * a magnifying glass with bones, dog hair, and dog food.
   * dog tags of different sizes, including some with squeakers.
   * a balance scale and dry dog food.

2. During a cooking activity, prepare dog biscuits. The recipe is listed under cooking.

Dramatic Play:

1. Pet Store

Using stuffed animals simulate a pet store. Include a counter complete with cash register and money. Post a large sign that says "Pet Store." Set out many stuffed dogs with collars and leashes. Children will enjoy pretending they have a new pet.

175

2. Veterinarian's Office

Use some medical equipment and stuffed dogs to create a veterinarian's office.

3. Pet Show

Encourage the children to bring a stuffed animal to school. Children can pretend that their stuffed animals can do tricks. Have ribbons available for them to look at and award to each other.

4. Dog House

Construct a dog house from a large cardboard box. Provide dog ears and tails for the children to wear as they imitate the pet.

Arts and Crafts:

1. Paw Prints

Make stamps out of erasers, sponges or with the child's fist.

2. Dog Puppets

Provide socks, paper bags, and/or paper plates to make dog puppets.

3. Dog Masks

Use fake fur ears and pipe cleaners for whiskers.

4. Bone Printing

Provide different meat bones, a tray of tempera paint and paper to make prints.

5. Bone Painting

Cut easel paper in bone shapes.

6. Dog Collages

Provide dog pictures cut out of magazines to make a collage.

Large Muscle:

1. Encourage the children to dramatize the following movements:

* a big dog
* a tiny dog
* a dog with heavy steps
* a dog with light steps
* a happy dog
* a sad dog
* a mad dog
* a loud dog
* a quiet dog
* a hungry dog
* a tired dog
* a curious dog
* a sick dog

2. Dog Hoops

Provide hoops for the children to jump through as they imitate dogs.

3. Scent Walk

Place prints of dog paws on the play yard leading to different activities. Encourage the child to crawl to each activity.

4. Tracks

If snow is available, make tracks with boots that have different treads. Encourage children to follow one track.

5. Bean Bag Bones

Provide round bean bags or make special bone-shaped bean bags. Encourage the children to throw them into a large dog food bowl.

Field Trips/Resource People:

1. Pet Store

Take a field trip to a pet store. While there ask the manager how to care for dogs. Observe the different types of cages, collars, leashes, food, and toys.

2. Veterinarian Office

Take a field trip to a veterinarian's office or animal hospital. Compare its similarities and differences to a doctor's office.

3. Kennel

Visit a kennel and observe the different sizes of cages and dogs.

4. Variety Store

Visit a variety store and observe pet accessories.

5. Grocery Store

Take a field trip to the grocery store and purchase the ingredients needed to make dog biscuits.

6. Dog Trainer

Invite an obedience trainer to talk about teaching dogs.

7. Additional Resource People

* veterinarian
* pet store owner
* parents (bring in family dogs)
* humane society representative
* representatiove from a kennel
* dog groomer
* person with a seeing eye dog (guide dog)

Math:

1. Dog Bones

Cut dog bone shapes of four different sizes from tagboard. Encourage the children to sequence them.

2. Classifying Dog Biscuits

Purchase three sizes of dog biscuits. Using dog dishes, have the children sort them according to size and type.

3. Weighing Biscuits

Using the scale, encourage the children to weigh different sizes and amounts of dog biscuits.

Social Studies:

1. Share Your Dog

Individually invite the parents to bring their child's pet to school.

2. Pictures of Dogs

Display pictures of different types of dogs.

3. Bulletin Board

Prepare a bulletin board with pictures of the children's dogs.

4. Slides

Take slides of field trips and of resource people. Share them at group time. (This slide series may be shared with parents at meetings or coffees.)

5. Dog Biscuits

Prepare dog biscuits and donate to the local animal shelter. (See Cooking.)

6. Chart

Make a chart including the children's name, type of pet, size of pet and the name of the pet. Count the number of dogs, cats, birds, etc. Discuss the most popular names.

7. Dogs

Using pictures or a real dog, talk about a dog's body. Some dogs have long noses so they can smell things very well; others have short hair to live in hot climates. Discuss why some dogs are good guard dogs. Discuss how dogs' tongues help them to cool off on hot days. Also talk about what else a dog's rough tongue is used for.

Group Time (games, language):

1. The Dog Catcher

Hide stuffed dogs or those cut from construction paper around the classsroom and have children find them.

2. Child-created Stories

Bring in a picture of a dog or stuffed dog. Encourage the children to tell you a story about the picture or the stuffed dog. While the child speaks, record the words. Place the story in the book corner.

3. Dog Chart

Make a chart listing the color of each child's dog. A variation would be to have the children state their favorite color of dog. This activity can be repeated using size.

4. Doggie, Doggie, Where's Your Bone?

Bring in a clean bone or a bone cut from construction paper. Sit the children in a circle. Choose one child to be the dog. Have the child pretending to be the dog sit in the middle. The doggie closes his eyes. A child from the circle sneaks up and takes the bone. Children call, "Doggie, Doggie, Where's Your Bone? Someone stole it from your home!" The "dog" gets three guesses to find out who has the bone.

5. The Lost Dog

(This is a variation of the "Dog Catcher" game.) Using the children's stuffed animals from home, have the children trade dogs so that each is holding another's pet. One child begins by hiding the dog he is holding while the other children cover their eyes. He tells the owner, "Your dog is lost, but we can help you find it." As the dog owner looks, he can put the pet he is holding on his carpet square to free both hands. The group gives "hot" and "cold" clues to indicate whether the child is close to or far away from the pet. When the child finds his pet, he is the next one to hide a pet.

Cooking:

1. Hot "Dog" Kebabs on a Stick

paper plates and napkins
skewers
1 package hot dogs

2 green peppers, cut up
cherry tomatoes

Place 2 pieces of green pepper, 2 cherry tomatoes, and 2 hotdog pieces on each child's plate. Show the children how to thread the ingredients on skewers. Bake the kabobs in a preheated oven for 15 minutes at 350 degrees.

2. Dog Biscuits

2 1/2 cups whole wheat flour
1/2 cup powdered dry milk
1/2 teaspoon salt
1/2 teaspoon garlic powder
6 tablespoons margarine, shortening, or
   meat drippings
1 egg
1 teaspoon brown sugar
1/2 cup ice water

Combine flour, milk, salt and flour. Cut in the shortening. Mix in egg. Add enough water until mixture forms a ball. Pat the dough to a half inch thickness on a lightly oiled cookie sheet. Cut with cutters and remove scraps. Bake 25 to 30 minutes at 350 degrees. This recipe may be varied by adding pureed soup greens, liver powder, etc.

3. Dogs-in-a-Blanket

cheese crust
   1/2 teaspoon salt
   pinch baking powder
   1 cup white flour
   1/4 cup shortening
   1/4 cup water
   1/4 cup finely shredded cheddar cheese
hot dogs

Stir the dry ingredients in a large bowl. Cut in shortening and then add 1/4 cup water. Stir with a fork and add more water only if necessary to work in flour. Add cheese and knead together. Cut the cheese pie crust in strips and wrap each around a whole or half of a hotdog. Bake at 350 degrees until crust is light brown.

Source: *Super Snacks*. Jean Warren. (Alderwood Manor, WA: Warren Publishing House, 1982).

4. Hush Puppies

vegetable oil
2 1/4 cups yellow cornmeal
1 teaspoon salt
2 tablespoons finely chopped onion

3/4 teaspoon baking soda
1 1/2 cups buttermilk

Heat oil (about 1 inch deep) to 375 degrees. Mix cornmeal, salt, onion and baking soda in a bowl. Add buttermilk. Drop by spoonfuls into hot oil. Fry until brown about 2 minutes.

Records:

The following records can be found in preschool educational catalogs:

1. **Children's Stories and Songs.** "I Had a Little Dog." Performed by Ed Mc Curdy.

2. **Children's Creative Play Songs,** Vol. 5. "Animals." Art Barduhn.

3. **The Small Singer** Vol. 2. "Kitty and Puppy." Roberta Mc Laughlin and Lucille Wood.

4. **Walk Like the Animals.** "Puppy Dog." Georgiana Liccione Stewart.

5. "Doggie In the Window," (Happy Time and Golden, 33 1/3 RPM; Golden, 45 RPM).

Books and Stories:

The following books and stories can be used to complement the theme:

1. **The Digging-est Dog.** Al Perkins. (New York: Random House, Inc., 1967).

2. **Harry the Dirty Dog.** Gene Zion. (New York: Harper and Row Publishers, 1956).

3. **The Very Little Dog.** Grace Skaar. (New York: Young Scott Books, 1949).

4. **The Pokey Little Puppy.** Janette Sebring Lowrey. (Racine, WI: Western Publishing Company, Inc., 1942).

5. **All About Dogs.** Grace Skaar. (New York: Young Scott Books, 1947).

6. **How Puppies Grow.** Millicent E. Salsam. (New York: Four Winds Press, 1971).

7. **The Blue Ribbon Puppies.** Crockett Johnson. (New York: Harper and Row Publishers, 1958).

8. **The Noisy Book.** Margaret Wise Brown. (New York: Harper and Row Publishers, 1939).

9. **Four Puppies.** Anne Heathers. (Racine, WI: Western Publishing Company, Inc., 1960).

10. **The Dog That Lost His Family.** Jean Lee Latham and Bee Lewi. (New York: Macmillan Company, 1961).

11. **Whistle for Willie.** Ezra Jack Keats. (New York: Viking Press, 1969).

12. **I Am a Puppy.** Ole Risom. (New York: Western Publishers, 1970).

13. **The Puppy Who Wanted a Boy.** Jane Thayer. (New York: William Morrow, 1958).

14. **Puppies.** Judith E. Rinard. (Washington, D.C.: National Geographic Society, 1982).

15. **Shaggy Dogs and Spotty Dogs, and Shaggy and Spotty Dogs.** Seymour Leichman. (New York: Harcourt, Brace, Jovanovich, 1973).

16. **Animal Doctors. What Do They Do?** Carla Greene. (New York: Harper and Row Publishers, 1967).

Puzzles:

The following puzzles are listed in preschool educational catalogs.

1. **"Dog"** 9 pieces. Judy/Instructo.

2. **"Children's Pets"** 5 pieces. Child Craft.

3. **"Little Pet Puzzles"** 5 pieces. Child Craft.

4. **"Left-Right, Inside-Outside Dogs"** 5 pieces. Child Craft.

5. **"Dog"** 9 pieces. Rolf Puzzles.

19 EASTER

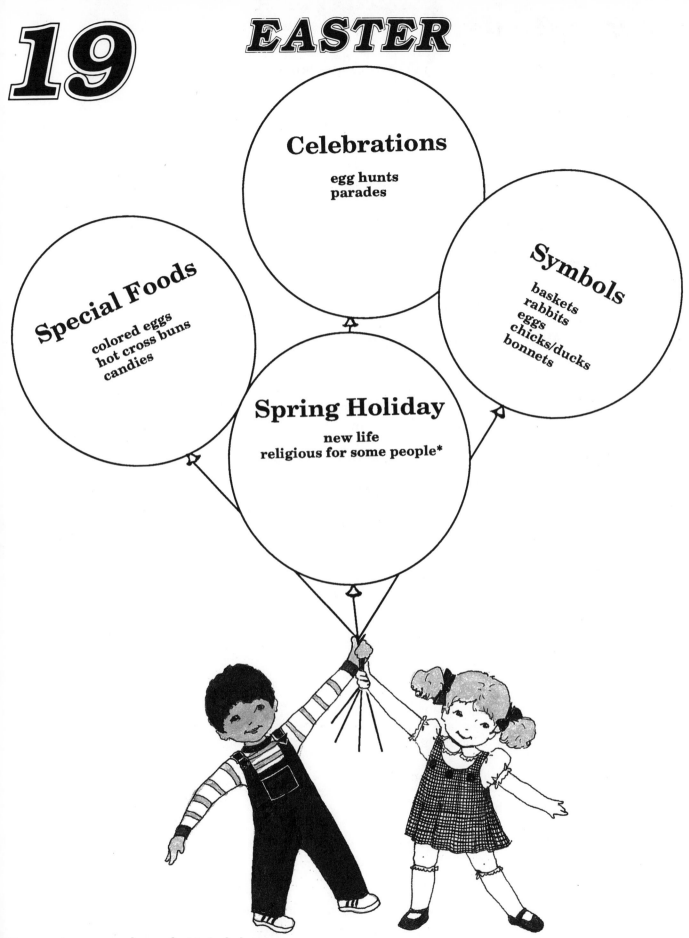

Celebrations
egg hunts
parades

Symbols
baskets
rabbits
eggs
chicks/ducks
bonnets

Special Foods
colored eggs
hot cross buns
candies

Spring Holiday
new life
religious for some people*

*Some center personnel may elect to include an
Easter theme with an emphasis on the celebration
opposed to the traditional religious emphasis.

Theme Goals:

Through participating in the experiences provided by this theme, the children may learn:

1. Easter traditions.

2. Easter symbols.

3. Boiled eggs can be dyed and decorated for Easter.

4. Care of rabbits.

Concepts for the Children to Learn:

1. Easter is a holiday.

2. Many families celebrate Easter.

3. At Easter eggs are decorated.

4. There are many symbols of Easter including baby animals, baskets, rabbits, eggs and new clothing.

5. Baskets filled with eggs and candy may be hidden.

6. Baby animals born in the Spring are a sign of new life.

7. Bonnets (hats) may be worn at Easter time.

Vocabulary:

1. **Easter**—a holiday in Spring.

2. **basket**—a woven container.

3. **hatch**—to break out of a shell.

4. **dye**—to change the color.

5. **duckling**—a baby duck.

6. **chick**—a baby chicken.

7. **lamb**—a baby sheep.

8. **bunny**—a baby rabbit.

9. **holiday**—a day of celebration.

10. **Spring**—the season of the year when plants begin to grow.

11. **bonnet**—a kind of hat.

Bulletin Board

The purpose of this bulletin board is to promote correspondence of sets to the written numeral. Construct baskets out of stiff tagboard. Write a numeral beginning with the number one on each basket as illustrated. Carefully, attach these to the bulletin board stapling all the way around the round bottom of the baskets. Construct many small Easter eggs. Encourage the children to deposit the corresponding amount of Easter eggs in the numbered baskets. Care needs to be taken when removing the eggs. The number of baskets should reflect the developmental level of the children. If available, you might want to try using lightweight Easter baskets. They are harder to hang up, but may prove to be more sturdy.

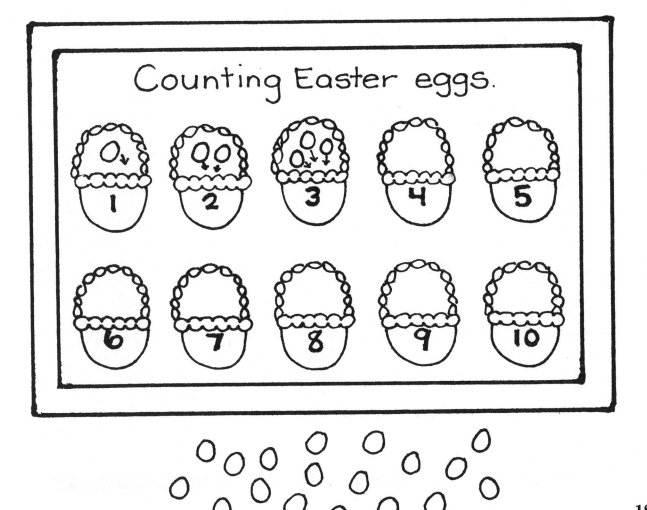

Parent Letter

Dear Parents,

"Here comes Peter Cottontail, hopping down the bunny trail..." Easter is on its way and it is also the theme we will explore this week. This is an exciting holiday for children. Through learning experiences planned for the unit, the children will find out about ways that families celebrate Easter and symbols that represent Easter. Included will be the Easter bunny and Easter baskets and foods that are associated with Easter.

At School This Week

Learning experiences planned to reinforce concepts of Easter include:

* a special visitor for the week— a rabbit! The children will assist in taking care of the rabbit.
* a hat shop in the dramatic play area with materials to create Easter bonnets.
* Easter grass and plastic eggs in the sensory table.
* an egg hunt! On Friday, we will search our play yard for hidden eggs and place them in our baskets.

At Home

To establish a sense of family history, recall family Easter celebrations that you have had in the past with your child. What special things does your family do together on this holiday? And, of course, dye some Easter eggs!

Be adventurous and try some dyes from natural materials. Natural dying is not new; natural dyes were the original Easter egg colors the world over. To make purple eggs purchase a box of frozen blackberries. Thaw and place in a saucepan. Add eggs and cover with water plus 1 tablespoon of vinegar. Bring the water to a boil and simmer for 20 minutes. Afterward, take the pan off the heat source and let stand for approximately 20 minutes.

To make gold eggs use powdered tumeric. Place eggs in a saucepan and add enough water to cover. Then add 3 tablespoons of tumeric and bring to a boil. Simmer for 20 minutes. Remove from heat source and cool.

To create pale green eggs, cut spinach and place in the bottom of a pan. Add enough water to cover and add eggs. Bring to a boil and simmer for 20 minutes. Remove from heat and allow to set for more intense color.

From all of us,

Music:

1. "Did You Ever See a Rabbit?"
(Sing to the tune of "Did You Ever See a Lassie?")

Did you ever see a rabbit, a rabbit, a rabbit?
Did you ever see a rabbit, a rabbit on
Easter morn?
He hops around so quietly
And hides all the eggs.
Did you ever see a rabbit, on Easter morn?

2. "Easter Bunny"
(Sing to the tune of "Ten Little Indians")

Where, oh, where is the Easter Bunny,
Where, oh, where is the Easter Bunny,
Where, oh, where is the Easter Bunny,
Early Easter morning?

Find all the eggs and put them in a basket,
Find all the eggs and put them in a basket,
Find all the eggs and put them in a basket,
Early Easter morning.

3. "Easter Eggs"
(Sing to the chorus of "Jingle Bells")

Easter eggs, Easter eggs,
Hidden all around.
Come my children look about
And see where they are found.

Easter eggs, Easter eggs
They're a sight to see.
One for Tom and one for Ann
And a special one for me!

Insert names of children in your classroom.

4. "Easter Eggs"
(Sing to the tune of "Mama's Little Baby Loves Shortnin'")

Easter eggs here and there,
Easter eggs everywhere
What's the color of the
Easter egg here?

Fingerplays:

FIVE LITTLE EASTER EGGS

Five little Easter eggs lovely colors
wore;

Mother ate the blue one and then there
were four.
Four little Easter eggs, two and two, you see;
Daddy ate the red one, and then there
were three.
Three little Easter eggs; before I knew
Sister ate the yellow one, then there were two.
Two little Easter eggs; oh what fun.
Brother ate the purple one, then there was
one.
One little Easter egg; see me run!
I ate the very last one, and then there
were none!

This could be a fingerplay or could be done
with colored finger puppet eggs with the
children holding a particular color going
down when that color is named.

Source: *Fingerplays that Motivate.* Don Peek.
(T.S. Denison and Company: Minneapolis,
1975).

KITTY AND BUNNY

Here is a kitty.
  (make a fist with one hand)
Here is a bunny.
  (hold up other hand with pointer and
  middle fingers up straight)
See his tall ears so pink and funny?
  (wiggle the two extended fingers)
Kitty comes by and licks his face;
  (extend thumb and wiggle near the bunny)
And around and around the garden they race.
  (make circular motions with hands)
And then without a single peep,
They both lie down and go to sleep.
  (fold hands)

Source: *Fingerplays that Motivate.* Don Peek.
(T.S. Denison and Company: Minneapolis,
1975).

EASTER BUNNY

Easter Bunny, Easter Bunny
  (make "ears" at head with arms
  outstretched)
Pink and white
Come fill my basket
  (make filling motion)
Overnight
  (pretend to sleep, lay head on hands)

Source: *Let Your Fingers Do the Talking.* Kathy Overholser. (T.S. Denison and Company: Minneapolis, 1979).

THE DUCK

I waddle when I walk.
  (hold arms elbow high and twist trunk
  side to side, or squat down)
I quack when I talk.
  (place palms together and open and close)
And I have webbed toes on my feet.
  (spread fingers wide)
Rain coming down
Makes me smile, not frown
  (smile)
And I dive for something to eat.
  (put hands together and make diving
  motion)

MY RABBIT

My rabbit has two big ears
  (hold up index and middle fingers for ears)
And a funny little nose.
  (join other three fingers for nose)
He likes to nibble carrots
  (move thumb away from other two fingers)
And he hops wherever he goes.
  (move whole hand jerkily)

Science:

1. Incubate and Hatch Eggs

Check the yellow pages of your telephone book to see if any hatcheries are located in your area.

2. Dying Eggs

Use natural products to make egg dye. Beets—deep red, yellow—onions (add soda to make bright yellow), cranberries—light red, spinach leaves—green, and blackberries—blue. To make dyed eggs pick two or three colors from the list. Make the dye by boiling the fruit or vegetable in small amounts of water. Let the children put a cool hard-boiled egg in a nylon stocking and dip it into the dye. Keep the egg in the dye for several minutes. Pull out the nylon and check the color. If it is dark enough, place the egg on a paper towel to dry. If children want to color the eggs with crayons before dying, you can show how the wax keeps liquid from getting on the egg.

3. Science Table Additions

* bird nests
* bird eggs
* different kinds of baskets
* an incubator
* newly planted seeds
* flowers still in bud (children can watch them open)
* pussy willows

4. Basket Guessing

Do reach-and-feel using a covered basket. Place an egg, a chick, a rabbit, a doll's hat, some Easter grass, etc. in a large Easter basket. Let the children place their hands into the basket individually and describe the objects they are feeling.

Dramatic Play:

1. Flower Shop

Plan a flower shop for the dramatic play area. Include spring plants, baskets and Easter lilies.

2. Egg Center

Create a colored egg center to be used during self-directed play. Some children paint plastic eggs, some sell the eggs, and others buy them.

3. Costume Shop

Place costumes for bunny use, Easter baskets and Easter eggs in the dramatic play area. The children can take turns hiding the eggs and going on hunts.

4. A Bird Nest

Place a nest with eggs in the dramatic play area. Also provide bird masks, a perch and other bird items in the area for use during self-initiated play.

5. Easter Clothes

Bring in Easter clothes for the children to dress up in. Suits, dresses, hats, purses, gloves, and dress-up shoes should be included.

6. Hat Shop

Make a hat shop. Place hats with ribbons, flowers, netting, and other decorations in the dramatic play area. The children can decorate the hats. If the children are interested, plan an Easter Parade.

Arts and Crafts:

1. Easter Collages

Collect eggshells, straw, Easter grass or plant seeds for making collages. Place on art table with sheets of paper and glue.

2. Colorful Collages

Use pastel-colored sand and glue to make collages.

3. Wet Chalk Eggs

Use wet chalk to decorate paper cut in the shape of eggs in pastel colors. Show the children the difference between wetting the chalk in vinegar and water. The vinegar color will be brighter.

4. Easel Ideas

Cut egg-shaped easel paper or basket-shaped paper. Clip to the easel. Provide pastel paints at the easel. To make the paint more interesting add glitter.

5. Milk Carton Easter Baskets

Cut off the bottom four inches of milk cartons. Provide precut construction or wallpaper to cover the baskets, and yarn. Include small bits of paper or bright cloth to glue on. Make a handle using a thin strip of paper that is stapled to the carton. Use the baskets for the children's snack.

6. Plastic Easter Baskets

Easter baskets can be made by using the green plastic baskets that strawberries and blueberries come in from the grocery store. Cut thin strips of paper that children can practice weaving through the holes. This activity is most successful with older children.

7. Color Mixing

Provide red, yellow and blue dyed water in shallow pans. Provide the children with medicine droppers and absorbant paper cut in the shape of eggs. Also the children can use medicine droppers to apply color to the paper. Observe what happens when the colors blend together.

8. Rabbit Ears

Construct rabbit ears out of heavy paper. Attach them to a band that can be worn around the head, fitting it for size. These ears may stimulate creative movement as well as dramatic play.

9. Shape Rabbit

Provide a large, a medium, and four small circles cut from white paper, as well as two tall thin triangles. Show the children how to put these shapes together to make a rabbit.

Sensory:

1. Sensory Table Activities

Add to the sensory table:

* cotton balls with scoops and measuring cups

* birdseed or beans
* straw or hay and plastic eggs
* plastic chicks and ducks with water
* Easter grass, eggs, small straw mats
* dirt with plastic flowers and/or leaves
* dyed, scented water and water toys
* sand, shovels and scoops

2. Clay Cutters

Make scented clay. Place on the art table with rabbit, duck, egg, and flower cookie cutters for the children to use during self-directed or self-initiated play.

Large Muscle:

1. Bunny Trail

Set up a bunny trail in the classroom. Place tape on the floor and have children hop over the trail. To make it more challenging, add a balance beam to resemble a bridge.

2. Eggs in the Basket

The children can practice throwing egg-shaped or regular bean bags into a large basket or bucket.

3. Rabbit Tag

Make the egg-shaped bean bags to play rabbit tag. To play the game, the children stand in a circle, with one child being the rabbit. The rabbit walks around the circle with a bean bag balanced on his head, and drops a second bean bag behind the back of another child. The second child must put the bean bag on his head and follow the rabbit around the circle once. Each child must keep the bean bag balanced—if it drops, it must be picked up and replaced on the head. If the rabbit is tagged, he chooses the next rabbit. If the rabbit returns to the empty spot in the circle, the second child becomes the rabbit. This is an unusual game in that the action is fairly slow, but it's still very exciting.

4. Egg Rolling

Place mats on the floor and have children roll across with their arms at their sides. For older children, you can place the mat on a slightly inclined plane and have children roll down, then try to have them roll back up which is more challenging.

Field Trips/Resource People:

1. The Farm

Take a trip to a farm to see the new baby animals.

2. The Hatchery

Visit a hatchery on a day that they are selling baby chicks.

3. Neighborhood Walk

Take a walk around the neighborhood and look for signs of new life.

4. Rabbit Visit

Bring some rabbits to school for the children to observe.

Math:

1. Egg Numerals

Collect five large plastic eggs, such as the kind that nylon stockings can be purchased in. Put numerals from one to five (or ten, for older children) on the eggs. Let the children place the correct number of cotton balls or markers into each egg.

2. Easter Seriation

Cut different sized tagboard eggs, chicks, ducks and rabbits. The children can place the items in a row from the smallest to the largest.

Social Studies:

1. Family Easter Traditions

During large group, ask the children what special activities their families do to celebrate Easter. Their families may go to church, eat together, have egg hunts, or do other things that are special on this day.

2. Sharing Baskets

Decorate eggs or baskets to give to a home for the elderly. If possible, take a walk and let the children deliver them.

Group Time (games, language):

1. The Last Bunny

This is a game for ten or more players. It is more fun with a large number. An Easter rabbit is chosen by counting out or drawing straws. All the other players stand in a circle. The Easter rabbit walks around the circle and taps one player on the back saying, "Have you seen my bunny helper?" "What does it look like?" asks the player and the Easter rabbit describes the bunny helper. He may say, "She is wearing a watch and blue shoes." The player tries to guess who it is. When he names the right person, the Easter rabbit says, "That's my helper!" and the other player chases the bunny helper outside and around the circle. If the chaser catches the bunny helper before he can return to his place the chaser becomes the Easter rabbit. If the bunny helper gets there first then the first Easter rabbit must try again. The Easter rabbit takes the place in the circle of whoever is the new Easter rabbit.

Source: *Games and How to Play Them.* Anne Rockwell. (Thomas Y. Crowell Co.: New York, 1973).

2. Outdoor Egg Hunt

Plan an egg hunt outdoors, if possible. Hide the boiled eggs that the children have decorated, candy eggs in wrappers, or small Easter candies in clear plastic bags.

The children can use the baskets they have made to collect their eggs. Then, weather permitting, eat the boiled eggs for a snack outdoors.

Cooking:

1. Decorating Cupcakes

Let the children use green frosting, dyed coconut shreds, and jelly beans to decorate cupcakes and put them into an Easter basket. As a last touch, add a pipe cleaner handle. Cake mixes can be used to make the cupcakes. Follow the directions on the box. Place paper liners in a muffin pan to insure easy removability.

2. Bunny Food

Carrot sticks, celery, and lettuce can be available for snack.

3. Egg Sandwiches

Use the boiled eggs the children have decorated to make egg salad or deviled eggs for snack time.

4. Carrot and Raisin Salad

4 cups grated carrots
1 cup raisins
1/2 cup mayonnaise or whipped salad dressing

Place ingredients in a bowl and mix thoroughly.

5. Bunny Salad

For each serving place one lettuce leaf on a plate. Put one canned pear half with the cut side down on top of the lettuce leaf. Add sections of an orange to represent the ears. Decorate the bunny face by adding grated carrots, raisins, nuts or maraschino cherries to make eyes, a nose and a mouth.

EASTER EGGS

Where did the custom of coloring Easter eggs come from? No one knows for sure. In any case, the Easter holiday centers around eggs for young children. Here are some projects you might like to try.

To hard cook eggs: Place eggs in a saucepan and add enough cold water to cover at least 1 inch above the eggs. Heat rapidly to boiling and remove from heat. Cover the pan and allow to stand for 22 to 24 minutes. Immediately cool the eggs in cold water.

* Make a vegetable dye solution by adding a teaspoon of vinegar to 1/2 cup of boiling water. Drop in food coloring and stir. The longer the egg is kept in the dye, the deeper the color will be.

* Add a teaspoonful of salad oil to a dye mixture and mix in the oil well. This results in a dye that produces swirls of color. Immerse the egg in the dye for a few minutes.

* Draw a design on an egg with a crayon before dying. The dye will not take to the areas with the crayon marks and the design will show through.

* Wrap rubber bands, string, yarn or narrow strips of masking tape around an egg to create stripes and other designs. Dip the egg in a dye and allow to dry before removing the wrapping.

* Drip the wax of a lighted birthday candle over an egg or draw a design on the egg using a piece of wax. Place the egg in dye. Repeat process again, if desired, dipping the egg in another color of dye. (Note: The lighted candle is to be used by an adult only.)

* Felt-tip markers can be used to decorate dyed or undyed eggs.

* Small stickers can be used on eggs.

* Craft items such as sequins, glitter and ribbons and small pom poms can be used with glue to decorate eggs.

* Apply lengths of yarns, string or thread to the eggs with glue, creating designs, and allow to dry.

* Egg creatures can be created by using markers, construction paper, feathers, ribbon, lace, cotton balls, fabric and buttons. To make an egg holder, make small cardboard or construction paper cylinders. A toilet paper or paper towel tube can be cut to make stands as well.

* Save the shells from the eggs to use for eggshell collages. Crumble the shells and sprinkle over a glue design that has been made on paper or cardboard.

Record:

The following record can be found in preschool educational catalogs:

Holiday Songs and Rhythms. Hap Palmer. (Educational Activities, Inc.: Freeport, NY). "Easter Time is Here Again."

Books and Stories:

The following books and stories can be used to complement the theme:

1. **The Easter Egg Artists.** Adrienne Adams. (New York: Scribner Publishing, 1976).

2. **The Runaway Bunny.** Margaret Wise Brown. (New York: Harper Brothers, 1942).

3. **Telka's Easter.** L. Budd. (Chicago: Rand McNally and Company, 1972).

4. **Bunny Trouble.** Hans Wilhelm. (New York: Scholastic Books, 1985).

5. **The Easter Cat.** Meinheit DeJong. (New York: Macmillan, 1971).

6. **Listen Rabbit.** Aileen Fischer. (New York: Crowell Company, 1964).

7. **The Easter Bunny that Overslept.** Priscilla and Otto Friedrich. (New York: Lathrop Publishing, 1957).

8. **Where is It?** Tana Hoban. (New York: Macmillan, 1974).

9. **Easter in November.** Lilo Hess. (New York: Crowell Company, 1964).

10. **Daddy Long Ears.** Robert Kraus. (New York: Windmill Books, 1970).

11. **The Whiskers of Ho Ho.** William Littlefield. (New York: Lathrop Publishing, 1958).

12. **The Egg Tree.** Katherine Milhous. (New York: Charles Scribner's Sons, 1950).

13. **Our Easter Book.** Jane Moncure. (Chicago: Childrens World, 1972).

14. **Happy Easter, Mother Duck.** Elizabeth Winthrop. (New York: Golden Press, 1985).

15. **The Candy Egg Bunny.** Lisa Wiel. (New York: Holiday House, 1975).

Puzzles:

The following puzzles can be found in preschool educational catalogs:

1. **"Pets"** Judy/Instructo.

2. **"Rabbit"** Judy/Instructo.

3. **"Hen and Chicks"** Judy/Instructo.

4. **"Sheep and Lambs"** Judy/Instructo.

5. **"Matchette"** Judy/Instructo.

6. **"Church"** Judy/Instructo.

20

FALL

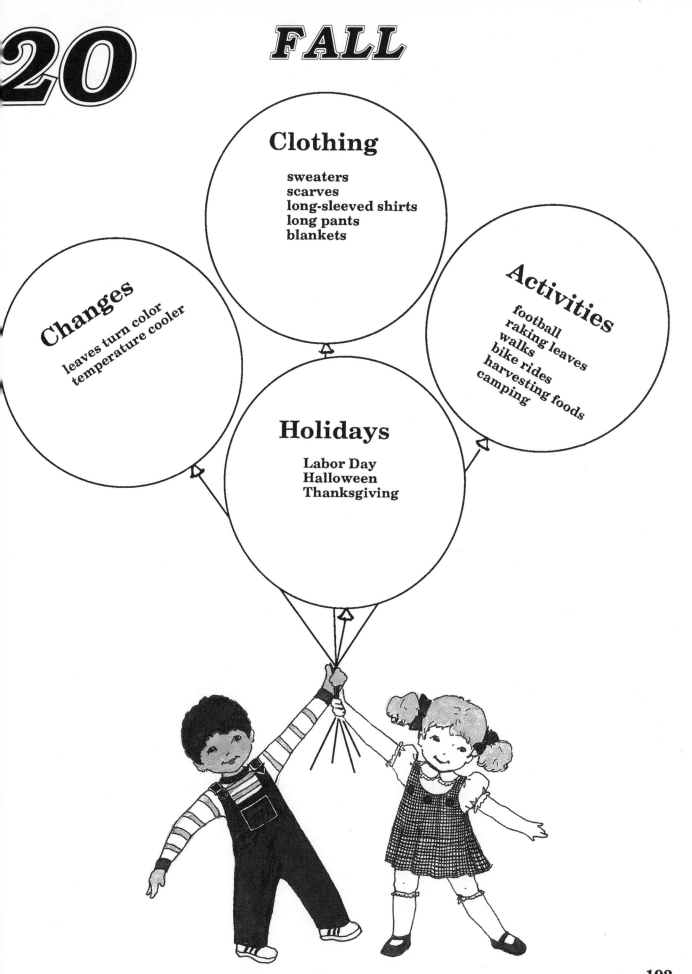

Clothing

sweaters
scarves
long-sleeved shirts
long pants
blankets

Changes

leaves turn color
temperature cooler

Activities

football
raking leaves
walks
bike rides
harvesting foods
camping

Holidays

Labor Day
Halloween
Thanksgiving

Theme Goals:

Through participating in the experiences provided by this theme, the children may learn:

1. Characteristics of fall weather.

2. Fall holidays.

3. Fall clothing.

4. Fall activities.

Concepts for the Children to Learn:

1. Fall is one of the four seasons.

2. Fall is the season between summer and winter.

3. Some trees change color in the fall.

4. In some places the weather becomes cooler in the fall.

5. The day becomes shorter in the fall.

6. Leaves fall from some trees in the fall.

7. Labor Day, Halloween and Thanksgiving are some fall holidays.

8. Scarfs and sweaters may need to be worn in the fall in some areas.

9. Pumpkins and apples can be harvested in the fall.

10. Football is a fall sport.

11. Blankets are usually needed on our beds in the fall in some places.

Vocabulary:

1. **fall**—the season between summer and winter.

2. **Halloween**—the holiday when people wear costumes and go trick or treating.

3. **Thanksgiving**—a holiday to express thanks.

4. **Labor Day**— a holiday to honor working people.

5. **season**—a time of the year.

Bulletin Board

The purpose of this bulletin board is to foster a positive self concept as well as develop skills of name recognition. Construct an acorn for each child. Print the children's names on the acorns. See illustration. Laminate and punch holes in the acorns. Children can hang their acorns on a push pin on the bulletin board when they arrive.

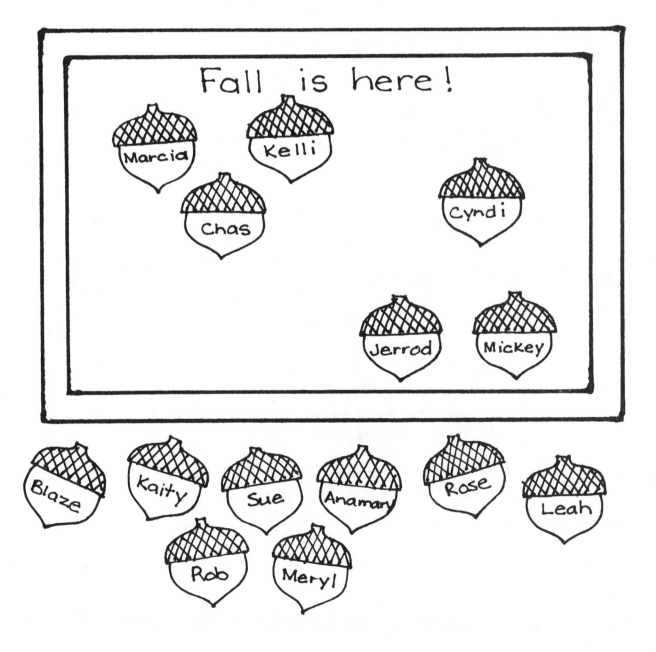

Parent Letter

Dear Parents,

Where we live, the days are getting shorter, the temperature is getting colder, and the leaves are changing color. It's the perfect time to introduce our next unit—fall. During the week children will become more aware of changes that take place in the fall and common fall activities.

At School This Week

A few of this week's learning experiences include:

* recording the temperature and the changing colors of the leaves.
* making leaf rubbings in the art area.
* raking leaves on our playground during outdoor time.

We will also be taking a fall walk around the neighborhood to observe the trees in their peak changes. We will be leaving Thursday at 10:00 a.m. Please feel free to join us. It will be a scenic tour.

At Home

To develop classification skills help your child sort leaves by their color, type or size.

Fingerplays promote language and vocabulary skills. This fingerplay is one we will be learning this week. Enjoy it with your child at home!

Autumn

Autumn winds begin to blow.
  (blow)
Colored leaves fall fast and slow.
  (make fast and slow motions with hands)
Twirling, whirling all around,
  (turn around)
'Til at last, they touch the ground.
  (fall to the ground)

Have a good week!

Music:

1. "Little Leaves"
(Sing to the tune of "Ten Little Indians")

One little, two little, three little leaves.
Four little, five little, six little leaves.
Seven little, eight little, nine little leaves.
Ten little leaves fall down.

2. "Happy Children Tune"
(Sing to the tune of "Did You Ever See a Lassie?"

Happy children in the autumn,
In the autumn, in the autumn.
Happy children in the autumn
Do this way and that.

While singing the song, children can keep time by pretending to rake leaves, jump in the leaves, etc.

3. "Pretty Leaves are Falling Down"
(Sing to the tune of: "London Bridges")

Pretty leaves are falling down, falling down, falling down.
Pretty leaves are falling down, all around the town.
  (wiggle fingers)

Let's rake them up in a pile, in a pile, in a pile.
Let's rake them up in a pile, all around the town.
  (make raking motions)

Let's all jump in and have some fun, have some fun, have some fun.
Let's all jump in and have some fun, all around the town.
  (jump into circle)

Fingerplays:

AUTUMN

Autumn winds begin to blow.
  (blow)
Colored leaves fall fast and slow.
(make fast and slow falling motions with hands)
Twirling, whirling all around
  (turn around)
'Til at last, they touch the ground.
  (fall to the ground)

LEAVES

Little leaves fall gently down
Red and yellow, orange and brown.
  (flutter hands as leaves falling)
Whirling, whirling around and around.
  (turn around)
Quietly without a sound.
  (put finger to lips)
Falling softly to the ground
  (begin to fall slowly)
Down and down and down and down.
  (lie on floor)

LITTLE LEAVES

The little leaves are falling down
  (use hands to make falling motion)
Round and round, round and round.
  (turn around)
The little leaves are falling down,
  (use hands to make falling motion)
Falling to the ground.
  (fall to ground)

TWIRLING LEAVES

The autumn wind blows—Oooo Oooo Oooo.
  (make wind sounds)
The leaves shake and shake then fly into the sky so blue.
  (children shake)
They whirl and whirl around them twirl and twirl around.
  (turn around in circles)
But when the wind stops, the leaves sink slowly to the ground.
Lower, lower, lower, and land quietly without a sound.
  (sink very slowly and very quietly)

Science:

1. Leaf Observation

Collect leaves from a variety of trees.
Place them and a magnifying glass on the science table for the children to explore.

2. Temperature Watch

Place a thermometer outside. A large cardboard thermometer can also be constructed out of tagboard with movable elastic or ribbon for the mercury. The children can match the temperature on the cardboard thermometer with the outdoor one.

3. Weather Calendar

Construct a calendar for the month. Record the changes of weather each day by attaching a symbol to the calendar. Symbols should include clouds, sun, snow, rain, etc.

4. Color Change Sequence

Laminate or cover with contact paper, several leaves of different colors. The children can sort, count and classify the leaves.

Dramatic Play:

1. Fall Wear

Set out warm clothes such as sweaters, coats, hats and blankets to indicate cold weather coming on. The children can use the clothes for dressing up.

2. Football

Collect football gear including balls, helmets and jerseys and play on the outdoor playground.

Arts and Crafts:

1. Fall Collage

After taking a walk to collect objects such as grass, twigs, leaves, nuts and weeds, collages can be made in the art area.

2. Leaf Rubbings

Collect leaves, paper and crayons and show the children how to place several leaves under a sheet of paper. Using the flat edge of crayon color rub over paper. The image of the leaves will appear.

3. Pumpkin Seed Collage

Wash and dry pumpkin seeds and place them in the art area with glue and paper. The children can make pumpkin seed collages.

4. Leaf Spatter Painting

Use a lid from a box that is approximately 9 inches x 12 inches x 12 inches. Cut a rectangle from top of lid leaving a 1 1/2 inch border. Invert the lid and place a wire screen over the opening. Tape the screen to the border. Arrange the leaves on a sheet of paper. Place the lid over the arrangement. Dip a toothbrush into thin tempera paint and brush across screen. When the tempera paint dries, remove the leaves.

Sensory:

Leaves

Place a variety of leaves in the sensory table. Try to include moist and dry examples for the children to compare.

Large Muscle:

Raking Leaves

Child-sized rakes can be provided. The children can be encouraged to rake leaves into piles.

Field Trips/Resource People:

1. Neighborhood Walk

Take a walk around the neighborhood when the leaves are at their peak of changing colors. Discuss differences in color and size.

2. Apple Orchard

Visit an apple orchard. Observe the apples being picked and processed. If possible let children pick their own apples from a tree.

3. Pumpkin Patch

Visit a pumpkin patch. Discuss and observe how pumpkins grow, their size, shape and color. Let the children pick a pumpkin to bring back to the classroom.

Math:

1. Weighing Acorns and Pine Cones

A scale, acorns, and pine cones for the children to weigh can be added to the science table.

2. Leaf Math

Out of construction paper or tagboard, prepare pairs of various shaped leaves. The children can match the identical leaves.

Social Studies:

Bulletin Board

Construct a bulletin board using bare branches to represent a tree. Cut out leaves from colored construction paper and print one child's name on each. At the beginning of the day, children can hang their name on the tree when they arrive.

Cooking:

1. Apple Banana Frosty

1 golden delicious apple, diced
1 peeled sliced banana
1/4 cup milk
3 ice cubes

Blend all the ingredients in a blender. Serves 4 children.

2. Apple Salad

6 medium apples
1/2 cup raisins
1/2 teaspoon cinnamon
1/2 cup chopped nuts
1/4 cup white grape juice

Peel and chop the apples. Mix well and add the remaining ingredients. Serves 10 children.

NATURE RECIPES

Cat tails

Use them in their natural color or tint by shaking metallic powder over them. Handle carefully. The cat tail is dry and feels crumbly. It will fall apart easily.

Crystal Garden

Place broken pieces of brick or terra cotta clay in a glass bowl or jar. Pour the following solution over this:

4 teaspoons water
1 teaspoon ammonia
4 teaspoons bluing
1 teaspoon Mercurochrome
4 teaspoons salt

Add more of this solution each day until the crystal garden has grown to the desired size. (Adult supervision required.)

Drying Plants for Winter Bouquets

Strip the leaves from the flowers immediately. Tie the flowers by their stems with string and hang them with the heads down in a cool dry place away from the light. Darkness is essential for preserving their color. Thorough drying takes about 2 weeks.

Preserving Fall Leaves

Place alternate layers of powdered borax and leaves in a box. The leaves must be completely covered. Allow them to stand for four days. Shake off the borax and wipe each with liquid floor wax. Rub a warm iron over a cake of paraffin, then press the iron over front and back of leaves.

Preserving Magnolia Leaves

Mix two parts of water with one part of glycerine. Place stems of the magnolia leaves in the mixture and let them stand for several days. The leaves will turn brown and last several years. Their surface may be painted or sprayed with silver or gold paint.

Pressing Wild Flowers

When gathering specimens, include the roots, leaves, flowers and seed pods. Place between newspapers, laying two layers of blotters underneath the newspaper and two on top to absorb the moisture. Change the newspapers three times during the week. Place between two sheets of corrugated cardboard and press. It usually takes seven to ten days to press specimens. Cardboard covered with cotton batting is the mounting base. Lay the flower on the cotton and cover with cellophane or plastic wrap to preserve the color.

Treating Gourds

Soak gourds for two hours in water. Scrape them clean with a knife. Rub with fine sandpaper. While still damp cut an opening to remove seeds.

Records:

The following records can be found in preschool educational catalogs:

1. **The Singing Calendar.** Dixie James and Linda Becht.

2. **Sing a Song of Holidays and Seasons.** Roberta McLaughlin and Lucille Wood. (Bowman Records).

Books and Stories:

The following books and stories can be used to complement the theme:

1. **Fall is Here.** Bertha Parker. (New York: Harper & Row, 1966).

2. **Autumn Harvest.** Alvin Tresselt. (New York: Lothrop, Lee & Shepard, 1951).

3. **What Happens in the Autumn.** Suzanne Venino. (Washington, D.C.: National Geographic Society, 1982).

4. **Autumn.** Lucille Wood. (New York: Bowman, 1971).

5. **The Bears' Autumn.** Keizaburo Tejima. (Chicago: Childrens Press, 1986).

Puzzles:

The following puzzles can be found in preschool educational catalogs.

1. **"Halloween"** 22 pieces. Judy/Instructo.

2. **"Thanksgiving"** 20 pieces. Judy/Instructo.

3. **"Apple Tree Seasons"** 6 pieces. Child Craft.

4. **"Sort the Seasons"** Child Craft.

21

FAMILIES

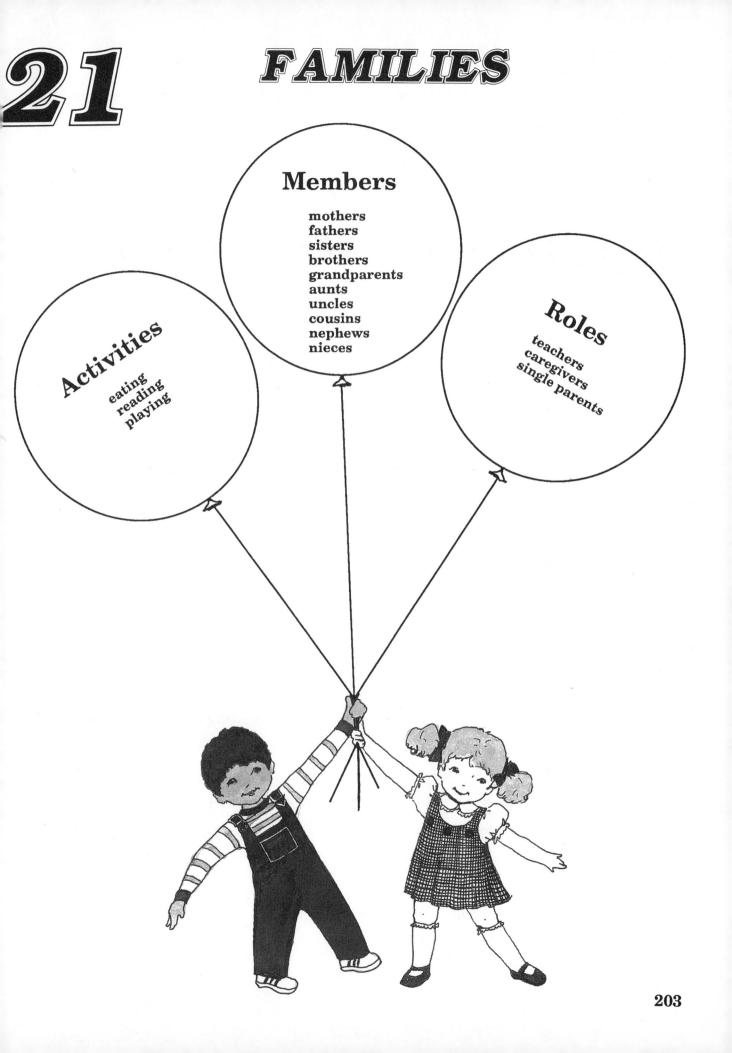

Members

mothers
fathers
sisters
brothers
grandparents
aunts
uncles
cousins
nephews
nieces

Activities

eating
reading
playing

Roles

teachers
caregivers
single parents

Theme Goals:

Through participating in the experiences provided by this theme, the children may learn:

1. The members in a family.
2. Roles of family members.
3. Family activities.

Concepts for the Children to Learn:

1. A family is a group of people who live together.
2. Mothers, fathers, sisters and brothers are family members.
3. Grandparents, aunts, uncles, cousins, nephews and nieces are family members.
4. Camping, eating, reading and watching television are all family activities.
5. Each family is a special group of people.
6. Families teach us about our world.
7. Family members care for us.
8. Some children live with one parent.

Vocabulary:

1. **mother**—female parent.
2. **father**—male parent.
3. **children**—young people.
4. **sister**—a girl having the same parents as another person.
5. **brother**—a boy having the same parents as another person.
6. **grandmother**—mother of a parent.
7. **grandfather**—father of a parent.
8. **cousins**—son or daughter of an uncle or aunt.
9. **aunt**—sister of a parent.
10. **uncle**—brother of a parent.
11. **nephew**—son of a brother or sister.
12. **niece**—daughter of a brother or sister.
13. **love**—feeling of warmth toward another.
14. **family**—people living together.

Bulletin Board

The purpose of this bulletin board is to foster awareness of various family sizes, as well as to identify family members. From tagboard construct a name card for each child. Print each child's name on one of the tagboard pieces. Then cut people figures as illustrated. Laminate the name cards and people. Staple the name cards to a bulletin board. Individually, the children can affix the people in their family behind their name using tape, sticky putty or a stapler.

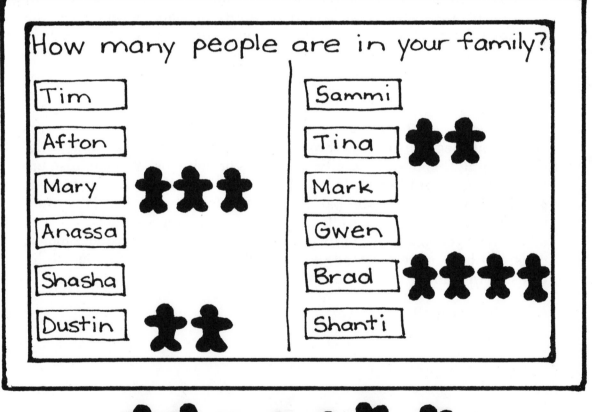

Parent Letter

Dear Parents,

This week we will be starting a unit on families. Through this unit, the children will develop an understanding of various family patterns. They will also discover what family members do for each other, as well as activities that families can participate in together.

At School This Week

A few of this week's highlights include:

* creating pictures of our families on a bulletin board.
* looking at photographs of classmates' families. To assist us with this unit, please send a picture of your family to school with your child. We will place the photograph in a special photo album to look at in the reading area.

At Home

There are several activities you can do at home to foster the concepts of this unit. Begin by looking through family photographs with your child. While doing this discuss family traditions or customs. You can also encourage your child to dictate a letter to you to write to a grandparent or other relative. Plan and participate in a family activity. This could be as simple as taking a walk together or going on a picnic.

We invite you and your family to visit us this week. This includes moms, dads, brothers, sisters, grandparents and other relatives! If you are interested in coming, please let me know!

From all of us,

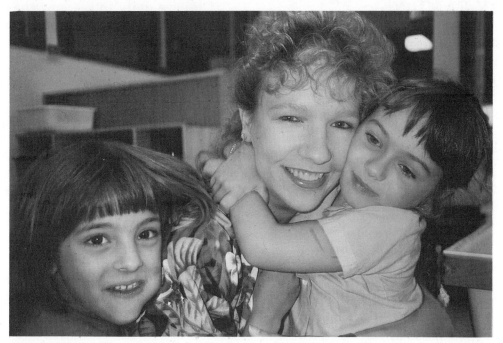

FIGURE 21 Families are loving and caring parts of our lives.

Music:

"Family Helper"
(Sing to the tune of "Here We are Together")

It's fun to be a helper, a helper, a helper.
It's fun to be a helper, just any time.
Oh, I can set the table, the table, the table.
Oh, I can set the table at dinner time.
Oh, I can dry the dishes, the dishes, the dishes.
Oh, I can dry the dishes, and make them shine.

Fingerplays:

MY FAMILY

If you peek in my room at night,
   (stand on toes as if peeking)
My family you will see,
   (nod head)
They kiss my face and tuck me in tight,
   (kiss into the air)
Why? Because they love me!
   (hug yourself)

SEE MY FAMILY

See my family? See them all?
   (hold up all five fingers)

Some are short
   (hold up thumb)
Some are tall
   (hold up middle finger)

Let's shake hands. "How do you do?"
   (grasp hands and shake)
See them bow? "How are you?"
   (bend fingers)

Father,
   (hold up middle finger)
Mother,
   (hold up pointer finger)
Sister,
   (hold up ring finger)
Brother
   (hold up thumb)
And me.
   (hold up pinky finger)

THIS IS THE MOTHER

This is the mother, kind and dear.
   (make a fist then point to the thumb)
This is the father sitting near.
   (show each finger in turn)
This is the brother strong and tall.
This is the sister, who plays with her ball.
This is the baby, the littlest of all.
See my whole family large and small?
   (wiggle all fingers)

I LOVE MY FAMILY

Some families are large.
   (spread arms out wide)
Some families are small.
   (bring arms close together)
But I love my family
   (cross arms over chest)
Best of all!

A GOOD HOUSE

This is the roof of the house so good.
   (make roof with hands)
These are the walls that are made of wood.
   (hands straight, palms parallel)
These are the windows that let in the light.
   (thumbs and forefingers form window)
This is the door that shuts so tight.
   (hands straight by side)
This is the chimney so straight and tall.
   (arms up straight)
Oh! What a good house for one and all!

All fingerplays taken from *Finger Frolics: Fingerplays for Young Children*. Cromwell, Faitel and Hibner. (Michigan: Partner Press, 1983).

Science:

1. Sounds

Tape different sounds from around the house that families hear daily such as a crying baby, brushing teeth, telephone ringing, toilet flushing, doorbell ringing, water running, electric shaver, alarm clock, etc. Play the tape for the children to identify the correct sound.

2. Feely Box

Place objects pertaining to a family into a box. Include items such as a baby rattle, a toothbrush, a comb, baby bottle, etc. The children feel the objects and try to identify them.

3. Animal Families

Gerbils or hamsters with young babies in a cage can be placed on the science table.

Observe daily to see how they raise their babies. Compare the animal behavior to the children's own families.

Dramatic Play:

1. Baby Clothing

Arrange the dramatic play area for washing baby dolls. Include a tub with soapy water, washcloths, drying towels, play clothes, brush and comb.

2. Family Picnic

Collect items to make a picnic basket. Include paper napkins, cups, plates, plastic eating utensils, etc.

3. Doll House

Set up a large doll house for children to play with. These can be constructed from cardboard. Include dolls to represent several members of a family.

Arts and Crafts:

1. Family Collage

The children can cut pictures of people from magazines. The pictures can be pasted on a sheet of paper to make a collage.

2. My Body

Trace each child's body on a large piece of paper. The children can use crayons and felt-tip markers to color their own body picture. When finished, display the pictures around the room or in the center's entrance.

Sensory:

1. Washing baby dolls in lukewarm, soapy water
2. Washing dishes in warm water
3. Washing doll clothes and hanging them up to dry
4. Cars and houses with sand

Large Muscle:

Neighborhood Walk

Take a walk through a neighborhood and have children identify different homes. Observe the colors and sizes of the homes.

Field Trips/Resource People:

Family Day

Invite moms, dads, sisters, brothers, grandfathers, grandmothers, and other family members to a tea at your center.

Math:

1. Families—Biggest to Smallest

Cut out from magazines several members of a family. The children can place the members from largest to smallest, and then smallest to largest. They can also identify each family member as the biggest and the smallest.

2. Family Member Chart

Graph the number of family members for each child's family in the classroom.

Social Studies:

Family Pictures

1. Display posters of families. Discuss at group time ways that families help and care for each other.

2. Ask each child to bring in a family picture. Label each child's picture and place on a special bulletin board with the caption "Our Families."

Group Time (games, language):

A Hundred Ways to Get There

During outdoor play or large group, form a large circle. Begin the game by choosing a child to cross the circle by skipping, hopping, jumping, crawling, running, etc. Once the circle has been crossed the child takes the place of another person who then goes across the circle in another manner. Each child can try to think of something new.

Cooking:

1. Peanut Butter and Jelly

Cut whole wheat bread into house shapes for snack one day. Put peanut butter, raisins, and jelly on the table with knives. Let children choose their own topping.

2. Gingerbread Families

Use the following recipe to create gingerbread families.

1 1/2 cups whole wheat pastry flour
1 teaspoon baking soda
1/2 teaspoon salt
1/2 teaspoon ginger
1 teaspoon cinnamon
1/4 cup oil
1/4 cup maple syrup
1/4 cup honey
1 large egg

Preheat oven to 350 degrees. Measure all of the dry ingredients into a bowl and mix well. Measure all wet ingredients into a second bowl and mix well. Add the two mixtures together. Pour the combined mixture into an 8-inch square pan and bake for 30 to 35 minutes. When cool, roll the gingerbread dough into thin slices and provide cookie cutters for children to cut their family. Decorate the figures with raisins, peanut butter, wheat germ, etc. Enjoy for snack time.

3. Raisin Bran Muffins

4 cups raisin bran cereal
2 1/2 cups all purpose flour
1 cup sugar
1/2 cup chopped walnuts
2 1/2 teaspoons baking soda
1 teaspoon salt
2 eggs, beaten

2 cups buttermilk
1/2 cup cooking oil

Stir the cereal, flour, sugar, nuts, baking soda and salt together in a large mixing bowl. In a separate bowl beat the eggs, buttermilk and oil together. Add this mixture to the dry ingredients and stir until moistened. The batter will be thick. Spoon the batter into greased or lined muffin cups, filling 3/4 full. Bake in a 375-degree oven for 20 to 25 minutes and remove from pans.

SNACK IDEAS

MILK

1. Dips (yogurt, cottage cheese, cream cheese)
2. Cheese (balls, wedges, cutouts, squares, faces, etc.)
3. Yogurt and fruit
4. Milk punches made with fruits and juices
5. Conventional cocoa
6. Cottage cheese (add pineapple, peaches etc.)
7. Cheese fondues (preheated, no open flames in classroom)
8. Shakes (mix fruit and milk in a blender)

MEAT

1. Meat strips, chunks, cubes (beef, pork, chicken, turkey, ham, fish)
2. Meat balls, small kabobs
3. Meat roll-ups (cheese spread, mashed potatoes, spinach, lettuce leaves or tortillas)
4. Meat salads (tuna, other fish, chicken, turkey, etc.) as spreads for crackers, stuffing for celery, rolled in spinach or lettuce
5. Sardines
6. Stuffing for potatoes, tomatoes, squash

EGGS

1. Hard boiled
2. Deviled (use different flavors)
3. Egg salad spread
4. Eggs any style that can be managed
5. Egg as a part of other recipes
6. Eggnog

FRUITS

1. Use standard fruits, but be adventurous: pomegranates, cranberries, pears, peaches, apricots, plums, berries, pineapples, melons, grapes, grapefruit, tangerines
2. Kabobs and salads
3. Juices and juice blends
4. In muffins, yogurt, milk beverages
5. Fruit "sandwiches"
6. Stuffed dates, prunes, etc.
7. Dried fruits (raisins, currents, prunes, apples, peaches, apricots, dates, figs)

VEGETABLES

1. Variety—Sweet and white potatoes, cherry tomatoes, broccoli, cauliflower, radishes, peppers, mushrooms, zucchini, all squashes, rutabaga, avocados, eggplant, okra, pea pods, turnips, pumpkin, sprouts, spinach
2. Almost any vegetable can be served raw with or without dip
3. Salads, kabobs, cutouts
4. Juices and juice blends
5. Soup in a cup (hot or cold)
6. Stuffed—celery, cucumbers, zucchini, spinach, lettuce, cabbage, squash, potatoes, tomatoes
7. Vegetable spreads
8. Sandwiches

DRIED PEAS AND BEANS

1. Peanuts, kidney beans, garbanzos, limas, lentils, yellow and green peas, pintos, black beans
2. Beans and peas mashed as dips or spreads
3. Bean, pea or lentil soup in a cup
4. Roasted soybean—peanut mix
5. Three-bean salad

PASTAS

1. Different shapes and thicknesses
2. Pasta with butter and poppy seeds
3. Cold pasta salad
4. Lasagne noodles (cut for small sandwiches)
5. Chow mein noodles (wheat or rice)

BREADS

1. Use a variety of grains—whole wheat, cracked wheat, rye, cornmeal, oatmeal, bran, grits, etc.
2. Use a variety of breads—tortillas, pocket breads, crepes, pancakes, muffins, biscuits, bagels, popovers, English muffins
3. Toast—plain, buttered, with spreads, cinnamon
4. Homemade yeast and quick breads
5. Fill and roll up crepes, pancakes
6. Waffle sandwiches

CEREALS, GRAINS, SEEDS

1. Granola
2. Slices of rice loaf or rice cakes
3. Dry cereal mixes (not pre-sweetened)
4. Seed mixes (pumpkin, sunflower, sesame, poppy, caraway, etc.)
5. Roasted wheat berries, wheat germ, bran as roll-ins, toppers, or as finger mix
6. Popcorn with toppers of grated cheese, flavored butters, mixed nuts
7. Stir into muffins or use as a topper

Records:

The following records can be found in preschool educational catalogs:

1. **A Place of Our Own.** Fred Rogers.

2. **Sounds Around Us.** "Around the House." (Glenview, Il: Scott Foresman and Company).

3. **The Sleepy Family.** (New York: Young People's Records).

4. **Small Voice, Big Voice with Dick, Laurie and Jed.** (Folkway Records and Service Corporation).

Book and Stories:

The following books and stories can be used to complement the theme:

1. **All Kinds of Families.** Norma Simon. (Chicago: Albert Whitman and Company, 1976).

2. **Hooray for Me.** Jeremy Charlip and Lillian Moore. (New York: Parents Press Magazine, 1975).

3. **When You Were a Baby.** Linda Hayward. (Racine, WI: Western Publishers, 1982).

4. **This is My Father and Me.** Dorka Raynor. (Chicago: Albert Whitman and Company, 1977).

5. **I Love My Mother.** Paul Zindel. (New York: Harper and Row, 1975).

6. **Grandma's Wheelchair.** Lorraine Henriod. (Chicago: Albert Whitman and Company, 1982).

7. **We Are Having a Baby.** Viki Holland. (New York: Scribner, 1972).

8. **Martin's Father.** Margrit Eichler. (New York: Lollipop Power, 1977).

9. **I'm in a Family.** JoAnn Stover. (New York: David McKay Company, 1966).

10. **Come Over to My House.** Theo LeSieg. (New York: Random House, 1966).

11. **He's My Brother.** Joe Lasker. (Chicago: Albert Whitman and Company, 1974).

12. **Tommy Builds a House.** Gunilla Wolde. (Boston: Houghton Mifflin Company, 1969).

13. **Mary Jo's Grandmother.** Janice May Udry. (Chicago: Albert Whitman and Company, 1970).

14. **Have You Seen My Brother?** Elizabeth Guilfoile. (New York: Follet Publishing Company, 1962).

15. **Cousins Are Special.** Susan Goldman. (Chicago: Albert Whitman and Company, 1978).

16. **People in My Family.** Bobbie Kalman. (New York: Crabtree Publishing Company, 1985).

17. **The New Baby.** Fred Rogers. (New York: G.P. Putnam's Sons, 1985).

18. **The Two of Them.** Aliki. (New York: Greenwillow Books, 1979).

19. **Grandparents Around the World.** Dora Raynor. (Chicago: Albert Whitman and Company, 1977).

20. **Kevin's Grandma.** Barbara Williams. (New York: Dutton, 1975).

21. **Messy Baby.** Jan Omerod. (New York: Lothrop, Lee and Shepard, 1985).

22. **My Mother's Getting Married.** Joan Drescher. (New York: Dial Press, 1986).

23. **Grandpa and Bo.** Kevin Henkes. (New York: Greenwillow Books, 1986).

24. **What Kind of Family is This? A Book About Step Families.** Barbara Seuling. (Racine, WI: Western Publishing Company, Inc., 1985).

25. **Daddy Doesn't Live Here Anymore.** Betty Boegehold. (Racine, WI: Western Publishing Company, 1985).

26. **Molly and Grandpa.** Sally G. Ward. (New York: Scholastic, 1986).

27. **Charlie and Grandma.** Sally G. Ward. (New York: Scholastic, 1986).

28. Teach Me About Brothers and Sisters. Joy Berry. (Chicago: Childrens Press, 1987).

29. Teach Me About Mommies and Daddies. Joy Berry. (Chicago: Childrens Press, 1987).

30. Teach Me About Relatives. Joy Berry. (Chicago: Childrens Press, 1987).

Puzzles:

The following puzzles can be found in preschool educational catalogs:

1. "House Puzzle" 16 pieces. Judy.

2. "Rubber Fit-In Figures of a Family" Judy.

3. "Washing Dishes" 24 pieces. Constructive Playthings.

4. "Washing the Car" 24 pieces. Constructive Playthings.

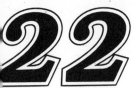

22 FARM ANIMALS

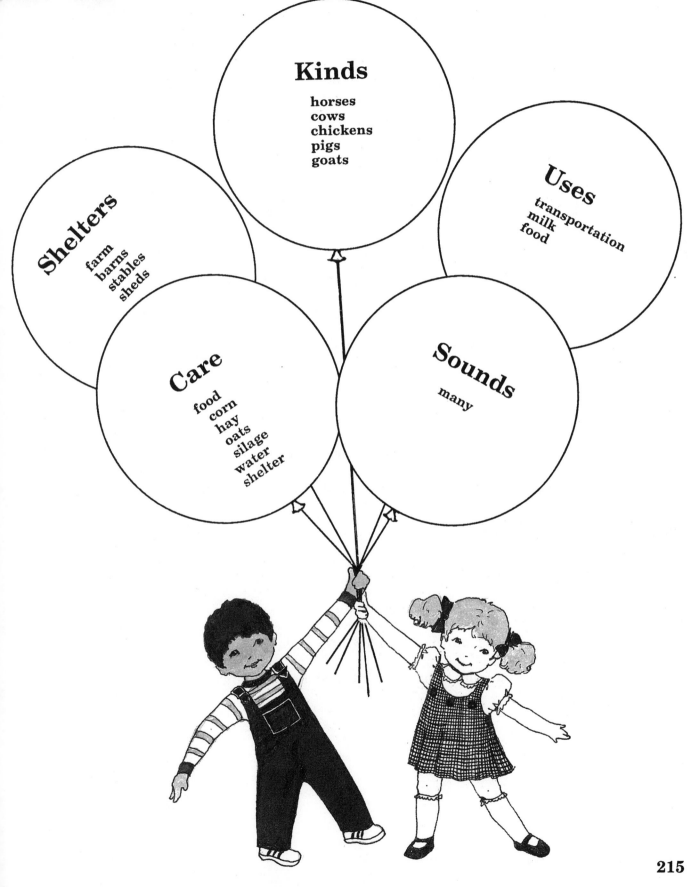

Kinds

horses
cows
chickens
pigs
goats

Uses

transportation
milk
food

Shelters

farm
barns
stables
sheds

Care

food
corn
hay
oats
silage
water
shelter

Sounds

many

Theme Goals:

Through participating in the experiences provided by this theme, the children may learn:

1. Names of farm animals.

2. Uses for farm animals.

3. Farm animal shelters.

4. Food for farm animals.

5. Sounds of farm animals.

Concepts for the Children to Learn:

1. A farm animal lives on a farm.

2. Barns, stables and sheds are homes for farm animals.

3. Horses are farm animals that can be used for transportation.

4. Cows, chickens, pigs and goats are farm animals.

5. Some cows and goats give milk.

6. Farm animals eat corn, hay, oats and silage.

7. A farmer cares for farm animals.

8. We can recognize some farm animals by their sounds.

Vocabulary:

1. **herd**—a group of animals.

2. **stable**—building for horses and cattle.

3. **farmer**—person who cares for farm animals.

4. **barn**—building to house animals and store grain.

Bulletin Board

The purpose of this bulletin board is to foster one-to-one correspondence skills and matching sets to written numerals. Out of tagboard construct red barns as illustrated. The number of barns constructed will depend upon the maturity of your group of children. Place a numeral on each red barn. Construct the same number of black barns by tracing around the red barns onto black construction paper. After cutting out, place small white circles (dots from paper punch) onto the black barns. Laminate all barns. Staple black barns to the board. Punch a hole in each red barn window. During self selected activity periods the children can hang red barns on push pins of corresponding black barns.

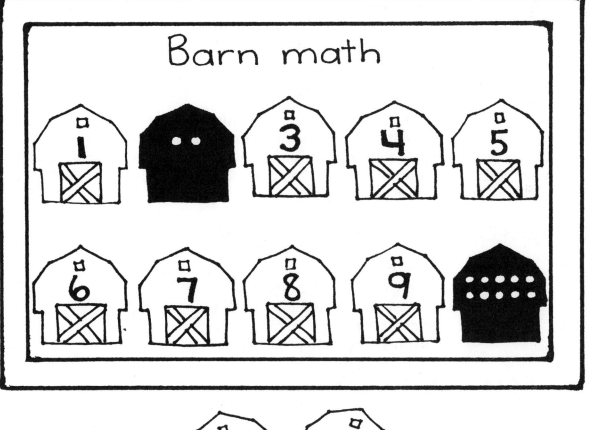

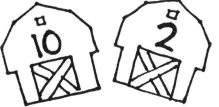

Parent Letter

Dear Parents,

This week at school we will be discussing farm animals. The children will be learning the many different ways that farm animals help us. They will also become aware of the difference between pets and farm animals. The children will also discover that farm animals need homes and food.

At School This Week

Some of the learning activities scheduled for this week include:

* making a barn out of a large cardboard box for the dramatic play area
* tasting different kinds of eggs, milk and cheese for breakfast one day
* observing and comparing the many grains and seeds farm animals eat at the science table
* dressing up like farmers and farm animals
* making buttermilk chalk pictures

At Home

There are many ways you can integrate this unit into your family life. To stimulate imagination and movement skills ask your child to imitate different farm animals by walking and making that animal's noise. Also, your child will be learning this rhyme at school. You can also recite it at home to foster language skills.

If I Were a Horse

If I were a horse, I'd gallop all around.
  (slap thighs and gallop in a circle)
I'd shake my head and say "Neigh, neigh."
  (shake head)
I'd prance and gallop all over town.

Have a good week!

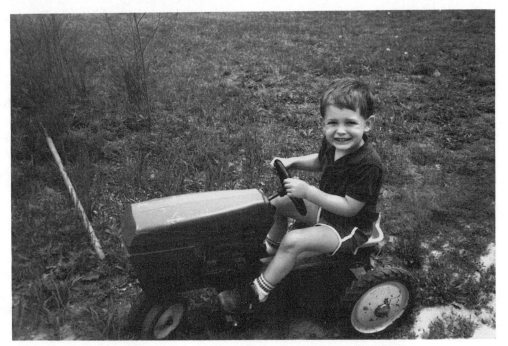
FIGURE 22 Farming is a tradition for many families.

Music:

1. **"Old Mac Donald Had a Farm"**
   (traditional)

2. **"The Animals on the Farm"**
   (Sing to the tune of "The Wheels on the Bus")

   The cows on the farm go moo, moo, moo.
   Moo, moo, moo, moo, moo, moo.
   The cows on the farm go moo, moo, moo
   all day long.

   The horses on the farm go nay, nay, nay.
   Nay, nay, nay, nay, nay, nay.
   The horses on the farm go nay, nay, nay
   all day long.

   (pigs—oink)
   (sheep—baa)
   (chicken—cluck)
   (turkeys—gobble)

3. **"The Farmer in the Dell"**
   (traditional)

   The farmer in the dell,
   The farmer in the dell,
   Hi-ho the dairy-o
   The farmer in the dell.

   The farmer takes a wife/husband.
   The farmer takes a wife/husband.
   Hi-ho the dairy-o
   The farmer in the dell.

   The other verses are:
   The wife/husband takes the child
   The child takes the nurse
   The nurse takes the dog
   The dog takes the cat
   The cat takes the rat
   The rat takes the cheese

   The final verse:
   The cheese stands alone.
   The cheese stands alone.
   Hi-ho the dairy-o
   The cheese stands alone.

Fingerplays:

THIS LITTLE COW

This little cow eats grass.
   (hold up one hand, fingers erect, bend
   down one finger)
This little cow eats hay.
   (bend down another finger)
This little cow drinks water.
   (bend down another finger)
And this little cow does nothing.
   (bend down another finger)
But lie and sleep all day.

IF I WERE A HORSE

If I were a horse, I'd gallop all around.
  (slap thighs and gallop in a circle)
I'd shake my head and say "Neigh, neigh."
  (shake head)
I'd prance and gallop all over town.

THIS LITTLE PIG

This little pig went to market.
  (point to one finger at a time)
This little pig stayed home.
This little pig had roast beef.
This little pig had none.
This little pig cried "Wee, wee, wee"
And ran all the way home.

EIGHT BABY PIGS

Two mother pigs lived in a pen.
  (thumbs)
Each had four babies and that made ten.
  (fingers of both hands)
These four babies were black and white.
  (fingers of one hand)
These four babies were black as night.
  (fingers of other hand)
All eight babies loved to play
  (wiggle fingers)
And they rolled in the mud all day!
  (roll hands)

THE FARM

The cows on the farm go, "Moo-oo, moo-oo;"
The rooster cries, "Cock-a-doodle-doo;"
The big brown horse goes, "Neigh, neigh;"
The little lamb says, "Baa" when he
wants to play.
The little chick goes, "Peep, peep, peep;"
The cat says, "Meow" when it's not asleep;
The pig says, "Oink" when they want to eat.
And we all say "Hello" when our friends
we meet.

Source of fingerplays: *Finger Frolics: Fingerplays for Young Children.* Cromwell Hibner, and Faitel (Partner Press, 1983).

Science:

1. Sheep Wool

Place various types of wool on a table for the children to observe. Included may be wool clippings, lanolin, dyed yarn, yarn spun into thread, wool cloth, wool articles such as mittens and socks.

2. Feathers

Examine various types of feathers. Use a magnifying glass. Discuss their purposes such as keeping animals warm and helping ducks to float on water. Add the feathers to the water table to see if they float. Discuss why they float.

3. Milk Tasting

Plan a milk tasting party. To do this, taste and compare the following types of milk products: cow milk, goat milk, cream, skimmed milk, whole milk, cottage cheese, sour cream, butter, margarine, buttermilk.

4. Eggs

Taste different kinds of eggs. Let children choose from scrambled, pouched, deviled, hard-boiled and fried. This could also be integrated as part of the breakfast menu.

5. Cheese Types

Observe, taste and compare different kinds of cheese. Examples include swiss, cheddar, colby, cottage cheese and cheese curds.

6. Egg Hatching

If possible, contact a hatchery to borrow an incubator. Watch the eggs hatch in the classroom.

7. Feels from the Farm

Construct a feely box containing farm items. Examples may include an ear of corn, hay, sheep wool, a turkey feather, hard boiled egg, etc.

Dramatic Play:

1. Farmer

Clothes and props for a farmer can be placed in the dramatic play area. Include items such as hats, scarves, overalls, boots, etc.

2. Saddle

A horse saddle can be placed on a bench in the classroom. The children can take turns sitting on it, pretending they are riding a horse.

3. Barn

A barn and plastic animals can be added to the classroom. The children can use blocks as accessories to make pens, cages, etc.

4. Veterinarian

Collect materials to make a veterinarian prop box. Stuffed animals can be used as patients.

Arts and Crafts:

1. Yarn Collage

Provide the children with several types and lengths of yarn. Include clipped yarn, yarn fluffs, frayed yarn in several different colors along with paper.

2. Texture Collage

On the art table provide several colors, shapes and types of fabric for creating a texture collage during the self-selected activity period for the children.

3. Grain and Seed Collage

Corn, wheat, hay, oats, barley, grains that farm animals eat, can be placed on the art table. Paper and glue or paste should also be provided.

4. Buttermilk Chalk Picture

Brush a piece of cardboard with 2 to 3 tablespoons of buttermilk or dip chalk in buttermilk. Create designs using colored chalk as a tool.

5. Farm Animal Mobiles

Cut pictures of farm aniamls from magazines and hang them from hangers or branches.

6. Eggshell Collages

Collect eggshells and crush into pieces. Place the eggshells in the art area for the children to glue on paper. Let dry. If desired, the shells can be painted. If preparation time is available, eggshells can be dyed with food coloring by teacher prior to the activity.

7. Sponge Prints

Cut farm animal shapes out of sponges. If a pattern is needed, cut out of a coloring book. Once cut, the sponge forms can be dipped into a pan of thick tempera paint and used as a tool to apply a design.

Sensory:

Add to the Sensory Table:

* different types of grain such as oats, wheat, barley, corn and measuring devices
* wool and feathers
* sand and plastic farm animals
* provide materials to make a barnyard. Include soil, hay, farm animals, barns, farm equipment toys, etc.

Large Muscle:

1. Trikes

During outdoor play, encourage children to use trikes and wagons for hauling.

2. Barn

Construct a large barn out of a large cardboard box. Let all the children help paint it outdoors. When dry, the children can play in it.

Field Trips/Resource People:

1. Farmer

Invite a farmer to talk to the children. If possible, have him bring a smaller farm animal for the children to touch and observe.

2. The Farm

Visit a farm. Observe the animals and machinery.

3. Milk Station

Visit a milk station if there is one in your area.

4. Grocery Store

Visit the dairy section of a grocery store. Look for dairy products.

Math:

1. Puzzles

Laminate several pictures of farm animals; coloring books are a good source. Cut the pictures into puzzles for the children.

2. Grouping and Sorting

Collect plastic farm animals. Place in a basket and let the children sort them according to size, color, where they live, how they move, etc.

Social Studies:

Farm Animal of the Day

Throughout the week let children take care of and watch baby farm animals. Suggestions include a piglet, chicks, small ducks, rabbit or lamb.

Group Time (games, language):

1. "Duck, Duck, Goose"

Sit the children in a circle. Then choose one child to be "it." This child goes around the circle and touches each of the other children on the shoulder and says "Duck, Duck, Goose." The child who is tapped as "goose" gets up and chases the other child around the circle. The first child who returns back to the empty spot sits down and the other child proceeds with the game of tapping children on the shoulder until someone else is tapped as the goose.

2. Thank You

Write a thank you note as a follow up activity after a field trip or a visit from a resource person.

Miscellaneous:

Transition

During transition time encourage the children to imitate different farm animals. They may gallop like a horse, hop like a bunny, waddle like a duck, move like a snake, etc.

Cooking:

1. Make Butter

Fill baby food jars half full with whipping cream. Allow the children to take turns shaking the jars until the cream separates. First it will appear like whipping cream, then like overwhipped cream and finally an obvious separation will occur. Then pour off liquid and taste. Wash the butter in cold water in a bowl several times. Drain off milky liquid each time. Taste and then wash again until nearly clear. Work the butter in the water with a wooden spoon as you wash. Add salt to taste. Let the children spread the butter on crackers or bread.

2. Make Cottage Cheese

Heat one quart of milk until lukewarm. Dissolve one rennet tablet in a small amount of the milk. Stir the rennet mixture into remaining milk. Let the mixture stand in a warm place until set. Drain the mixture through a strainer lined with cheesecloth. Bring the corners of the cloth together and squeeze or drain the mixture. Rinse the mixture with cold water and drain again. Add a small amount of butter and salt.

3. Purple Cow Drink Mix

1/2 gallon milk
1/2 gallon grape juice
6 ice cubes
blender

Mix the ingredients in a blender for one minute. Drink. Enjoy! This recipe will serve approximately 20 children.

4. Animal Crackers

Serve animal crackers and peanut butter for snack.

5. Hungry Cheese Spread

1 8-ounce goat cheese or 8-ounce soft
  cream cheese
1/4 cup soft butter
1 teaspoon salt
1 tablespoon paprika
1 teaspoon dry mustard
1 1/2 tablespoons caraway seeds

Blend the cheese and butter in the mixing bowl. Add the remaining ingredients. Mix them well. Put the blended cheese into a small serving bowl. Chill in the refrigerator for at least 30 minutes before serving.

Source: *Many Hands Cooking*. Terry Touff Cooper and Marilyn Ratner. (New York: Thomas Y. Crowell Company, 1974).

6. Corn Bread

2 cups cornmeal
1 teaspoon salt
1/2 teaspoon baking soda
1 1/2 teaspoons baking powder
1 tablespoon sugar
2 eggs
1 1/2 cups buttermilk
1/4 cup cooking oil

Heat oven to 400 degrees. Sift cornmeal, salt, soda, baking powder and sugar into a bowl. Stir in unbeaten eggs, buttermilk and cooking oil until all ingredients are mixed. Pour the batter into a greased 9 inch x 9 inch pan or corn stick pans. Bake for 30 minutes until lightly browned.

Record:

The following record can be found in preschool educational catalogs:

Look At My World. "My Pony Stop and Go." Kathy Lecinski Poelker, Look at Me Company.

Books and Stories:

The following books and stories can be used to complement the theme:

1. **Big Red Barn.** Margaret W. Brown. (Reading, MA: Addison-Wesley, 1956).

2. **The Big Book of Farm Animals.** Jane Carruth. (New York: P. Dalton and Company, Inc., 1973).

3. **The Milk Makers.** Gail Gibbons. (New York: Macmillan, 1985).

4. **The New Baby.** Edith Newlin Chase. (New York: Scholastic, 1984).

5. **Baby Animals on the Farm.** Rebecca Heller. (New York: Western Publishing Company, Inc., 1981).

6. **Brown Cow Farm.** Dahlov Ipcar. (New York: Doubleday and Company, Inc., 1959).

7. **What Do the Animals Say?** Grace Skaar. (New York: Young Scott Books, 1968).

8. **Good Morning Farm.** Betty Ren Wright. (New York: Western Publishing Company, 1973).

9. **Wake Up, Farm!** Alvin R. Tresselt. (New York: Lothrop, Lee and Shephard, 1949).

10. **Don't Count Your Chicks.** Ingri Aulaire. (New York: Doubleday Doran and Company, 1951).

11. **Picture Book Farm.** Lucy Hawkinson. (Chicago: Childrens Press, 1971).

12. **Farmer Brown.** Dick Brura. (Los Angeles: Price, Stern, Sloan, 1984).

13. **Farm Alphabet Book.** Jane Miller. (New York: Scholastic, 1981).

14. **Animals That Give People Milk.** Terrance W. McCabe and Harley W. Mitchell. (Chicago: National Dairy Council, 1970).

15. **Baby Farm Animals.** Merrill Windsor. (Washington, DC: National Geographic Society, 1984).

16. **A Visit to the Dairy Farm.** Sandra Ziegler. (Chicago: Childrens Press, 1987).

Puzzles:

The following puzzles can be found in preschool educational catalogs:

1. **"Farm Animals"** Judy/Instructo.

2. **"Barn"** Judy/Instructo.

3. **"Cow"** Judy/Instructo.

4. **"Horse"** Judy/Instructo.

5. **"Rooster"** Judy/Instructo.

6. **"Chickens"** Judy/Instructo.

7. **"Pig and Piglets"** Judy/Instructo.

8. **"Horse and Foal"** Judy/Instructo.

9. **"Cow and Calf"** Judy/Instructo.

FEELINGS

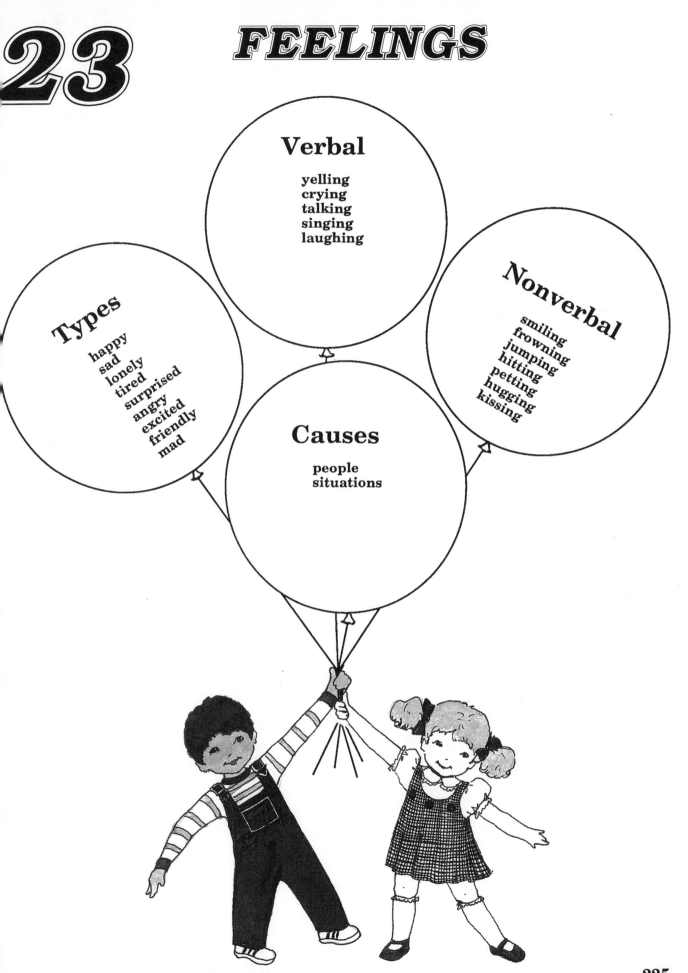

Verbal

yelling
crying
talking
singing
laughing

Nonverbal

smiling
frowning
jumping
hitting
petting
hugging
kissing

Types

happy
sad
lonely
tired
surprised
angry
excited
friendly
mad

Causes

people
situations

Theme Goals:

Through participating in the experiences provided in this theme, the children may learn:

1. Types of feelings.

2. Verbal expressions of feelings.

3. Nonverbal expression of feelings.

4. Causes for our feelings.

Concepts for the Children to Learn:

1. Everyone has feelings.

2. Feelings show how we feel.

3. Feelings change.

4. Happy, sad, excited and surprised are types of feelings.

5. Happy people usually smile.

6. Sad people sometimes cry.

Vocabulary:

1. **feelings**—expressed emotions.

2. **happy**—a feeling of being glad.

3. **smile**—a facial expression of pleasure or happiness.

4. **surprise**—a feeling from something unexpected.

5. **sad**—the feeling of being hurt or unhappy.

6. **afraid**—the feeling of being unsure of or frightened about something.

Bulletin Board

The purpose of this bulletin board is to help the children become aware of feelings, as well as recognize their printed names. Prepare individual name cards for each child. Then prepare different expression faces such as happy, sad and mad. Staple faces to top of bulletin board. See the illustration for an example. If available, magnetic strips may be added to the bulletin board under faces and pieces affixed to name cards, or push pins may be placed on the board and holes punched in name cards. The children may place their names under the face they decide they feel as they arrive at school. Later during large group time, the board can be reviewed to see if any of the children's feelings have changed.

How do you feel?

☺ happy   ☹ sad   😠 mad

Beth   Tomas   Ted   Jane
Derek Marie
Bruce

Elyse   Meghan   Pete   Jenny   Caryn
Sylvia   Steven   Morgan
Cathy   Lauren   Stacey   Kelly

Parent Letter

Dear Parents,

This week we will be starting a unit on emotions and feelings. Throughout each day, the children experience many feelings ranging from happiness to sadness. The purpose of this unit is to have the children develop an understanding of feelings. Feelings are something we all share, and feelings are acceptable. We will also be exploring ways of expressing different feelings.

At School This Week

Some of the learning experiences planned for this week include:

* listening and discussing the book *Alexander and the Terrible, Horrible, No Good, Very Bad, Day* by Judith Viorst.
* singing songs about our feelings.
* drawing and painting to various types of music.

Our Special Visitor

"Clancy the Clown" will be visiting the children on Thursday at 3:00 p.m. The children are all looking forward to this special visitor. You are encouraged to join us and share their excitement.

At Home

To help your child identify situations that elicit feelings, have your child cut or tear pictures from discarded magazines that depict events or situations that make your child feel happy or sad. These pictures can then be glued or pasted on paper to create a feelings collage.

Talking with your child about your feelings will encourage parent-child communication. Tell your child what things make you feel various ways. Then ask your child to share some feelings.

Have a Happy Week!

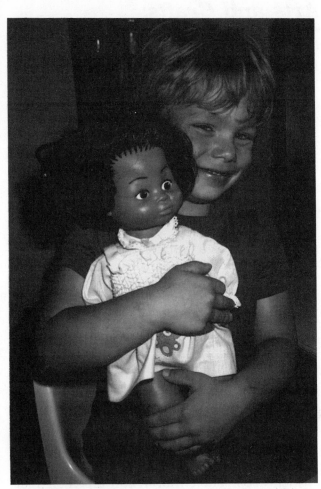

FIGURE 23 Enjoyment is just one of many feelings.

Music:

1. **"Feelings"**
(Sing to the tune of "Twinkle, Twinkle Little Star")

I have feelings.
You do, too
Let's all sing about a few.

I am happy.
   (smile)
I am sad.
   (frown)
I get scared.
   (wrap arms around self)
I get mad.
   (make a fist and shake it)

I am proud of being me.
   (hands on hips)
That's a feeling too you see.

I have feelings.
   (point to self)
You do, too.
   (point to someone else)
We just sang about a few.

2. **"If You're Happy and You Know It"**
(traditional)

If you're happy and you know it
Clap your hands.
   (clap twice)
If you're happy and you know it
Clap your hands.
   (clap twice)
If you're happy and you know it
Then your face will surely show it.
If you're happy and you know it
Clap your hands.
   (clap twice)

For additional verses, change the emotions and actions.

Fingerplays:

FEELINGS

Smile when you're happy.
Cry when you are sad.
Giggle if it's funny.
Get angry if you're mad.

Source: *Everyday Circle Times*. Dick Wilems.

I LOOKED INSIDE MY LOOKING GLASS

I looked inside my looking glass
To see what I could see.
It looks like I'm happy today,
Because that smiling face is me.

STAND UP TALL

Stand up tall
Hands in the air.
Now sit down
In your chair.
Clap your hands
And make a frown.
Smile and smile.
Hop like a clown.

Science:

1. Sound Tape

Tape various noises that express emotions; suggestions include sounds such as laughter, cheering, growling, shrieking, crying, etc. Play these sounds for the children letting them identify the emotion. They may also want to act out the emotion.

2. Communication Without Words

Hang a large screen or sheet with a bright light behind it. The children can go behind the screen and act out various emotions. Other children guess how they are feeling.

3. How Does It Feel?

Add various pieces of textured materials to the science table. Include materials such as soft fur, sandpaper, rocks, and cotton. Encourage the children to touch each object and explain how it feels.

Dramatic Play:

1. Flower Shop

Plastic flowers, vases and wrapping paper can be placed in the dramatic play area. Make a sign that says "Flower Shop." The children may want to arrange, sell, deliver and receive flowers from one another.

2. Post Office

Collect discarded greeting cards and envelopes. The children can stamp and deliver the cards to one another.

3. Puppet Center

A puppet center can be added to the dramatic play area. Include a variety of puppets and a stage.

Arts and Crafts:

1. Drawing to Music

Play various types of music including jazz, classical and rock and let the children draw during the self-selected activity period. Different tunes and melodies might make us feel a certain way.

2. Playdough

Playdough is a wonderful way to vent feelings. Prepare several types and let the children feel the different textures. Color each type a different color. Add a scent to one and to another add a textured material such as sawdust, rice or sand. A list of playdoughs can be found later in this theme.

3. Footprints

Mix tempera paint. Pour the paint into a shallow jelly roll pan approximately 1/4 inch deep. The children can dip their feet into the pan. After this, they can step directly onto paper. Using their feet as an application tool, footsteps can be made. This activity actually could be used to create a mural which could be hung the center's lobby.

Sensory:

Texture Feelings

Various textures can create feelings. Let the children express their feelings by adding the following to the sensory table:

* cotton
* water (warm or with ice)
* black water
* blue water
* sand
* pebbles
* dirt with scoops
* plastic worms with water

Large Muscle:

1. Mirrors

The children should sit as pairs facing each other. Select one child to make a "feeling face" at the partner. Let the other child guess what feeling it is. A variation of this activity would be to have partners face each other. When one child smiles, the partner is to imitate his feelings.

2. Simon Says

Play Simon Says using emotions:
"Simon Says walk in a circle feeling happy..."
"Simon Says walk in a circle feeling sad..."

Field Trips/Resource People:

1. A Clown

Invite a clown to the center. You may ask the clown to dress and apply makeup for the children. After the clown leaves provide makeup for the children.

2. Musician

Invite a musician to play a variety of music for the children to express feelings.

3. Florist

Invite a florist to visit your classroom and show how flowers are arranged. Talk about why people send flowers. If convenient the children could visit the florist, touring the greenhouses.

Math:

Face Match

Cut faces of people from magazines, and collect two small boxes. On one shoebox draw a happy face. On the other box, draw a sad face. The children can sort the pictures accordingly.

Social Studies:

Pictures

Share pictures of individuals engaged in different occupations such as doctors, firefighters, beauticians, florists, nurses, bakers, etc. Discuss how these individuals help us and how they make us feel.

Group Time (games, language):

Happy Feeling

Discuss happiness. Ask each child one thing that makes him happy. Record each answer on a "Happiness Chart." Post the chart for the parents to observe as they pick up their children.

Cooking:

1. Happy Rolls

1 package of fast-rising dry yeast
1 cup warm water
1/3 cup sugar
1/3 cup cooking oil
3 cups flour
a dash of salt

Measure the warm water and pour it into a bowl. Sprinkle the yeast on top of the water. Let the yeast settle into the water. Mix all of the ingredients in a large bowl. Place the dough on a floured board to knead it. Demonstrate how to knead, letting each of the children take turns kneading the bread. This is a wonderful activity to work through emotions. After kneading it for about 10 minutes, put the ball of dough into a greased bowl. If kneaded sufficiently, the top of the dough should have blisters on it. Cover the bowl and put in the sun or near heat. Let it rise for about an hour or until doubled. Take the dough out of the bowl. Punch it down, knead for several more minutes and then divide the dough into 12 to 15 pieces. Roll each piece of dough into a ball. Place each ball on a greased cookie sheet. Let the dough rise again until doubled. Bake at 450 degrees for 10 to 12 minutes. A happy face can be drawn on the roll with frosting.

2. Berry "Happy" Shake—Finland

10 fresh strawberries or 6 tablespoons sliced strawberries in syrup, thawed
2 cups cold milk
1 1/2 tablespoons sugar or honey

Wash the strawberries (if fresh) and cut out the stems. Cut the strawberries into small pieces. (If you are using frozen strawberries, drain the syrup into a small bowl or cup and save it. Pour the milk into the mixing bowl. Add the strawberries. If you are using fresh strawberries, add the sugar or honey. If you are using frozen strawberries, add 3 tablespoons of the strawberry syrup instead of sugar. Beat with the egg beater for 1 minute. Pour the drink into the glasses.

Source: *Many Hands Cooking.* Terry Touff Cooper and Marilyn Ratner. (New York: Thomas Y. Crowell Company, 1974).

3. Danish Smile Berry Pudding

1 10-ounce package frozen raspberries, thawed
1 10-ounce package frozen strawberries, thawed
1/4 cup cornstarch
2 tablespoons sugar
1/2 cup cold water
1 tablespoon lemon juice
slivered almonds

Puree berries in blender or press through sieve. Mix cornstarch and sugar in 1 1/2-quart saucepan. Gradually stir in water; add puree. Heat to boiling, stirring constantly. Boil and stir 1 minute. Remove from heat. Stir in lemon juice. Pour into dessert dishes or serving bowl. Cover and refrigerate at least 2 hours. Sprinkle with almonds; serve with half-and-half if desired. Makes 6 servings.

Source: *Betty Crocker's International Cookbook.* (New York: Random House, 1980).

RECIPES FOR DOUGHS AND CLAYS

Clay Dough

3 cups flour
3 cups salt
3 tablespoons alum

Combine ingredients and slowly add water, a little at a time. Mix well with spoon. As mixture thickens, continue mixing with your hands until it has the feel of clay. If it feels too dry, add more water. If it is too sticky, add equal parts of flour and salt.

Play Dough

2 cups flour
1 cup salt
1 cup hot water
2 tablespoons cooking oil
4 teaspoons cream of tartar
food coloring

Mix well. Knead until smooth. This dough may be kept in a plastic bag or covered container and used again. If it gets sticky, more flour may be added.

Favorite Playdough

Combine and boil until dissolved:

2 cups water
1/2 cup salt
food coloring or tempera paint

Mix in while very hot:

2 tablespoons cooking oil
2 tablespoons alum
2 cups flour

Knead (approximately 5 minutes) until smooth. Store in covered airtight containers.

Oatmeal Dough

2 cups oatmeal
1 cup flour
1/2 cup water

Combine ingredients. Knead well. This dough has a very different texture, is easily manipulated, and looks different. Finished projects can be painted when dry.

Baker's Clay #1

1 cup cornstarch
2 cups baking soda
1 1/2 cups cold water

Combine ingredients. Stir until smooth. Cook over medium heat, stirring constantly until mixture reaches the consistency of slightly dry mashed potatoes.

Turn out onto plate or bowl, covering with damp cloth. When cool enough to handle, knead thoroughly until smooth and pliable on cornstarch-covered surface.

Store in tightly closed plastic bag or covered container.

Baker's Clay #2

4 cups flour
1 1/2 cups water
1 cup salt

Combine ingredients. Mix well. Knead 5 to 10 minutes. Roll out to 1/4-inch thickness. Cut with decorative cookie cutters or with a

knife. Make a hole at the top.

Bake at 250 degrees for 2 hours or until hard. When cool, paint with tempera paint and spray with clear varnish or paint with acrylic paint.

Cloud Dough

3 cups flour
1 cup oil
scent (oil of peppermint, wintergreen, lemon, etc.)
food coloring

Combine ingredients. Add water until easily manipulated (about 1/2 cup).

Sawdust Dough

2 cups sawdust
3 cups flour
1 cup salt

Combine ingredients. Add water as needed. This dough becomes very hard and is not easily broken. It is good to use for making objects and figures which one desires to keep.

Salt Dough

4 cups salt
1 cup cornstarch

Combine with sufficient water to form a paste. Cook over medium heat, stirring constantly.

Peanut Butter Playdough

2 1/2 cups peanut butter
2 tablespoons honey
2 cups powdered milk

Mix well with very clean hands. Keep adding powdered milk until the dough feels soft, not sticky. This is a dough that can be eaten.

Variations:

1. Cocoa or carob powder can be added for chocolate flavor.
2. Raisins, miniature marshmallows, or chopped peanuts may be added or used to decorate finished shapes.

Each child can be given dough to manipulate and then eat.

Cooked Clay Dough

1 cup flour
1/2 cup cornstarch
4 cups water
1 cup salt
3 or 4 pounds flour
coloring if desired

Stir slowly and be patient with this recipe. Blend the flour and cornstarch with cold water. Add salt to the water and boil. Pour the boiling salt and water solution into the flour and cornstarch paste and cook over hot water until clear. Add the flour and coloring to the cooked solution and knead. After the clay has been in use, if too moist, add flour; if dry, add water. Keep in covered container. Wrap dough with damp cloth or towel. This dough has a very nice texture and is very popular with all age groups. May be kept 2 or 3 weeks.

Play Dough

5 cups flour
2 cups salt
4 tablespoons cooking oil
add water to right
consistency

Powdered tempera may be added in with flour or food coloring may be added to finished dough. This dough may be kept in plastic bag or covered container for approximately 2 to 4 weeks. It is better used as playdough rather than leaving objects to harden.

Used Coffee Grounds

2 cups used coffee grounds

1/2 cup salt
1 1/2 cups oatmeal

Combine ingredients and add enough water to moisten. Children like to roll, pack and pat this mixture. It has a very different feel and look, but it's not good for finished products. It has a very nice texture.

Mud Dough

2 cups mud
2 cups sand
1/2 cup salt

Combine ingredients and add enough water to make pliable. Children like to work with this mixture. It has a nice texture and is easy to use. This cannot be picked up to save for finished products easily. It can be used for rolling and cutouts.

Soap Modeling

2 cups soap flakes

Add enough water to moisten and whip until

consistency to mold. Use soap such as Ivory Flakes, Dreft, Lux, etc. Mixture will have very slight flaky appearance when it can be molded. It is very enjoyable with all age groups and is easy to work. Also, the texture is very different from other materials ordinarily used for molding. It may be put up to dry, but articles are very slow to dry.

Soap and Sawdust

1 cup whipped soap
1 cup sawdust

Mix well together. This gives a very different feel and appearance. It is quite easily molded into different shapes by all age groups. May be used for 2 to 3 days if stored in tight plastic bag.

Records:

The following records can be found in preschool educational catalogs:

1. **Tickles You.** Gary and Bill Rosenshontz

2. **Happy Hour.** Hap Palmer

Books and Stories:

The following books and stories can be used to complement the theme:

1. **When the New Baby Comes I'm Moving Out.** Martha Alexander. (New York: The Dial Press, 1979).

2. **Where Is Daddy?** Beth Goff. (Boston: Beacon Press, 1969).

3. **The Happy Day.** Ruth Krouss. (New York: Harper and Row, 1968).

4. **Benjie on His Own.** Joan M. Lexau. (New York: The Dial Press, 1970).

5. **Frog and Toad are Friends.** Arnold Lobel. (New York: Harper and Row, 1970).

6. **New Day.** C.L. Keyworth. (New York: Morrow, 1986).

7. **Sometimes I Like To Cry.** Elizabeth and Henry Stanton. (Chicago: Albert Whitman and Company, 1978).

8. **David's Waiting Day.** Bernadette Watts. (New York: Prentice-Hall, Inc., 1977).

9. **Jack is Glad, Jack is Sad.** Charlotte Steiner. (New York: Alfred A. Knopf, 1962).

10. **Alexander and the Terrible, Horrible, No Good, Very Bad Day.** Judith Viorst. (New York: Atheneum, 1972).

11. **It's Mine—A Fable.** Leo Lionni. (New York: Alfred A. Knopf, 1986).

12. **Things I Hate.** Harriet Wittels and Joan Greisiman. (New York: Behavioral Publication, 1973).

13. **Ira Sleeps Over.** Bernard Waber. (New York: Scholastic, 1972).

14. **Love.** Jane Blek Mancure. (Chicago: Childrens Press, 1980).

15. **Kindness.** Jane Belk Mancure. (Chicago: Childrens Press, 1980).

16. **Caring.** Jane Belk Mancure. (Chicago: Childrens Press, 1980).

17. **How Do I Feel?** Norma Simon. (Chicago: Albert Whitman and Company, 1978).

18. **Darlene.** Eloise Greenfield. (New York: Methuen, 1980).

Puzzles:

The following puzzles can be found in preschool educational catalogs:

1. **"Color Balloons"** Judy/Instructo.

2. **"Girl"** Judy/Instructo.

3. **"Boy"** Judy/Instructo.

24 FIRE FIGHTERS

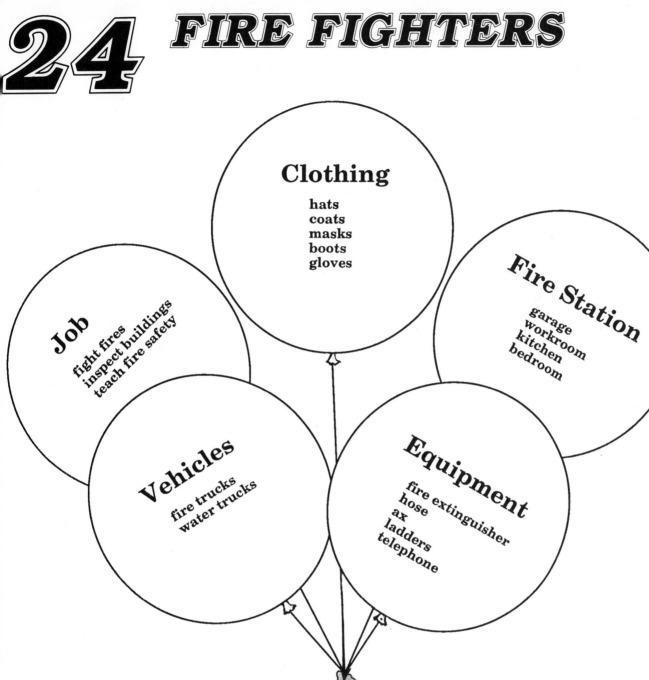

Clothing

hats
coats
masks
boots
gloves

Job

fight fires
inspect buildings
teach fire safety

Fire Station

garage
workroom
kitchen
bedroom

Vehicles

fire trucks
water trucks

Equipment

fire extinguisher
hose
ax
ladders
telephone

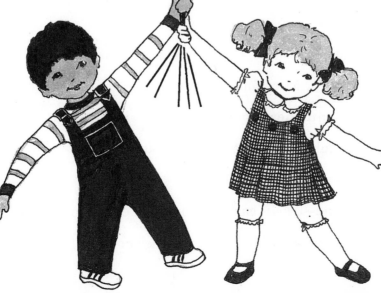

Theme Goals:

Through participating in the experiences provided by this theme, the children may learn:

1. The firefighter's job.

2. Firefighter's clothing.

3. Vehicles used by firefighters.

4. Firefighting equipment.

5. Areas inside of a fire station.

Concepts for the Children to Learn:

1. Men and women who fight fires are called firefighters.

2. Firefighters help keep our community safe.

3. Firefighters wear special hats and clothing.

4. The fire station has a garage, kitchen, workroom and sleeping rooms.

5. The fire station has a special telephone number.

6. Ladders and water hoses are needed to fight fires.

7. Fire and water trucks are driven to fires.

8. Firefighters check buildings to make sure they are safe.

9. Firefighters teach us fire safety.

10. Fire extinguishers can be used to put out small fires.

11. Fire drills teach us what to do in case of a fire.

Vocabulary:

1. **fire alarm**—a sound warning people about fire.

2. **fire drill**—practice for teaching people what to do in case of a fire.

3. **fire extinguisher**—equipment that puts out fires.

4. **hose**—a tube that water flows through.

5. **helmet**—a protective hat.

6. **fire engine**—trucks carrying tools and equipment needed to fight fires.

7. **fire station**—a building that provides housing for fire fighters and fire trucks.

Bulletin Board

The purpose of this bulletin board is to develop an awareness of clothing worn by firefighters and to reinforce color matching skills. From tagboard construct five firefighter hats. Color each hat a different color. Then construct five firefighter boots from tagboard. Color coordinate boots to match the hats. Laminate all of the pieces. Staple hats in two rows across the top of the bulletin board as illustrated. Staple boots in a row across the bottom of the bulletin board. Affix matching yarn to each hat. Children can match each hat to its corresponding colored boot by winding the string around a push pin in the top of the boot.

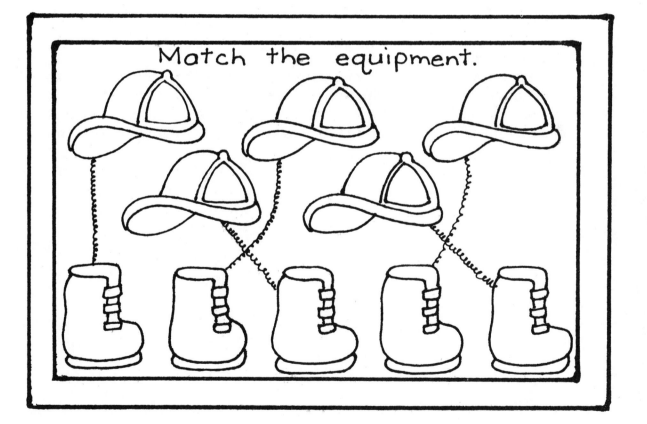

Parent Letter

Dear Parents,

Because next week is Fire Prevention Week, we have decided that it would be fun and educational to focus on some very important community helpers—firefighters. The children will become more aware of the role of the firefighter, clothing worm by firefighters and parts of the fire station. We will also be talking about how to use the telephone to call the emergency fire number.

At School This Week

We have many activities planned for the week! On Monday, we will paint a large box to create our own fire engine to use during the week in the dramatic play area. On Tuesday, a real fire engine will visit the parking lot, so the children can see how many tools firefighters need to take along on the job. We'll also be making fire helmets, and practicing our fire drill procedures.

At Home

To ensure your family's safety, talk with your child about what would happen in the event of a fire at your house. You can do this calmly, without frightening your child. Practice taking a fire escape route from the child's bedroom, the playroom, kitchen and other rooms of your house. Establish a meeting place so that family members can go to the same location in the event of a fire.

Have a good week!

The cars move to clear the way.
The children run and yell.
  (run and yell)
The fire fighters roll out the heavy hose.
  (pretend to roll out hose)
They put up ladders with a bang.
  (pretend to climb ladders)
They fight the fire and then start back.
And the bell goes "clang clang clang."
  (make soft, slow bell noises that fade
  out)

TEN BRAVE FIREFIGHTERS

Ten brave firefighters sleeping in a row.
  (fingers curled to make sleeping men)
Ding, dong, goes the bell
  (pull down on the bell cord)
And down the pole they go.
  (with fists together make hands slide
  down the pole)
Off on the engine, oh, oh, oh!
  (pretend you are steering the fire engine
  very fast)
Using the big hose, so, so, so.
  (make a nozzle with fist to use hose)
When all the fire's out, home so slow.
Back to bed, all in a row.
  (curl all fingers again for sleeping men)

Source: Adapted from *Finger Frolics*. Liz
Cromwell and Dixie Hibner. (Mt. Ranier,
MD: Gryphon House, 1976).

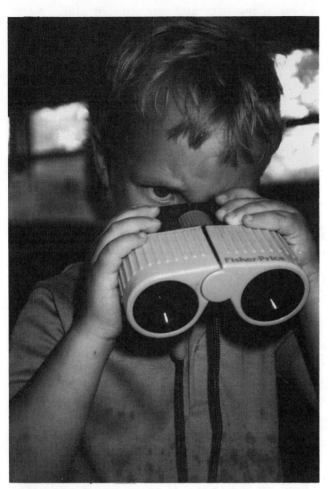

**FIGURE 24 Spotting fires is the job of
Forest Rangers.**

Music:

"Down By the Station"

Down by the station early in the morning
See the great big fire trucks all in a row.
Hear the jangly fire bell sound a loud
alarm now—
Chug chug, clang clang, off we go!

Fingerplays:

THE FIRE TRUCK

The big red fire truck rushes down the
street.
"Clang clang clang" goes the bell.
  (make bell and siren noises.)

Dramatic Play:

1. Firefighters

Place firefighting clothes such as hats,
boots, coats for children to wear.
Sometimes fire station personnel will
allow schools to borrow some of their
clothing and equipment. Also provide a
bell to use as an alarm. A vacuum cleaner
hose or a length of garden hose can be included to represent a water hose to extend
play.

2. Fire Truck

A fire truck can be cut from a cardboard refrigerator box. The children may want to paint the box yellow or red. A steering wheel and chairs may be added.

Art and Crafts:

1. Firefighters' Hats

Provide materials for the children to make fire hats. The hats can be decorated with foil, crayons or paint. The emergency number 911 may be printed on the crown.

2. Charcoal Drawings

Provide real charcoal at the easels to be used as an application tool.

3. Crayon Melting

Place waxed crayons and paper on the art table for the children to create a design during self-initiated or self-directed play. Place a clean sheet of paper over the picture. Apply a warm iron. Show the children the effect of heat. This activity needs to be carefully supervised. The caption "crayon melting" may be printed on a bulletin board. On the board place the children's pictures, identifying each by name in the upper left hand corner.

Sensory:

1. Fill the sensory table with water. Provide cups and rubber tubing to resemble hoses and funnels.

2. Place sand in the sensory table. Add fire engines, firefighter dolls and popsicle sticks to make fences and blocks to make buildings or houses.

Large Muscle:

1. Firefighter's Workout

Lead children in a firefighter's workout. Do exercises like jumping jacks, knee bends, leg lifts and running in place. Ask children why they think firefighters need to be in good physical condition for their jobs.

2. Obstacle Course

Make an obstacle course. Let children follow a string or piece of tape under chairs or tables, over steps and across ladders. This activity can be planned for indoors or outdoors.

Field Trips/Resource People:

1. Fire Station

Take a trip to a fire station. Observe the clothing worn by firefighters, the building, the vehicles and the tools.

2. Firefighter

Invite a firefighter to bring a fire truck to your school. Ask the firefighter to point out the special features such as the hose, siren, ladders, light and special clothing kept on the truck. If permissable and safe, let the children climb onto the truck.

Math:

1. Sequencing

Cut a piece of rubber tubing into various lengths. The children can sequence the pieces from shortest to longest.

2. Emergency Number

Contact your local telphone company for trainer telephones to use. If developmentally appropriate, teach the children how to dial a local emergency number.

Social Studies:

1. Safety Rules

Discuss safety rules dealing with fire. Let children generate ideas about safety. Discuss why fire drills are a good idea.

2. Fire Inspection Tour

Tour the classroom or building looking for fire extinguishers, emergency fire alarm boxes and exits.

3. Fire Drill

Schedule a fire drill. Prior to the drill talk to the children about fire drill procedures.

Group Time (games, language):

Language Experience

Review safety rules. Write the rules on a large piece of paper. These rules can also be included in a parent letter as well as posted in the classroom.

Cooking:

Firehouse Baked Beans

Purchase canned baked beans. To the beans, add cut-up hot dogs and extra catsup. Heat and serve for snack.

Records:

The following records can be found in preschool educational catalogs:

1. **Little Firemen.** Young People's Records.

2. **Men Who Come to Our House.** "Let's Be Firemen." Young People's Records.

3. **Look At My World.** "At the Firehouse." Kathy Lecinski Poelker. Look at Me Company.

Books and Stories:

The following books and stories can be used to complement the theme:

1. **The Fire Cat.** Esther Holden Averill. (New York: Harper and Row, 1960).

2. **Safety First-Fire.** Eugene Baker. (New York: Creative Press, 1980).

3. **Country Fireman.** Jerrold Beim. (New York: William Morrow, 1980).

4. **The Little Fireman.** Margaret Brown. (Reading, MA: Addison-Wesley, 1952).

5. **Curious George at the Fire Station.** Margaret Rey and Alan J. Shalleck. (New York: Scholastic, 1985).

6. **The Little Fire Engine.** Graham Greene. (New York: Doubleday and Company, 1973).

7. **The Fireman.** William Kotzwinkel. (New York: Pantheon Books, 1969).

8. **Your World: Let's Visit the Fire Station.** Billy N. Pope. (Dallas: Taylor Publishing Company, 1966).

9. **Careers with the Fire Department.** Johanna Pottersen. (New York: Lerner, 1975).

10. **Firegirl.** Gibson Rich. (Old Westbury, NY: Feminist Press, 1972).

11. **What It's Like to be a Fireman.** Arthur Shay. (New York: Reilly and Lee, 1971).

12. **The Big Book of Real Fire Engines.** George J. Zaffo. (New York: Grosset and Dunlap, 1958).

13. **Fire.** Marie Rius. (Woodbury, NY: Barron's, 1985).

Puzzles:

The following puzzles are listed in preschool educational catalogs.

1. **"Traffic"** Childcraft Knob Puzzles.

2. **"Fire Engine"** Childcraft.

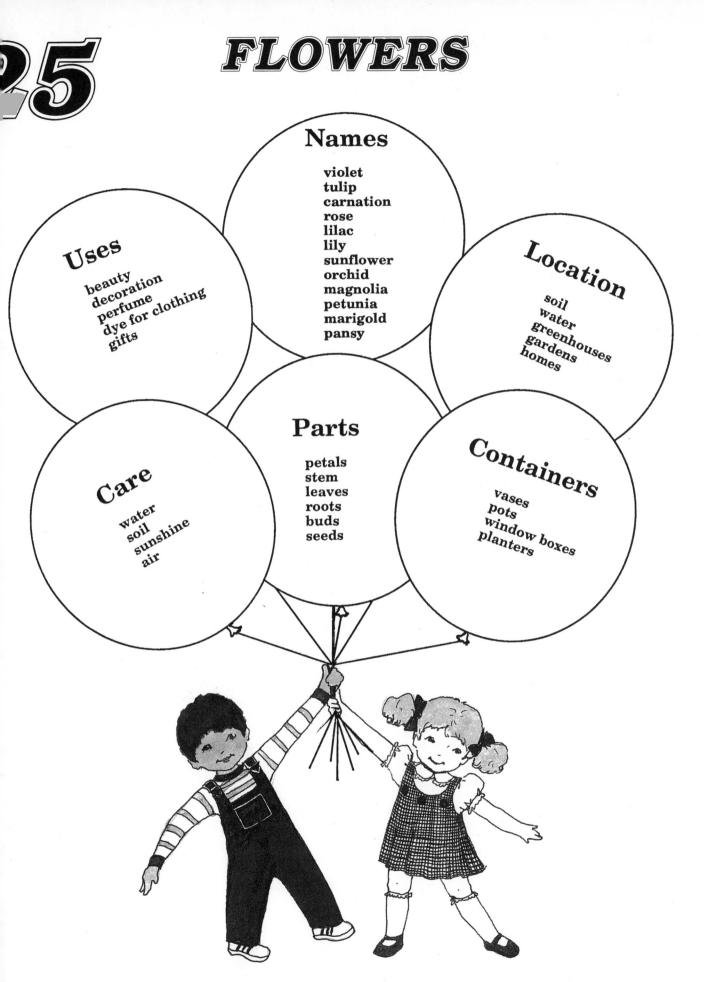

FLOWERS

25

Names
- violet
- tulip
- carnation
- rose
- lilac
- lily
- sunflower
- orchid
- magnolia
- petunia
- marigold
- pansy

Uses
- beauty
- decoration
- perfume
- dye for clothing
- gifts

Location
- soil
- water
- greenhouses
- gardens
- homes

Care
- water
- soil
- sunshine
- air

Parts
- petals
- stem
- leaves
- roots
- buds
- seeds

Containers
- vases
- pots
- window boxes
- planters

Theme Goals:

Through participating in the experiences provided by this theme, the children may learn:

1. Parts of the flower.

2. Flowers have names.

3. Places flowers grow.

4. Uses of flowers.

5. Containers that hold flowers.

6. Care of flowers.

Concepts for the Children to Learn:

1. A flower is a plant.

2. Flowers add beauty to our world.

3. Flowers can be used for decoration.

4. Most flowers have a smell.

5. Vases, pots, window boxes and planters are all flower containers.

6. Flowers need soil, water, sunshine and air to grow.

7. Sometimes flowers are given to people for special reasons, such as holidays, birthdays or if someone goes to the hospital.

Vocabulary:

1. **flower**—part of a plant that blossoms.

2. **petal**—colored part of a flower.

3. **seed**—produces a new plant.

4. **stem**—the trunk of the plant.

5. **leaves**—growth from the stem.

6. **greenhouse**—a glass house for growing plants.

Bulletin Board

The purpose of this bulletin board is to develop color matching skills, as well as foster the correspondence of sets to written numerals. A math skills bulletin board can be created by cutting large numerals out of tagboard. Color each number a different color. Next, create tulips out of tagboard. The number will be dependent upon the maturity of the children. Color one tulip the same color as the numeral one. Color two tulips the same color as the numeral two. Continue with the numerals three and four. The children can hang the appropriate number of tulips on the bulletin board next to each numeral. The children can also match the colored tulips next to the corresponding colored numeral to make this activity self-correcting.

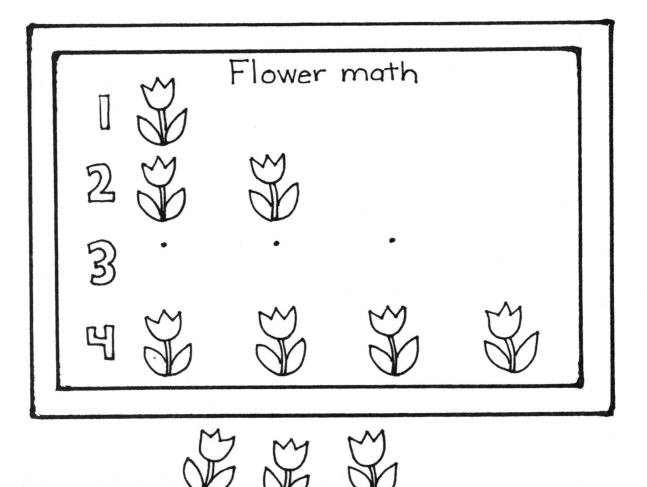

Parent Letter

Dear Parents,

Hello! As spring arrives and all the flowers begin to bloom, we will begin a unit on flowers. Through this unit the children will learn about the care, uses and parts of a flowering plant.

At School This Week

Some of the learning experiences planned to help the children make discoveries about flowers include:

* listening to the story *Dandelion* by Ladislav Svatos.
* observing and measuring the growth of various flowers.
* visiting a floral shop.
* playing a flower beanbag toss game.

At Home

You can integrate the concepts included in this unit into your home in many ways. If you are planning to plant a garden in your yard this spring, let your child help you. It might even be fun to section off a small part of your garden for your child to grow flowers and care for them. Another activity would be to examine the plants and flowers you have growing in your house. Also, let your child send flowers to someone that is special.

To develop language skills, we will be learning this fingerplay in school. Let your child teach it to you.

Daisies

One, two, three, four, five
  (pop up fingers, one at a time)
Yellow daisies all alive.
Here they are all in a row.
  (point to fingers standing)
The sun and the rain will help them grow.
  (make a circle with fingers, flutter fingers for rain)

Have a great week!

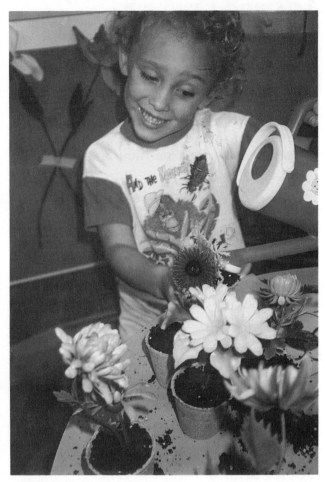

FIGURE 25 Growing flowers is a learning activity.

Music:

"Flowers"
   (Sing to the tune of "Pop! Goes the Weasel")

   All around the forest ground
   There's flowers everywhere.
   There's pink, yellow and purple, too.
   Here's one for you.

Fingerplays:

MY GARDEN

   This is my garden
      (extend one hand forward, palm up)
   I'll rake it with care
      (raking motion with fingers)
   And then some flower seeds
      (planting motion)
   I'll plant in right there.

The sun will shine
   (make circle with hands)
And the rain will fall
   (let fingers flutter down to lap)
And my garden will blossom
   (cup hands together extend upward slowly)
And grow straight and tall.

DAISIES

One, two, three, four, five
   (pop up fingers, one at a time)
Yellow daisies all alive.
Here they are all in a row.
   (point to fingers standing)
The sun and the rain will help them grow.
   (make a circle with fingers, flutter
   fingers for rain)

FLOWER PLAY

If I were a little flower
Sleeping underneath the ground,
   (curl up)
I'd raise my head and grow and grow
   (raise head and begin to grow)
And stretch my arms and grow and grow
   (stretch arms)
And nod my head and say,
   (nod head)
"I'm glad to see you all today."

Science:

1. **Flowers**

   Place a variety of flowers on the science
   table. Encourage the children to compare
   the color, shape, size and smell of each
   flower.

2. **Planting Seeds**

   Plant flower seeds in a styrofoam cup.
   Save the seed packages and mount on a
   piece of tagboard. Place this directly
   behind the containers on the science table.
   Encourage the children to compare their
   plants. When the plant starts growing
   compare the seed packages to the plant
   growth.

3. Carnation

Place a white carnation in a vase containing water with red food coloring added. Watch the tips of the carnation petals gradually change colors. Repeat the activity using other flowers and colors of water.

4. Observing and Weighing Bulbs

Collect flower bulbs and place in the science table. Encourage the children to observe the similarities and differences. A balance scale can also be added.

5. Microscopes

Place petals from a flower under a microscope for the children to observe.

Dramatic Play:

1. Garden

Aprons, small garden tools, a tin of soil, seeds, watering cans, pots and vases can all be provided. Pictures of flowers with names on them can be hung in the classroom.

2. Gardener

Gather materials for a gardener prop box. Include gloves, seed packets, sun hat, hoe, stakes for marking, watering cans, etc.

3. Flower Shop

In the dramatic play area, set up a flower shop complete with plastic flowers, boxes, containers, watering cans, misting bottle and cash register. Artificial corsages would also be a fun addition.

4. Flower Arranging

Artificial flowers and containers can be placed in the dramatic play area. The children can make centerpieces for the lunch table. Also, a centerpiece can be made for the science table, the lobby and the secretary or director.

Arts and Crafts:

1. Muffin Cup Flowers

For younger children, prepare shapes of flowers and leaves. The older children may be able to do this themselves. Attach the stems and leaves to muffin tin liners. Add a small amount of perfume to the flower for interest.

2. Collage

Cut pictures of flowers from seed catalogs. With these flowers, create a collage.

3. Easel

Cut easel paper into flower shapes.

4. Seed Collages

Place a pan containing a variety of seeds in the middle of the art table. In addition, supply glue and paper for the children to form a collage.

5. Egg Carton Flowers

Cut the sections of an egg container apart. Attach pipe cleaners for stems and decorate with watercolor markers.

6. Flower Mobile

Bring in a tree branch and hang from the classroom ceiling. Let the children make flowers and hang them on the branch for decoration.

7. Paper Plate Flowers

Provide snack-sized paper plates, markers, crayons and colored construction paper. The children may use these materials to create a flower.

Sensory:

Add to the sensory table:

* soil and plastic flowers
* water and watering cans

Field Trips/Resource People:

1. Florist

Arrange to visit a local floral shop. Observe the different kinds of flowers. Then watch the florist design a bouquet or corsage.

2. Walk

Walk around the neighborhood observing different types and colors of flowers.

Math:

1. Flower Growth

Prepare sequence cards representing flowers at various stages of growth. Encourage the children to sequence them.

2. Flower Match

Cut pictures of flowers from magazines or seed catalogs. If desired, mount the pictures. The children can match them by kind, size, color and shape.

3. Measuring Seed Growth

Plant several types of seeds. At determined intervals, measure the growth of various plants and flowers. Maintain a chart comparing the growth.

Group Time (games, language):

Hide the Flower

Choose one child to look for the flower. Ask him to cover his eyes. Ask another child to hide a flower. After the flower is hidden and the child returns to the group, instruct the first child to uncover his eyes and find the flower. Clues can be provided. For examples, if the child aproaches the area where the flower is hidden, the remainder of the children can clap their hands.

Cooking:

1. Fruit Candy

Some fruits start with a flower. Discuss which of the following fruits begin with a flower from the ingredients below.

1 pound dried figs
1 pound dried apricots
1/2 pound dates
2 cups walnuts
1/2 cup raisins
1/2 cup coarsely chopped walnuts

Put fruits and 2 cups of walnuts through a food grinder. Mix in the half cup of chopped walnuts and press into a buttered 9 inch x 13 inch pan. Chill and enjoy!

2. China—Egg Flower Soup

Watch an egg turn into a flower. Chinese cooks say that the cooked shreds of egg afloat in this soup look like flower petals.

1 tablespoon cornstarch
2 tablespoons cold water
1 egg
3 cups clear canned chicken broth
1 teaspoon salt
1 teaspoon chopped scallion or parsley
  (optional)

Put the cornstarch into a small bowl and gradually add water, stirring it with a fork until you no longer see any lumps. Break the egg into another small bowl and beat it with the fork. Pour the broth into the saucepan. Bring it to a boil over high heat. Add the salt. Give the cornstarch and water mixture a quick stir with the fork. Add it to the soup. Stir the soup with a spoon until it thickens and becomes clear (about one minute). Slowly pour the beaten egg into the soup. The egg will cook in the hot soup and form shreds. When all the egg has been added, stir once. Turn off the heat. Pour the soup into 4 soup bowls. Top if desired with chopped scallion or parsley for decorations.

Source: *Many Hands Cooking*. Terry Touff Cooper and Marilyn Ratner. (New York: Thomas Y. Crowell Company, 1974).

3. Dandelion Salad

6 cups young dandelion leaves, picked before flower blossoms

croutons, hard-boiled eggs, vegetables (optional)
dressing

Thoroughly wash the dandelion greens, removing stems and roots. Tear the leaves into small pieces and place in bowls. Add optional ingredients. Toss with salad dressing.

Record:

The following record can be found in preschool educational catalogs:

Science in a Nutshell. "Dandelion Seed" Ilene Follman and Helen Jackson. Kimbo Educational.

Books and Stories:

The following books and stories can be used to complement the theme:

1. **Flower: The Story of a Seed and How it Grew.** Mary Louise Downer. (New York: William R. Scott, 1974).

2. **Where Does Your Garden Grow?** Augusta Goldin. (New York: Thomas Y. Crowell Inc., 1967).

3. **The Carrot Seed.** Ruth Krauss. (New York: Harper and Row, 1945).

4. **The Reason For a Flower.** Ruth Heller. (New York: Scholastic, 1983).

5. **Seeds and More Seeds.** Millicent E. Selsam. (New York: Harper and Row, 1959).

6. **What is a Flower?** Jennifer W. Day. (New York: Golden, 1975).

7. **Dandelion.** Ladislav Svatos. (New York: Doubleday and Company, 1967).

8. **My Garden Grows.** Aldren Watson. (New York: Harper and Row, 1962).

9. **The Plant Sitter.** Gene Zion. (New York: Scholastic Book Services, 1959).

10. **The Rose In My Garden.** Arnold Lobel. (New York: Greenwillow Books, 1984).

11. **Let's Look at Flowers.** Harriet Huntington. (New York: Doubleday, 1969).

12. **The Floor of the Forest.** Ada and Frank Graham. (New York: Golden Press, 1974).

13. **Wildflower.** Millicent E. Selsam. (New York: Doubleday, 1964).

Puzzles:

The following puzzles can be found in preschool educational catalogs:

1. **"Tulip"** 9 pieces. Judy/Instructo.

2. **"Growing Flower"** Puzzle People.

3. **"Flower Pot"** 5 pieces. Judy/Instructo.

26 FRIENDS

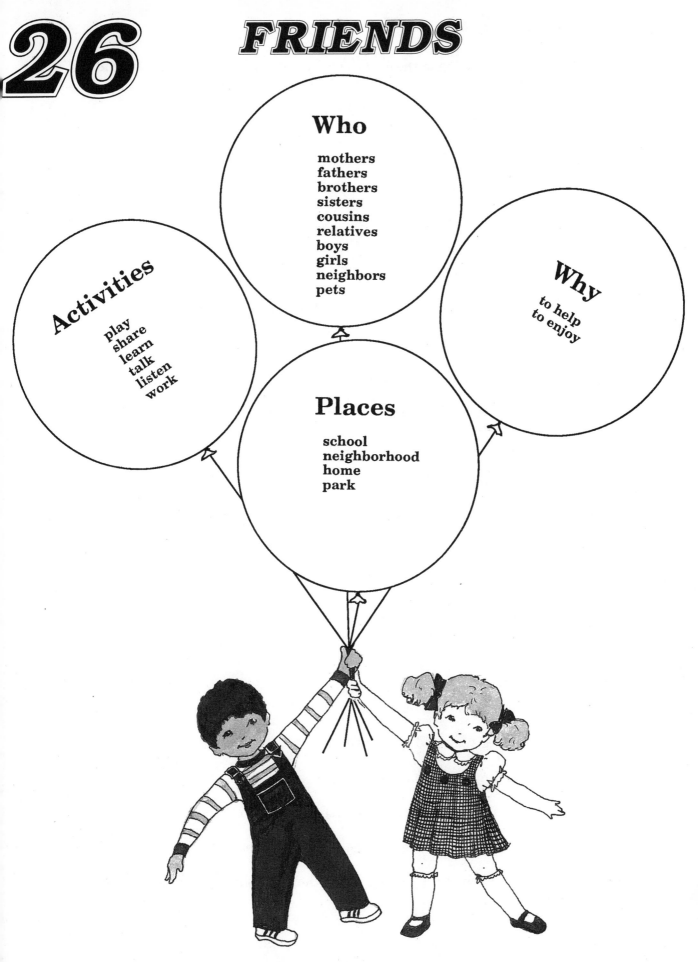

Who
mothers
fathers
brothers
sisters
cousins
relatives
boys
girls
neighbors
pets

Activities
play
share
learn
talk
listen
work

Why
to help
to enjoy

Places
school
neighborhood
home
park

Theme Goals:

Through participating in the experiences provided by this theme, the children may learn:

1. Who friends are.

2. Why we have friends.

3. Activities we can do with our friends.

4. Places we can make friends.

Concepts for the Children to Learn:

1. A friend is someone who I like and who likes me.

2. My friends are special to me.

3. We have friends at school.

4. Our brothers and sisters can be our friends.

5. Friends can help us with our work.

6. We play with our friends.

7. We share and learn with friends.

8. Friends talk and listen to us.

9. A pet can be a friend.

10. Friends can be boys or girls.

Vocabulary:

1. **friend**—a person we enjoy.

2. **sharing**—giving and taking turns.

3. **like**—feeling good about someone or something.

4. **giving**—sharing something of your own with others.

5. **cooperating**—working together to help someone.

6. **togetherness**—being with one another and sharing a good feeling.

7. **pal or buddy**—another word for friend.

Bulletin Board

The purpose of this bulletin board is to help the children with name recognition of their own and their friends' names. The bulletin board can also be used by the teacher as an attendance check. Prepare the board by constructing name cards for each child as illustrated. Then laminate and punch holes in each card. When the children arrive at school they can attach their name card to the bulletin board with a push pin.

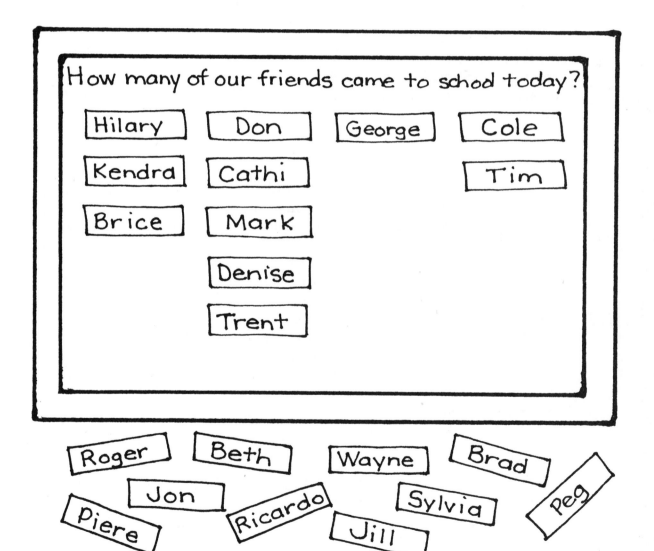

Parent Letter

Dear Parents,

This week at school we will be starting a unit on friends, which will include discovering people of all ages and even animal friends. The children have made many new friends at school with whom they are learning to share, cooperate, work and play. Through this unit, the children will become more aware of what a friend is and activities friends can do together.

At School This Week

Highlights of this week's learning experiences include:

* making friendship fortune cookies.
* sending notes to pen pals.
* creating a friendship chain with strips of paper.
* looking at pictures of our friends at school in our classroom photo album.

At Home

Your child may enjoy looking at photo albums of family and friends. Perhaps a friend could be invited to come and play with your child.

Here is a poem about friends we will be learning to promote an enjoyment of language and poetry.

Friends

I like my friends.
So when we are at play,
I try to be very kind,
and nice in every way.

Have a good week!

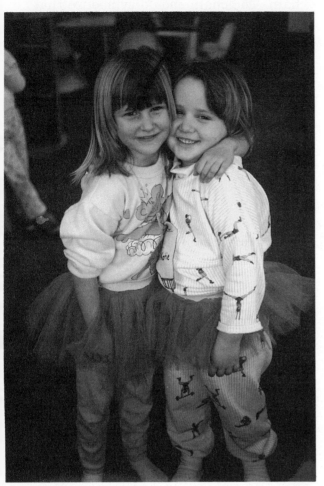

FIGURE 26 Friends are important people.

Music:

1. **"Do You Know This Friend of Mine"?**
(Sing to the tune of "The Muffin Man")

Do you know this friend of mine,
This friend of mine,
This friend of mine?
Do you know this friend of mine?
His name is _____.

Yes, we know this friend of yours,
This friend of yours,
This friend of yours.
Yes, we know this friend of yours.
His name is _____.

2. **"The More We Are Together"**
(Sing to the tune of "Have You Ever Seen a Lassie?")

The more we are together, together,
together,

The more we are together, the happier
we'll be.
For your friends are my friends, and my
friends are your friends.
The more we are together the happier we'll be.

We're all in school together, together,
together,
We're all in school together, and happy
we'll be.
There's Mary and Peter and Janet and
Joshua
There's ____ and ____ and ____ and ____.
We're all in school together and happy
we'll be.

Insert names of children in your classroom.

3. **"Beth Met a Friend"**
(Sing to the tune of "The Farmer in the Dell")

Beth met a friend,
Beth met a friend,
When she came to school today,
Beth met a friend.

Insert names of children in your classroom
for each verse.

Fingerplays:

FRIENDS

I like my friends.
So when we are at play,
I try to be very kind
and nice in every way.

FIVE LITTLE FRIENDS
(hold up five fingers; subtract one with
each action)

Five little friends playing on the floor,
One got tired and then there were four.
Four little friends climbing in a tree,
One jumped down and then there were three.
Three little friends skipping to the zoo,
One went for lunch and then there were two.
Two little friends swimming in the sun,
One went home and then there was one.
One little friend going for a run,
Decided to take a nap and then there were
none.

259

Science:

1. Comparing Heartbeats

Provide stethoscopes for the children to listen to their friends' heartbeats.

2. Fingerprints

Ink pads and white paper can be provided for the children to make fingerprints. Also, a microscope can be provided to encourage the children to compare their fingerprints.

3. Friends' Voices

Tape the children's voices throughout the course of the day. The following day, leave the tape recorder at the science table. The children can listen to the tape and try to guess which classmate is talking.

4. Animal Friends

Prepare signs for the animal cages listing the animal's daily food intake and care.

Dramatic Play:

1. Puppet Show

Set up a puppet stage with various types of puppets. The children can share puppets and act out friendships using the puppets in various situations.

2. A Tea Party

Provide dress-up clothes, play dishes and water in the dramatic play area.

Arts and Crafts:

1. Friendship Chain

Provide strips of paper for the older children to print their name on. For those children who are not interested or unable, print their names for them. When all the names are on the strips of paper, the children can connect them to make a chain. The chain should symbolize that everyone in the class is a friend.

2. Friendship Collage

Encourage the children to find magazine pictures of friends. These pictures can be pasted on a large sheet of paper for a collage. Later the paper can be used for decoration and discussion in the center lobby.

3. Friendship Exchange Art

Provide each child with a piece of construction with "To: _____" printed in the upper left corner and "From: _____" printed on the bottom. The teacher assists the children in printing their names on the bottom and the name of the person to their right on the top of the paper. Using paper scraps, tissue paper squares, fabric scraps and glue, each child will construct a picture for a friend. When finished, have each child pass the paper to the friend it was made for.

Sensory:

The sensory table is an area where two to four children can make new friends and share. Materials that can be added to the sensory table include:

* shaving cream
* playdough
* sand with toys
* water with boats
* wood shavings
* silly putty
  Mix equal parts of white glue and liquid starch. Food coloring can be added for color. Store in an airtight container.
* dry pasta dry with scoops and a balance scale
* goop
  Mix water and cornstarch. Add cornstarch to the water until you get the consistency that you want.

Large Muscle:

1. Double Balance Beam

Place two balance beams side by side and encourage two children to hold hands and cross together.

2. Bowling Game

Set up pins or plastic bottles. With a ball, have the children take turns knocking down the pins.

3. Outdoor Obstacle Course

Design an obstacle course outdoors that is specifically designed for two children to go through at one time. Use balance beams, climbers, slides, etc. Short and simple obstacle courses seem to work the best.

Field Trips/Resource People:

1. The Zoo

Take a trip to the zoo to observe animals.

2. The Nursing Home

Visit a nursing home allowing the children to interact with elderly friends.

3. Resource People

Invite the following community helpers into the classroom:

* police officer
* trash collecter
* janitor/custodian
* fire fighter
* doctor, nurse, dentist
* assistant director or principal
* principal or director

Math:

1. Group Pictures

Take pictures of the children in groups of 2, 3, 4, etc. Make seperate corresponding number cards. The children then can match the correct numeral to the picture card.

2. Friend Charts

Take individual pictures of the children and chart them according to hair color, eye color, etc. Encourage the children to compare their looks to the characteristics of their friends.

Social Studies:

Friends Bulletin Board

Ask the children to bring pictures of their friends into the classroom. Set up a bulletin board in the classroom where these pictures can be hung for all to see. Remind the children that friends can be family members and animals too.

Cooking:

1. Pound Cake Brownies

3/4 cup butter or margarine, softened
1 cup sugar
3 eggs
2 1-ounce squares unsweetened chocolate, melted and cooled
1 teaspoon vanilla
1 1/4 cups all-purpose flour
1/2 teaspoon baking powder
1/4 teaspoon salt
1/2 cup chopped nuts

Cream butter and sugar; beat in eggs. Blend in chocolate and vanilla. Stir flour with baking powder and salt. Add to creamed mixture. Mix well. Stir in nuts. Spread in a greased 9 x 9 x 2 inch baking pan. Bake at 350 degrees for 25 to 30 minutes. Cool. If desired, sift powdered sugar over the top. Cut into bars. Yields 24 bars.

TRANSITION ACTIVITIES

Clean-Up

"Do You Know What
    Time It is?"
(Sing to the tune of "The
    Muffin Man")

Oh, do you know what
    time it is,
What time it is, what
    time it is?
Oh, do you know what
    time it is?
It's almost clean-up
    time. (Or, its time to
    clean up.)

"Clean-up Time"
(Sing to the tune of
    "London Bridge")

Clean-up time is already
    here,
Already here, already here.
Clean-up time is already
    here,
Already here.

"This is the Way"
(Sing to the tune of
    "Mulberry Bush")

This is the way we pick
    up our toys,
Pick up our toys, pick up
    our toys.
This is the way we pick
    up our toys,
At clean-up time each day.

"Oh, It's Clean-up Time"
(Sing to the tune of "Oh,
    My Darling
    Clementine")

Oh, its clean-up time,
Oh, it's clean-up time,
Oh, it's clean-up time
    right now.
It's time to put the toys
    away,

It is clean-up time right
    now.

"A Helper I Will Be"
(Sing to the tune of "The
    Farmer in the Dell")

A helper I will be.
A helper I will be.
I'll pick up the toys and
    put them away.
A helper I will be.

**"We're Cleaning Up
    Our Room"**
(Sing to the tune of "The
    Farmer in the Dell")

We're cleaning up our
    room.
We're cleaning up our
    room.
We're putting all the
    toys away.
We're cleaning up our
    room.

"It's Clean-up Time"
(Sing to the chorus of
    "Looby Loo")

It's clean-up time at the
    preschool.
It's time for boys and girls
To stop what they are
    doing
And put away their toys.

"Time to Clean-up"
(Sing to the tune of "Are
    You Sleeping?")

Time to clean-up.
Time to clean-up.
Everybody help.
Everybody help.
Put the toys away, put
    the toys away.
Then sit down. (Or, then
    come here.)

Specific toys can be men-
    tioned in place of *toys*.

"Clean-up Time"
(Sing to the tune of "Hot
    Cross Buns")

Clean-up time.
Clean-up time.
Put all of the toys away.
It's clean-up time.

ROUTINES

"Passing Around"
(Sing to the tune of
    "Skip to My Loo")

Brad, take a napkin and
    pass them to Sara.
Sara, take a napkin and
    pass them to Tina.
Tina, take a napkin and
    pass them to Eric,
Passing around the
    napkins.

Fill in appropriate
    child's name and
    substitute napkin for
    any object that needs
    to be passed at meal
    time.

"Put Your Coat On"
(Sing to the tune of "Oh,
    My Darling
    Clementine")

Put your coat on.
Put your coat on.
Put your winter coat on
    now.
We are going to play
    outside.
Put your coat on right
    now.

Change coat to any
    article of clothing.

RAINY DAY ACTIVITIES

1. Get Acquainted Game

The children sit in circle formation. The teacher begins the game by saying, "My name is —————— and I'm going to roll the ball to —————— ." Continue playing the game until every child has a turn. A variation of the game is have the children stand in a circle and bounce the ball to each other. This game is a fun way for the children to learn each other's names.

2. Hide the Ball

Choose several children and ask them to cover their eyes. Then hide a small ball, or other object, in an observable place. Ask the children to uncover their eyes and try to find the ball. The first child to find the ball hides it again.

3. Which Ball is Gone?

In the center of the circle, place six colored balls, cubes, beads, shapes, etc. in a row. Ask a child to close his eyes. Then ask another child to remove one of the objects and hide it behind him. The first child uncovers his eyes and tells which colored object is missing from the row. The game continues until all the selections have been made. When using with older children, two objects may be removed at a time to further challenge their abilities.

4. "What Sound is That?"

The purpose of this game is to promote the development of listening skills. Begin by asking the children to close their eyes. Make a familiar sound. Then ask a child to identify it. Sources of sound may include:

tearing paper	blowing a pitch pipe	raising or lowering
sharpening a pencil	dropping an object	window shades
walking, running,	moving a desk or	leafing through
shuffling feet	chair	book pages
clapping hands	snapping fingers	cutting with
sneezing, coughing	blowing nose	scissors
tapping on glass,	opening or closing	snapping rubber
wood or metal	drawer	bands
jingling money	stirring paint in	ringing a bell
opening a window	a jar	clicking the tongue
pouring water	clearing the throat	crumpling paper
shuffling cards	splashing water	opening a box
blowing a whistle	rubbing sandpaper	sighing
banging blocks	together	stamping feet
bouncing ball	chattering teeth	rubbing palms
shaking a rattle	sweeping sound	together
turning the lights on	such as a brush or	rattling keys
knocking on a door	broom	

A variation of this game could be played by having a child make a sound. Then the other children and the teacher close their eyes and attempt to identify the sound. For older children this game can be varied with the production of two sounds. Begin by asking the children if the sounds are the same or different. Then have them identify the sounds. **I-1**

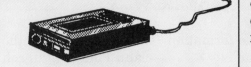

5. "Near or Far?"

The purpose of this game is to locate sound. First, tell the children to close their eyes. Then play a sound recorded on a cassette tape. Ask the children to identify the sound as being near or far away.

6. Descriptions

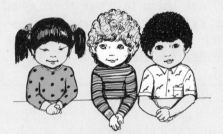

The purpose of this game is to encourage expressive language skills. Begin by asking each child to describe himself. Included with the description can be the color of his eyes, hair, and clothing. The teacher might prefer to use an imaginative introduction such as: "One by one, you may take turns sitting up here in Alfred's magic chair and describe yourself to Alfred. " Another approach may be to say, "Pretend that you must meet somebody at a very crowded airport who has never seen you before. How would you describe yourself so that the person would be sure to know who you are?"

A variation for older children would be to have one of the children describe another child without revealing the name of the person he is describing. To illustrate, the teacher might say, "I'm thinking of someone with shiny red hair, blue eyes, many freckles, etc...." The child being described should stand up.

7. Mirrored Movements

The purpose of this game is to encourage awareness of body parts through mirrored movements. Begin the activity by making movements. Encourage the children to mirror your movements. After the children understand the game, they may individually take the leader role.

8. Little Red Wagon Painted Red

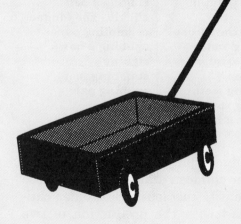

As a prop for the game, cut a red wagon with wheels out of construction paper. Then cut rectangles the same size as the box of the red wagon. Include purple, blue, yellow, green, orange, brown, black, and pink colors.

Sing the song to the tune of **"Skip to My Lou."**

*Little red wagon painted **red**.*
*Little red wagon painted **red**.*
*Little red wagon painted **red**.*
What color would it be?

Give each child a turn to pick and name a color. As the song is sung, let the child change the wagon color.

9. Police Officer Game

Select one child to be the police officer. Ask him to find a lost child. Describe one of the children in the circle. The child who is the police officer will use the description as a clue to find the "missing child."

10. Mother Cat and Baby Kits

Choose one child to be the mother cat. Then ask the mother cat to go to sleep in the center of the circle, covering his eyes. Then choose several children to be kittens. The verse below is chanted as the baby kittens hide in different parts of the classroom. Following this, the mother cat hunts for them. When all of the kittens have been located, another mother cat may be selected. The number of times the game is repeated depends upon the children's interest and attention span.

Mother cat lies fast asleep.

To her side the kittens creep.

But the kittens like to play.

Softly now they creep away.

Mother cat wakes up to see.

No little kittens. Where can they be?

11. Memory Game

Collect common household items, a towel and tray. Place the items on the tray. Show the tray containing the items. Cover with a towel. Then ask the children to recall the names of the items on the tray. To assure success, begin the activity with only two or three objects for young children. Additional objects can be added depending upon the developmental maturity of the children.

12. Cobbler, Mend My Shoes

Sit the children in a circle formation. Then select one child to sit in the center. This child gives a shoe to a child in the circle, and then closes his eyes. The children in the circle pass the shoe around behind them while the rhyme is chanted. When the chant is finished, the shoe is no longer passed. The last child with the shoe in his hand holds the shoe. Then the child sitting in the center tries to guess who has the shoe.

Cobbler, cobbler, mend my shoe

Have it done by half past two

Stitch it up and stitch it down

Now see with whom the shoe is found

13. Huckle Buckle Beanstalk

Ask the children to sit in a circle. Once seated, tell them to close their eyes. Then hide a small ball in an obvious place. Say, "Ready." Encourage all of the children to hunt for the object. Each child who spots it, returns to a place in the circle and says "Huckle buckle beanstalk." No one must tell where he has seen the ball until all the children have seen it.

14. What's Different?

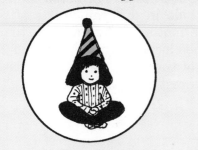

Sit all of the children in circle formation. Ask one child to sit in the center. The rest of the children are told to look closely at the child sitting in the center. Then the children are told to cover their eyes while you change some detail on the child in the center. For example, you may place a hat on the child, untie his shoe, remove a shoe, roll up one sleeve, etc. The children sitting in the circle act as detectives to determine "what's different?"

15. Cookie Jar

Sit the children in a circle formation on the floor with their legs crossed. Together they repeat a rhythmic chant while using alternating leg-hand clap to emphasize the rhythm. The chant is as follows.

Someone took the cookies from the cookie jar.

Who took the cookies from the cookie jar?

Mary took the cookies from the cookie jar.

Mary took the cookies from the cookie jar?

Who, me? (Mary)

Yes, you. (all children)

Couldn't be. (Mary)

Then who ? (all children)

―――――― *took the cookies from the cookie jar.* (Mary names another child.)

Use each child's name.

16. Hide and Seek Tonal Matching

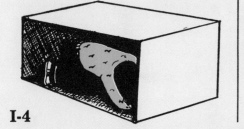

Sit the children in a circle formation. Ask one child to hide in the room while the other children cover their eyes. The children in the circle sing, "Where is ―――― hiding?" The child who is hiding responds by singing back, "Here I am." With their eyes remaining closed, the children point in the direction of the hiding child. All open eyes and the child emerges from his hiding place.

17. Listening and Naming

This game is most successful with a small group of children. The children should take turns shutting their eyes and identifying sounds as you tap with a wooden dowel on an object such as glass, triangle, drum, wooden block, cardboard box, rubber ball, etc.

18. Funny Shapes

Ask each child to choose a partner. One partner must make a large shape with his/her body. The other partner must follow the directions of movement. Roles reverse for the second set of directions. Provide directions such as:

1. Make a big shape.

go *over*
go *under*
go *through*
go *around*

2. Make a small shape.

go *over*
go *under*
go *through*
go *around*

19. Drop the Handkerchief

Direct the children to stand in a circle formation. Ask one child to run around the outside of the circle, dropping a handkerchief behind another child. The child who has the handkerchief dropped behind him/her must pick it up and chase the child who dropped it. The first child tries to return to the vacated space by running before he is tagged.

20. "If You Please"

This game is a simple variation of Simon Says. Ask the children to form a circle around a leader who gives directions, some of which are prefaced with "if you please." The children are to follow only the "if you please" directions, ignoring any that do not begin with "if you please." Directions to be used may include walking forward, hopping on one foot, bending forward, standing tall, etc. This game can be varied by having the children follow the directions when the leader says "do this" and not when he says "do that." Play only one version of this game on a single day. Too much variety will confuse the children.

21. Duck Duck Goose

Ask the children to squat in a circle formation. Then ask one child to walk around the outside of circle, lightly touching each child's head and saying "Duck, Duck." When he touches another child and says "Goose," that child chases him around the circle. If the child who was "it" returns to the "goose's" place without being tagged, he remains. When this happens, the tapped child is "it."

22. Fruit Basket Upset

Ask the children to sit in circle formation on chairs or on carpet squares. Then ask one child to sit in the middle of the circle as the chef. Hand pictures of various fruit to the rest of the children. Then to continue the game, ask the chef to call out the name of a fruit. The children holding that particular fruit exchange places. If the chef calls out "fruit basket upset," all of the children must exchange places including the chef. The child who doesn't find a place is the new chef. A variation of this game would be bread basket upset. For this game use pictures of breads, rolls, bagels, muffins, breadsticks, etc.

23. Bear Hunt

This is a rhythmic chant which may easily be varied. Start by chanting each line, encouraging the children to repeat the line.

Teacher: *Let's go on a bear hunt.*

Children: *(Repeat. Imitate walk by slapping knees alternately.)*

Teacher:
I see a wheat field.
Can't go over it;
Can't go under it.
Let's go through it.
(arms straight ahead like you're parting wheat)

I see a bridge.
Can't go over it;
Can't go under it.
Let's swim.
(arms in swimming motion)

I see a tree.
Can't go over it;
Can't go under it.
Let's go up it.
(climb and look)

I see a swamp.
Can't go over it;
Can't go under it.
Let's go through it.
(pull hands up and down slowly)

I see a cave.
Can't go over it;
Can't go under it.
Let's go in.
(walking motion)

I see two eyes. I see two ears.
I see a nose. I see a mouth.
It's a BEAR!!!
(Do all in reverse very fast)

24. "Guess Who?"

Individually tape the children's voices. Play the tape during group time, and let the children identify their classmates' voices.

25. Shadow Fun

Hang a bed sheet up in the classroom for use as a projection screen. Then place a light source such as a slide, filmstrip or overhead projector a few feet behind the screen. Ask two of the children to stand behind the sheet. Then encourage one of the two children to walk in front of the projector light. When this happens, the children are to give the name of the person who is moving.

26. If This Is Red — Nod Your Head

Point to an object in the room and say "If this is green, shake your hand. If this is yellow, touch your nose." If the object is not the color stated, children should not imitate the requested action.

27. Freeze

Encourage the children to imitate activities such as washing dishes, cleaning house, dancing, etc. Approximately every 10 to 20 seconds, call out "Freeze!" When this occurs, the children are to stop whatever they are doing and remain frozen until you say "Thaw" or "Move." A variation of this activity would be to use music. When the music stops, the children freeze their movements.

28. Spy the Object

Designate a large area on the floor as home base. Then select an object and show it to the children. Ask the children to cover their eyes while you place the object in an observable place in the room. Then encourage the children to open their eyes and search for the object. As each child spies the object he quietly returns to the home base area without telling. The other children continue searching until all have found the object. After all the children are seated, they may share where the object is placed.

29. Who Is Gone?

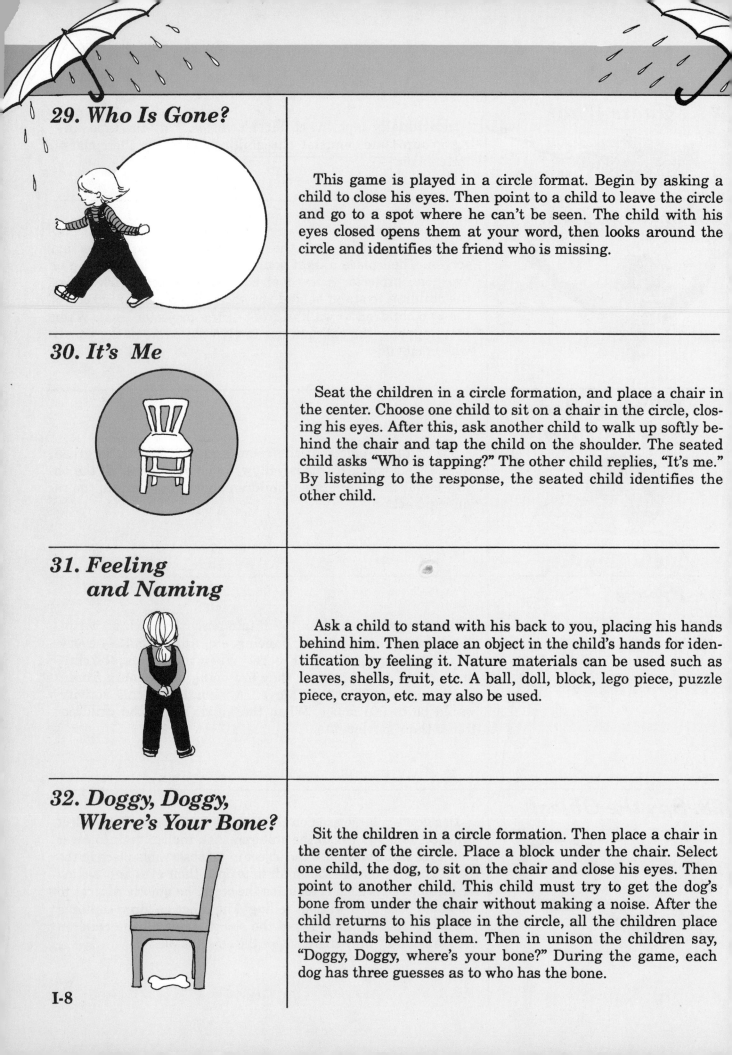

This game is played in a circle format. Begin by asking a child to close his eyes. Then point to a child to leave the circle and go to a spot where he can't be seen. The child with his eyes closed opens them at your word, then looks around the circle and identifies the friend who is missing.

30. It's Me

Seat the children in a circle formation, and place a chair in the center. Choose one child to sit on a chair in the circle, closing his eyes. After this, ask another child to walk up softly behind the chair and tap the child on the shoulder. The seated child asks "Who is tapping?" The other child replies, "It's me." By listening to the response, the seated child identifies the other child.

31. Feeling and Naming

Ask a child to stand with his back to you, placing his hands behind him. Then place an object in the child's hands for identification by feeling it. Nature materials can be used such as leaves, shells, fruit, etc. A ball, doll, block, lego piece, puzzle piece, crayon, etc. may also be used.

32. Doggy, Doggy, Where's Your Bone?

Sit the children in a circle formation. Then place a chair in the center of the circle. Place a block under the chair. Select one child, the dog, to sit on the chair and close his eyes. Then point to another child. This child must try to get the dog's bone from under the chair without making a noise. After the child returns to his place in the circle, all the children place their hands behind them. Then in unison the children say, "Doggy, Doggy, where's your bone?" During the game, each dog has three guesses as to who has the bone.

"Time To Go Outside"
(Sing to the tune of "When Johnny Comes Marching Home")

When it's time for us to
   go outside
To play, to play,
We find a place to put
   our toys
Away, away.
We'll march so quietly to
   the door.
We know exactly what's
   in store
When we go outside to
   play for a little while.

"We're Going On A Walk"
(Sing to the tune of "The Farmer in the Dell")

We're going for a walk.
We're going for a walk.
Hi-ho, the dairy-o,
We're going for a walk.

Additional verses:
What will we wear?

What will we see?
How will we go?
Who knows the way?

"Find A Partner"
(Sing to the tune of "Oh, My Darling Clementine")

Find a partner, find a
   partner,
Find a partner right
   now.
We are going for a walk.
Find a partner right
   now.

"Walk Along"
(Sing to the tune of "Clap Your Hands")

Walk, walk, walk along,
Walk along to the
   bathroom.
_____ and _____
   walk along,
Walk along to the
   bathroom.

Change walk to any other
   types of movement—
   jump, hop, skip, crawl.

"We're Going...."
(Sing to the tune of "Go In and Out the Window")

We're going to the
   bathroom,
We're going to the
   bathroom,
We're going to the
   bathroom,
And then we'll wash our
   hands.

"It's Time To Change"
(Sing to the tune of "Hello, Everybody")

It's time to change, yes
   indeed,
Yes indeed, yes indeed.
It's time to change, yes
   indeed
Time to change groups.
   (Or, Time to go
   outside.)

Records:

The following records can be found in preschool educational catalogs:

1. **Free to Be You and Me.** Marlo Thomas and Friends. Aristal Records.

2. **Getting to Know Myself.** Hap Palmer.

3. **Ideas, Thoughts and Feelings.** Hap Palmer.

4. **Look at My World.** Kathy Lecinski Poelker. Look at Me Company.

5. **Let's Be Together Today.** Fred Rogers.

Books and Stories:

The following books and stories can be used to complement the theme:

1. **A Friend is Someone Who Likes You.** Joan Anglund. (New York: Harcourt, Brace, Jovanovich, 1966).

2. **A Friend Can Help.** Terry Berger. (Chicago: Childrens Press, 1974).

3. **Let's Be Friends.** Bernice Byrant. (Chicago: Childrens Press, 1954).

4. **The Three Funny Friends.** Mary Chalmers. (New York: Harper and Row, 1961).

5. **May I Bring a Friend?** B.S. De Regniers. (New York: Atheneum Publishing Company, 1972).

6. **The Snowy Day.** Ezra Jack Keats. (New York: Viking Press, 1975).

7. **Steffie and Me.** Phyllis Hoffman. (New York: Harper and Row, 1970).

8. **Special Friends.** Terry Berger. (New York: Messner, 1979).

9. **Best Friends.** Mirian Cohen. (New York: Macmillan Publishing Company, 1971).

10. **Will I Have a Friend?** Mirian Cohen. (New York: Macmillan Publishing Company, 1967).

11. **Hi, Mrs. Mallory!** Ianthe Thomas. (New York: Harper and Row, 1979).

12. **Frog and Toad Are Friends.** Arnold Lobel. (New York: Harper and Row, 1969).

Puzzles:

The following puzzles can be found in preschool educational catalogs:

1. **"Children at Play"** 5 pieces. Constructive Playthings.

2. **"Riding Bike"** 15 pieces. Judy/Instructo.

3. **"Playing Ball"** 20 pieces. Judy/Instructo.

4. **"Playground and Kids Puzzle"** Lauri.

5. **"Quiet Time"** 12 pieces. Judy/Instructo.

6. **"Swing Time"** 14 pieces. Judy/Instructo.

7. **"Swing & Slide"** 9 pieces. (ABC School Supply).

27 FRUITS AND VEGETABLES

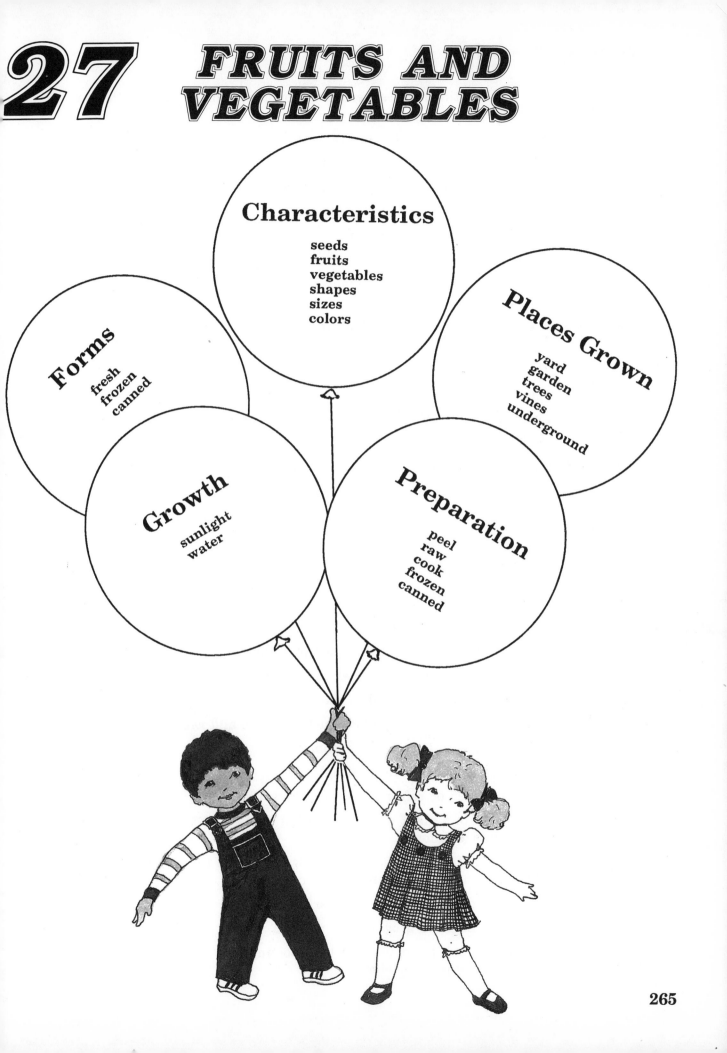

Characteristics

seeds
fruits
vegetables
shapes
sizes
colors

Places Grown

yard
garden
trees
vines
underground

Forms

fresh
frozen
canned

Growth

sunlight
water

Preparation

peel
raw
cook
frozen
canned

Theme Goals:

Through participating in the experiences provided by this theme, the children may learn:

1. Names of common fruits and vegetables.
2. Purposes of fruits and vegetables.
3. Places fruits and vegetables are grown.
4. Preparation of fruits and vegetables.
5. Tastes of fruits and vegetables.
6. Fruit or vegetable seeds.
7. Preparation of fruits or vegetables.

Concepts for the Children to Learn:

1. There are many kinds of fruits and vegetables.
2. Fruits and vegetables come in many shapes, sizes and colors.
3. Fruits and vegetables need sunlight and water to grow.
4. Fruits and vegetables can be bought fresh, frozen or canned.
5. Some people grow fruits and vegetables in gardens.
6. Fruits and vegetables have different names.
7. Most fruits and vegetables can be eaten raw or cooked.
8. Some fruits and vegetables we eat with skin; some we need to peel first.
9. Fruits have seeds.

Vocabulary:

1. **fruit**—usually a sweet tasting part of a plant.
2. **vegetable**—part of a plant that can be eaten.
3. **garden**—ground used to grow plants.
4. **produce**—agriculture products such as fruits and vegetables.
5. **vine**—plant with long slender stem.
6. **cooked**—prepare food by heating.
7. **frozen**—chilled or refrigerated to make solid.
8. **seeds**—part of a plant used for growing a new crop and are edible in some plants (sunflower, pumpkin).
9. **roots**—part of a plant that grows downward into the soil and are edible in some plants (potatoes, carrots).
10. **soil**—portion of earth; dirt used for growing.
11. **sprout**—to begin to grow.
12. **stems**—part of a plant used for transporting food and water and edible in some plants (celery).

Bulletin Board

The purpose of this bulletin board is to observe the growth of a lima bean seed. To prepare the bulletin board, place a moist paper towel in a small plastic bag and place a lima bean on top of the towel for each child. Staple each bag to the bulletin board as illustrated; place each child's name by his bag. Sprouting will occur faster if seeds have been pre-soaked overnight. Additional watering may be needed throughout the unit.

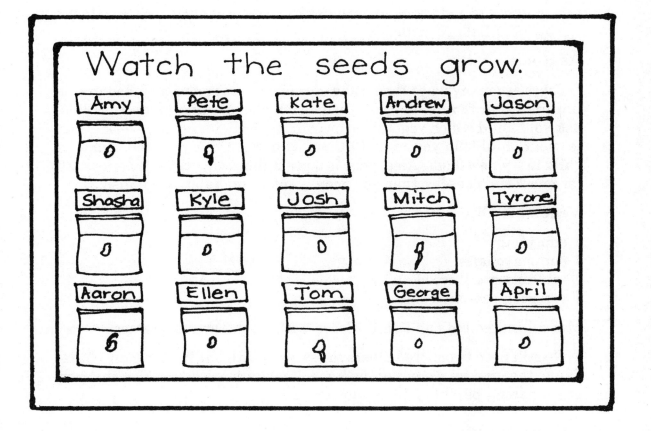

Parent Letter

Dear Parents,

Hello again! We hope that everyone in your family is healthy and happy. Speaking of health, we are starting a new unit this week on fruits and vegetables. Through the experiences planned for this unit, the children will become aware of many fruits and vegetables and how they are grown. Also they will discover how many fruits and vegetables taste.

At School This Week

Some of the many fun-filled learning activities scheduled for this week are:

* planting lima bean seeds to sprout. Take a look at our bulletin board this week.
* playing the role of a gardener/farmer in the dramatic play area.
* matching pictures of vegetables to where they are grown (trees, vines, underground, etc.)
* having a fruit and vegetable tasting party during snack.
* visiting a produce section at the grocery store.
* listening to a story called *What Was It Before It Was Orange Juice?* by Jane Belk Moncure.

At Home

There are many ways that you can integrate concepts included in this unit into your family life. To help develop memory and language skills, ask your child which vegetables or fruit he tried during the week. Then let your child help you prepare them at home. Cooking often tempts a child to try new foods. Also, here is a great dip recipe we will be making for snack on Tuesday that you may want to make at home also.

Vegetable Dip

1 cup yogurt
1 cup mayonaise
1 tablespoon dill weed
1 teaspoon seasoned salt

Mix all ingredients and chill. Serve with fresh raw vegetables.

We still need two more helpers to assist us with our field trip on Thursday to the grocery store. Let me know if you are available. The children enjoy having parents join in our activities.

Have a great week!

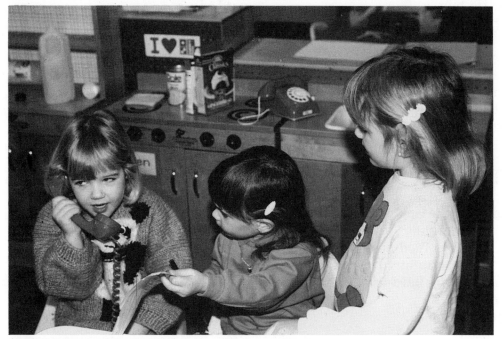

FIGURE 27 "Hello! Farmer Brown? Is the corn ripe yet?

Music:

1. **"The Vegetable Garden"**
   (Sing to the tune of "Mulberry Bush")

   Here we go 'round the vegetable garden,
   The vegetable garden, the vegetable
   garden,
   Here we go round the vegetable garden,
   So early in the morning.

   Other verses:
   This is the way we pull the weeds...
   This is the way we water the plants...
   This is the way we eat the vegetables...

2. **"Vegetables"**
   (Sing to the tune "Mary Had a Little
   Lamb")

   I'm a tomato, red and round,
   Red and round, red and round.
   I'm a tomato, red and round,
   Seated on the ground.

   I'm a corn stalk, tall and straight,
   Tall and straight, tall and straight.
   I'm a corn stalk, tall and straight
   And I taste just great.

Fingerplays:

MY GARDEN

This is my garden
   (extend one hand forward, palm up)
I'll rake it with care
   (make raking motion on palm with three
   fingers of other hand)
And then some seeds
   (planting motion)
I'll plant in there.
The sun will shine
   (make circle with arms)
And the rain will fall
   (let fingers flutter down to lap)
And my garden will blossom
   (cup hand together, extend upward slowly)
And grow straight and tall.

DIG A LITTLE HOLE

Dig a little hole.
   (dig)
Plant a little seed.
   (drop seed)
Pour a little water.
   (pour)
Pull a little weed.
   (pull and throw)

269

Chase a little bug.
  (chasing motion with hands)
Heigh-ho, there he goes.
  (shade eyes)
Give a little sunshine
  (circle arms over head)
Grow a little bean!
  (hands grow upward)

APPLE TREE

Way up high in the apple tree
  (hold arms up high)
Two little apples smiled at me.
  (look at 2 hands up high)
I shook that tree as hard as I could.
  (shake arms)
Down came the apples,
  (arms fall)
Mmm, were they good!
  (rub tummy)

BANANAS

Bananas are my favorite fruit.
  (make fists as if holding banana)
I eat one every day.
  (hold up one finger)
I always take one with me
  (act as if putting one in pocket)
When I go out to play.
  (wave good-bye)
It gives me lots of energy
  (make a muscle)
To jump around and run.
  (move arms as if running)
Bananas are my favorite fruit.
  (rub tummy)
To me they're so much fun!
  (point to self and smile)

VEGETABLES AND FRUITS

The food we like to eat that grows
On vines and bushes and trees.
Are vegetables and fruits my friends
Like cherries, grapes and peas.
Apples and oranges and peaches are fruits
And so are tangerines,
Lettuce and carrots are vegetables,
Like squash and beans.

Science:

1. Cut and Draw

Cut out or draw many different fruits and vegetables from tagboard or construction paper scraps. Also make a tree, a vine, and some soil. Have children classify the fruit to where it's grown on a tree, on vines or underground.

2. Tasting Center

Cut small pieces of various fruits and set up a tasting center. Encourage the children to taste and compare different fruits and vegetables.

3. Tasting Party

Plan a vegetable tasting party. Cut small pieces of vegetables. Also, have children taste raw vegetables compared to the same vegetable cooked.

4. Identify by Smelling

Place one each of several fruits and vegetables in small cups and cover with aluminum foil. Punch a small hole in the top of the aluminum foil. Then have the children smell the cups and try to identify each fruit or vegetable.

5. Growing a Seed

Give each child a plastic sealable bag, a moistened paper towel and a lima bean. Demonstrate how to place the bean in the paper towel and close bag. After the children have finished planting their bean, place each child's bag on a bulletin board. Check the bulletin board on a daily basis to see when the seed sprouts.

6. Carrot Tops in Water

Cut off the top of a carrot and place it in a shallow dish of water. Observe what happens day to day. Given time the top of the carrot should sprout.

7. Colored Celery Stalks

Place celery stalks into water colored with food coloring. Observe what happens to the leaves of celery.

Dramatic Play:

Grocery Store

Plan a grocery store containing many plastic fruits and vegetables, a cash register, grocery bags and play money if available. The children can take turns being a produce clerk, cashier and price tagger.

Arts and Crafts:

1. Fruit and Vegetable Collage

Make a fruit and vegetable collage. Have children draw or cut their favorite fruits and vegetables from magazines and paste on paper.

2. Seeds

Save several seeds from fruits and vegetables for the children to make a seed collage. When seeds are securely glued children can also paint them if desired. The collage can be secured to a bulletin board.

3. Cutting Vegetable and Fruit Shapes

Cut easel paper into a different shape of fruit or vegetable every day.

4. Mold with Playdough

The children can mold and create fruits and vegetables out of clay and playdough. Another option would be to color and scent the playdough. Examples might include orange-smelling orange, lemon-smelling yellow, banana-smelling yellow.

5. Potato Prints

Cut potatoes in half. The children can dip in paints and stamp the potatoes on a large sheet of paper.

6. Paint with Celery Leaves

Mix some thin temepra paint. Use celery leaves as a painting tool.

Sensory:

Preparing Fruits and Vegetables

Wash vegetables and fruits to prepare for eating at snack time.

Large Muscle:

Place hoes, shovels, rakes, and watering cans around the outdoor sand area.

Field Trips/Resource People:

1. Grocery Store

Take a trip to the grocery store to visit the produce department. Ask the clerk to show the children how the food is delivered.

2. Visiting a Farm

Visit a farm. Ask the farmer to show the children the fruits and vegetables grown on the farm.

3. Visit a Farmers' Market

Visit a farmers' market. Purchase fruits and vegetables that can be used for snacks.

4. Visit an Orchard

Visit an apple or fruit orchard. Observe how the fruit is grown. If possible, pick some fruit to bring back to the classroom.

Math:

1. Fruit and Vegetable Match

Cut out various fruits and vegetables from a magazine. Trace their shapes onto tagboard. Have children match the fruit or vegetable to the correct shape on the tagboard.

2. Seriation

Make five sizes of each vegetable or fruit you want to use. Have children place in order from smallest to largest, or largest to smallest.

3. Measuring

The children can measure their bean sprouts. Maintain a small chart of their measurements.

4. Parts and Wholes

Cut apples in half at snack time to introduce the concepts of parts and whole.

5. Grouping Pictures

Cut picures of fruits and vegetables for the children to sort according to color, size and shape.

Social Studies:

1. Field Trip to a Garden

Plan a field trip to a large garden. Point out different fruits and vegetables. If possible, have the children pull radishes and carrots.

2. Hang Pictures

On a bulletin board in the classroom hang pictures of fruits and vegetables.

3. Fruit and Vegetable Book

The children can make a fruit and vegetable book. Possible titles include "My favorite fruit is," "My favorite vegetable is," "I would like to grow," and "I would most like to cook." The children can paste pictures or adhere stickers to the individual pages.

Group Time (games, language):

1. Carrot, Carrot, Corn

Play Duck, Duck Goose, but substitute Carrot, Carrot, Corn.

2. Hot Potato

The children sit in a circle and the teacher gives one child a potato. Teacher then plays lively music and the children pass potato around the circle. When the music suddenly stops, the child with the potato must stand up and say the name of a fruit or vegetable. Encourage children to think of a fruit or vegetable that hasn't been named yet. Play the game until almost all fruits and vegetables have been named.

Cooking:

1. Vegetable Dip

1 cup plain yogurt
1 cup mayonnaise
1 tablespoon dill weed
1 teaspoon seasoned salt

Mix all the ingredients together and chill. Serve with fresh raw vegetables.

2. Ants on a Log

Cut celery into pieces and spread with peanut butter. Top with raisins, coconut or grated carrots. (Celery is difficult for younger children to chew.)

3. Applesauce

4 apples
1 tablespoon water
2 tablespoons brown sugar or honey

Wash the apples and cut into small pieces. Dip the pieces into water and roll in brown sugar or honey. Serves 8.

4. Banana Rounds

4 medium bananas
1/2 cup yogurt

3 tablespoons honey
1/8 teaspoon nutmeg
1/8 teaspoon cinnamon
1/4 cup wheat germ

The children can participate by peeling the bananas and slicing into "rounds." Measure the spices, wheat germ and honey. Blend this mixture with yogurt and bananas. Chill prior to serving. Serves 8.

5. Middle East Date and Banana Dessert

4 ounces (1 cup) pitted dates, cut up
2 bananas, thinly sliced
2 to 3 teaspoons finely shredded lemon
  peel
1/2 cup half and half
sliced almonds (optional)

Alternate layers of dates and bananas in serving dish or dessert dishes. Sprinkle with lemon peel. Pour half and half over top. Cover and refrigerate at least 4 hours. Just before serving sprinkle with almonds. Makes 3 to 4 servings.

Source: *Betty Crocker's International Cookbook.* (New York: Random House, 1980).

6. Finnish Strawberry Shake

20 fresh strawberries
4 cups milk
3 tablespoons sugar

Wash strawberries and remove stems. Cut strawberries into small pieces. Combine milk, sugar and strawberries in a large mixing bowl or blender. Beat with an egg-beater or blend for 2 minutes. Pour strawberry shakes into individual glasses. Makes 4 to 8 servings.

Variation: Raspberries or other sweet fruit may be used instead.

7. Banana Sandwiches

1/2 or 1 banana per child
peanut butter

Peel the bananas and slice them in half lengthwise. Spread peanut butter on one half of the banana and top with the other half.

COOKING VOCABULARY

The following vocabulary words can be introduced through cooking experiences:

bake	garnish	scrape
beat	grate	scrub
boil	grease	shake
broil	grill	shread
brown	grind	sift
chop	heat	simmer
cool	knead	spread
core	marinate	sprinkle
cream	measure	squeeze
cube	mince	stir
cut	mix	strain
dice	pare	stuff
dip	peel	tear
drain	pit	toast
freeze	pour	whip
frost	roast	
fry	roll	

Record:

The following record can be found in preschool educational catalogs:

Learning Basic Skills Through Music—Health and Safety. #EA-AR526R
Hap Palmer.

Books and Stories:

The following books and stories can be used to complement the theme:

1. **The Carrot and Other Root Vegetables.** Millicent E. Selsam. (New York: William Morrow and Company, 1970).

2. **The Tomato and Other Fruit Vegetables.** Millicent E. Selsam. (New York: William Morrow and Company, 1970).

3. **The Carrot Seed.** Ruth Krauss. (New York: Harper and Row, 1945).

4. **What Was It Before It Was Orange Juice?** Jane Belk Moncure. (Chicago: Childrens Press, 1985).

5. **From Seed to Salad.** Hanah Lyons Johnson. (New York: William Morrow and Company, 1978).

6. **Eat the Fruit, Plant the Seed.** Millicent E. Selsam. (New York: William Morrow and Company, 1980).

7. **Vegetables From Stems and Leaves.** Millicent E. Selsam. (New York: William Morrow and Company, 1972).

8. **Stone Soup.** Marcia Brown. (New York: C. Scribner's Sons, 1947).

9. **From Seed to Pear.** Ali Mitgutsch. (Minneapolis MN: Carolrhoda, 1981).

10. **Blueberries For Sal.** Robert Mc Closkey. (New York: The Viking Press, 1948).

11. **Fruit is Ripe For Timothy.** Alice Rothschild. (New York: Young Scott Books, 1963).

12. **Rain Makes Applesauce.** Julian Scheer. (New York: Holiday House, 1970).

13. **Good Lemonade.** Frank Asch. (New York: Franklin Watts, 1976).

14. **I Like Vegetables.** Sharon Lerner. (Minneapolis, MN: Lerner Publications Company, 1967).

15. **More Potatoes!** M. Selsam. (New York: Harper and Row, 1972).

Puzzles:

The following puzzles can be found in preschool educational catalogs:

1. **"Fruits"** Puzzle People.

2. **"Vegetables"** Puzzle People.

3. **"Fruits"** 5 pieces. Judy/Instructo.

4. **"Vegetables"** 5 pieces. Judy/Instructo.

5. **"Fruits and Vegetable Puzzle"** 16 pieces. Rolf.

GARDENS

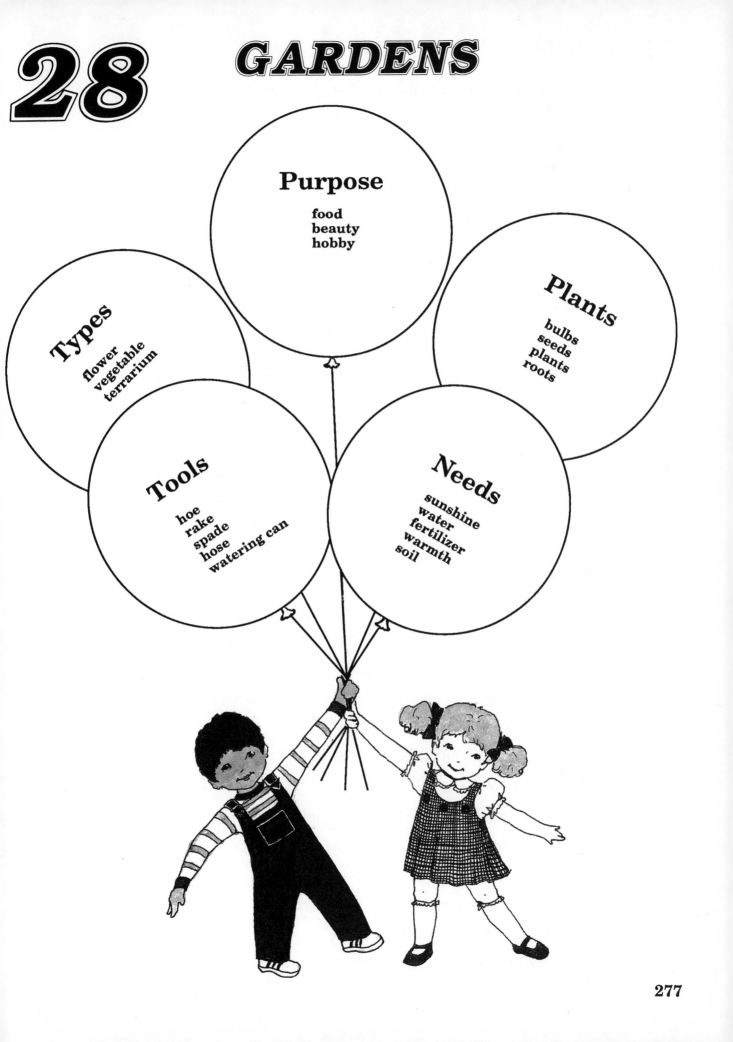

Purpose

food
beauty
hobby

Types

flower
vegetable
terrarium

Plants

bulbs
seeds
plants
roots

Tools

hoe
rake
spade
hose
watering can

Needs

sunshine
water
fertilizer
warmth
soil

Theme Goals:

Through participating in the experiences provided by this theme, the children may learn:

1. Purposes of gardens.

2. Types of gardens.

3. Tools used for gardening.

4. Care of gardens.

5. Types of plants grown in a garden.

Concepts for the Children to Learn:

1. Plants are living things.

2. Plants need sunshine, water, soil, fertilizer and warmth to grow.

3. Gardens produce food and beautiful flowers.

4. We plant gardens by placing bulbs, seeds, plants or roots in the ground.

5. Weeds are plants that do not bear fruit. They take water and food from our garden plants.

6. Fruits, vegetables and flowers can be planted in our gardens.

Vocabulary:

1. **bulb**—a type of seed.

2. **flower**—part of the plant that has colored petals.

3. **garden**—a place to grow plants.

4. **greenhouse**—building for growing plants and flowers.

5. **leaf**—flat green part of a plant.

6. **rake**—a tool with teeth or prongs.

7. **soil**—top of the ground.

8. **root**—part of the plant that grows into the ground.

9. **seed**—part of the plant from which a new plant will grow.

10. **stem**—part of the plant that holds the leaves and flowers.

11. **vegetable**—a plant that can be eaten.

12. **hoe**—a tool with a thin blade.

13. **weed**—plant that is not needed.

Bulletin Board

The purpose of this bulletin board is to foster visual discrimination skills. To prepare the bulletin board, construct five or six watering cans out of tagboard. Color each one a different color with felt-tip markers and hang on the bulletin board. Attach a string to each watering can. Next, construct the same number of small rakes out of tagboard. Color each one using the same colors as you used for the watering cans. Attach a push pin to the top of each rake. The children can match each watering can to the corresponding colored rake by winding the string around the correct push pin.

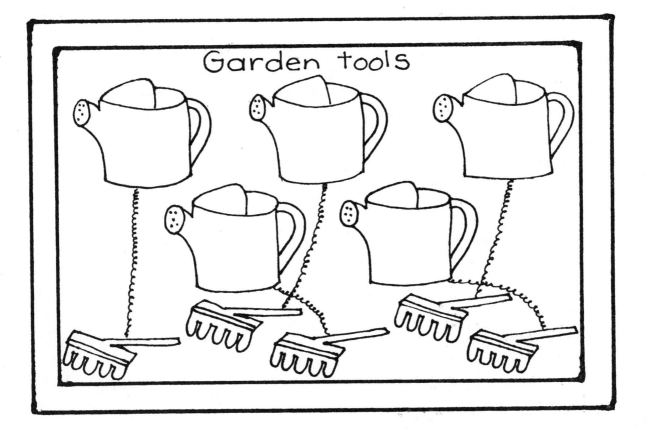

Parent Letter

Dear Parents,

"Mary, Mary, quite contrary, how does your garden grow?" That familiar nursery rhyme sums up the theme for this week—gardens! We will be exploring flower and vegetable gardens, as well as finding out about the work involved in planning and maintaining gardens and garden tools.

At School This Week

Some of the learning experiences planned to foster concepts related to gardens include:

* a flower shop set up in the dramatic play area.
* dramatizing the story of *The Big Turnip*.
* preparing a section of our play yard for a garden. The children will help decide which seeds to plant.
* mud in the sensory table.

At Home

If you have a garden, ask your child to help you water, weed and care for it. If you don't have a garden, take a walk and observe how many plants you can find that are cared for by people. What are the plants? How are they cared for?

Cut the tops of carrots off 1/4 inch from the stem to make a carrot-top garden. Place carrot tops in a shallow pie tin and pour 1/4 inch of water in the tin. Soon roots will appear, the greens will grow and your child will be able to observe the growth.

Have a good week!

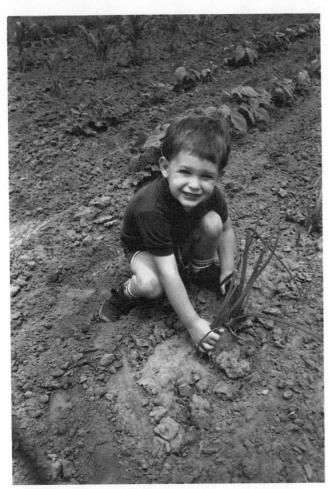

FIGURE 28 Gardens are fun to plant.

Music:

1. **"I Have a Little Pussy"**
(Each line sung on one note of the C-rising scale)

C I have a little pussy
D So very soft and gray.
E She lives down in the meadow
F Not very far away.
G She'll always be a pussy.
A She'll never be a cat.
B Because she's a pussy willow.
C Now, what do you think of that?

(Go down the scale)
C Meow
B Meow
A Meow
G Meow
F Meow
E Meow
D Meow

C Meow
Scat cat!

2. **"A Little Seed"**
(Sing to the tune "I'm a Little Teapot")

Here's a little seed in the dark, dark ground.
Out comes the warm sun, yellow and round.
Down comes the rain, wet and slow.
Up comes the little seed, grow, grow, grow!

Fingerplays:

SEEDS

Some little seeds have parachutes
To carry them around
(cup hand downward)
The wind blows them swish, swish, swish.
(flip fingers outward from parachute)
Then gently lays them on the ground.
(let hand gently float down and rest on lap)

RELAXING FLOWERS

Five little flowers standing in the sun
(hold up five fingers)
See their heads nodding, bowing one by one?
(bend fingers several times)
Down, down, down comes the gentle rain
(raise hands, wiggle fingers and lower arms to simulate falling rain)
And the five little flowers lift their heads up again!
(hold up five fingers)

HOW IT HAPPENS

A muddy hump,
(make a fist using both hands)
A small green lump,

(poke up thumbs together as one)
Two leaves and then
Two leaves again
   (raise forefinger of each hand from fist,
   then middle fingers)
And shooting up, a stem and cup.
   (put elbows, forearms, and hands
   together, fingers slightly curved)
One last shower,
   (rain movements with spread arms   and
   fingers)
Then a flower.
   (elbows, forearms together with hands
   wide apart, palms up)

LITTLE FLOWERS

The sun comes out and shines so bright
   (join hands over head in circle)
Then we have a shower.
   (wiggle fingers coming down)
The little bud pushes with all its might
   (one hand in fist; other hand clasped
   over, move hands up slowly)
And soon we have a flower.
   (join thumbs and spread fingers for
   flower)

MR CARROT

Nice Mr. Carrot
Makes curly hair.
   (hand on head)
His head grows underneath the ground,
   (bob head)
His feet up in the air.
   (raise feet)
And early in the morning
I find him in his bed
   (close eyes, lay head on hands)
And give his feet a great big pull
   (stretch legs out)
And out comes his head.

Science:

1. Growing Grass

Germinate grass seeds by placing a damp sponge in a pie tin of water and sprinkling seeds on the sponge. The children will notice tiny sprouts after a few days. Experiment by putting one sponge in the freezer, one near a heat source and one in a dark closet. Discuss what happens to each group of seeds.

2. Plants Contain Water

Cut off 1/4 inch from the bottom of a celery stalk. Fill a clear vase with water containing food coloring. Place the celery stalk in the vase. Encourage the children to observe color changes in the celery stalk. This activity can be repeated using a white carnation.

3. Planting Seeds

Purchase bean and radish seeds. If space permits, plant outdoors. Otherwise, place soil in planters indoors. Plant the seeds with the children. Identify the plants by pasting the seed packages on the planters. This will help the children to recognize the plants as they emerge from the soil.

4. The Science Table

Place a magnifying glass with different types of seeds and bulbs on the science table. During the week add fresh flowers, plant leaves and dried plants.

5. Rooting a Sweet Potato

To root a sweet potato in water, push toothpicks halfway into the potato. Then place the potato in a glass of water with the toothpicks resting on the top rim. Make sure the end of the potato is immersed in water. Place the glass where it will receive adequate light. Maintain the water level so that the bottom of the potato is always immersed. Note that in a few weeks roots will grow out of the sides and bottom of the potato, and leaves will grow out of the top. The plant can be left in the water or replanted in soil. This activity provides the children an opportunity to observe root growth.

6. Worm Farm

Collect the following materials: large clear jar with a wide mouth, soil, earthworms, gravel, food for worms (lettuce, cornmeal, cereals). Place gravel and soil in the jar. Add the worms. Add food on the top of the dirt and keep the soil moist but not wet. Tape black construction paper around outside of jar. The paper can be temporarily removed to observe the worms and see their tunnels.

Dramatic Play:

1. Flower Shop

Introduce a flower shop by gathering plastic flowers and plants. If desired, flowers can be made from tissue paper and pipe cleaners. Collect different kinds of vases and also styrofoam or sponge blocks so the children can make flower arrangements. A cash register, aprons, money and sacks can also be provided to encourage play.

2. Gardening Center

Gather tools, gloves, hats, seeds and plastic flowers or plants. The children can pretend to plant and grow seeds. Provide seed catalogs and order blanks for children to choose seeds to order.

3. Fruit Stand

Set up a fruit stand by using plastic fruits and vegetables. Aprons, a cash register, market baskets or bags and play money can also be used to encourage play. The children can take turns being the owner and the shopper.

4. Sandbox

The children can experiment with gardening tools in the sandbox.

Arts and Crafts:

1. Collage

Make collages using all types of seeds and beans. This activity can also be used by cutting pictures from seed catalogs.

2. Leaf Rubbings

Take the children on a leaf walk. The children choose a couple of large leaves to bring back to school. Place the leaves between two sheets of paper and rub with flat, large crayons across the top sheet of paper.

3. Stencils

Cut stencils out of tagboard of various shaped leaves or vegetables (see patterns). Laminate the stencils. The children can use crayons, pencils or marking pens to make the leaf or vegetable outlines. These stencils can be used as the front of the "soup and salad" party invitations listed under social studies activities.

4. Decorating Vases

Collect tin cans or milk cartons for the children to use as vases. If cans are used, file the sharp edges or cover them with masking tape. The children can decorate the containers with colored paper, gift wrapping paper or wall paper. Greeting cards may also be useful for this activity.

Sensory:

1. Sensory Activities

In the sensory table place:

* soil
* seeds
* plastic plants
* beans
* measuring cups
* balance scales
* worms
* miniature garden tools
* cut grass or hay

2. Fill and Guess

After showing and discussing several kinds of fruits or vegetables with children, place the fruits or vegetables in a bag. Individually let children reach in and touch one item. See if they can guess what it is before pulling it out of the bag. Older children may also be able to describe the item.

Large Muscle:

Leaf Jumping

This is an active skill game that can be played indoors or outdoors. Cut out large cardboard leaves and arrange them in an irregular line, as they might appear on a stem. The closer they are together, the harder the game will be. Beginning at one end, each player tries to jump over the leaves without touching them. Older children may try to skip or hop over the leaves.

Field Trips/Resource People:

1. Field Trips

Take a field trip to:

* a flower garden
* a vegetable garden
* a flower shop
* a farmers' market
* a greenhouse
* a conservatory
* a park
* the produce section of a grocery store
* a natural food store

2. Resource People

* gardeners
* florist to demonstrate flower arranging

Math:

1. Sorting Beans

Mix together several shapes and colors of large, dried beans. The children can sort the beans by size and color.

2. Inchworm Measuring

A good introduction for this activity is the story *Inch by Inch* by Leo Lionni. Cut 2 or 3 dozen inchworms out of felt. Then cut out flowers of various heights—with long or short stems. Encourage the children to place worms along stem from bottom to top of flower. How many inchworms tall is each flower? After this, have the children count the inchworms.

Social Studies:

1. Salad and Soup Party

The children can plan and participate in a salad and soup party for their parents. The groceries will need to be purchased, cleaned and prepared.

2. Plant Hunt

Go on a hunt to discover how many non-flowering plants such as algae, fungi, lichens, mosses and ferns are found in the school yard. Make a display. How are these plants different from garden plants?

Group Time (games, language):

1. Huckle Buckle Bean Stalk

A small object such as a plastic flower or acorn may be used for hiding. All the players cover their eyes, except the one who hides the object. After it is hidden, the players stand up and begin to look for it. When one locates it, he doesn't let others know the placement. Instead he quietly takes a seat saying "Huckle Buckle Bean Stalk." The game continues until all players have located the object. The first child to find the object usually hides it the next time. This game is appropriate for older children.

2. The Big Turnip—Creative Dramatics

First tell the story of the *Big Turnip*. Then pass out an identifying piece of clothing for each character. Hats work well for people and collars or signs for the animals. Retell the story, letting the children act the story out. Use as many characters as you have children. This would be a good outdoors activity.

Cooking:

1. Vegetable Soup

Begin with consomme or soup base. Add whatever vegetables, beans, etc. children want to add and can help to prepare. Make soup a day ahead so that all of the vegetables will be cooked thoroughly.

2. Indian—Cucumbers and Tomatoes with Yogurt

2 medium cucumbers
2 green onions with tops, chopped
1 teaspoon salt
2 tomatoes chopped
1/2 clove garlic, finely chopped
2 tablespoons snipped parsley
1/2 teaspoon ground cumin
1/8 teaspoon pepper
1 cup unflavored yogurt

Cut cucumbers lengthwise into halves. Scoop out seeds. Chop cucumbers. Mix cucumbers, green onions and salt. Let stand 10 minutes. Add tomatoes. Mix remaining ingredients except yogurt. Toss with cucumber mixture. Cover and refrigerate at least 1 hour. Drain thoroughly. Just before serving, fold in yogurt. Makes 6 servings.

Source: *Betty Crocker's International Cookbook.* (New York: Random House, 1980).

3. Lettuce or Spinach Rollups

On clean lettuce or spinach leaves, spread softened cream cheese or cottage cheese. If desired, sprinkle with grated carrots or chopped nuts. Roll them up. Chill and serve.

4. Carrot Cookies

1/2 cup honey
1 egg
1/2 cup margarine
1 cup whole wheat flour
1 1/4 teaspoons baking powder
1/4 teaspoon salt
1/2 cup rolled oats
1/2 cup wheat germ
1/2 cup grated raw carrots
1/2 cup raisins
1/2 cup nuts (optional)
1 teaspoon vanilla

Mix all ingredients in a bowl. Drop mixture by spoonsful onto a lightly greased cookie sheet. Flatten each ball slightly. Bake in a 350-degree oven for approximately 12 minutes.

Records:

The following records can be found in preschool educational catalogs:

1. **Walter the Waltzing Worm.** Hap Palmer

2. **Baby Beluga.** Raffi. "Oats and Beans and Barley Grow" and "Over in the Meadow"

3. **American Folk Songs.** Pete Seeger "Jimmy Crack Corn"

Stories and Books:

The following books and stories can be used to complement the theme:

1. **The Tiny Seed.** Eric Carle. (New York: Thomas Y. Crowell Company, 1970).

2. **The Plant Sitter.** Gene Zion. (New York: Harper and Row, 1959).

3. **Dandelion.** Ladislav Svatas. (New York: Doubleday and Company, 1976).

4. **Pumpkin Pumpkin.** Jeanne Titherington. (New York: Greenwillow Books, 1986).

5. **The Scarebunny.** Dorothy Kunhardt. (New York: Golden Press, 1985).

6. **Seeds and More Seeds.** Millicent Selsam. (New York: Harper and Row, 1959).

7. **I Found a Leaf.** Sharon Lerner. (New York: Lerner Publications, 1964).

8. **Who Goes There in My Garden?** Ethel Collier. (New York: Young Scott Books, 1963).

9. **The Turnip.** Janina Domanska. (New York: Macmillan Publishing Company, 1969).

10. **Apples.** Nonny Hogrogian. (New York: Macmillan Publishing Company, 1972).

11. **Where Does Your Garden Grow?** August Goldin. (New York: Thomas Y. Crowell, 1967).

12. **Busy Seeds.** Irma Simonton Black. (New York: Holiday House Inc., 1970).

13. **A Gardening Book: Indoors and Outdoors.** Anne B. Walsh. (New York: Atheneum, 1976).

14. **My Garden Grows.** Aldren Watson. (New York: Harper and Row, 1962).

15. **Inch by Inch.** Leo Lionni. (New York: Astor-Honor, 1962).

16. **Willie's Garden.** Myra McGee. (Emmaus, PA: Rodale Press, 1977).

17. **Let's Grow a Garden.** Gyo Fujikawa. (Japan: Zoeisha Publications, Limited, 1978).

18. **The Carrot Seed.** Ruth Krauss. (New York: Harper and Row, 1945).

Puzzles:

The following puzzles can be found in preschool educational catalogs:

1. **"Garden Tools"** 6 pieces. Constructive Playthings.

2. **"Fruits"** 5 pieces. Constructive Playthings.

3. **"Vegetables"** 5 pieces. Constructive Playthings.

4. **"Fruits"** 4 pieces. Constructive Playthings.

5. **"Color Worms"** 26 pieces. Puzzle People.

6. **"Garden"** Critter Puzzle.

7. **"Garden"** 8 pieces. Acre Toys.

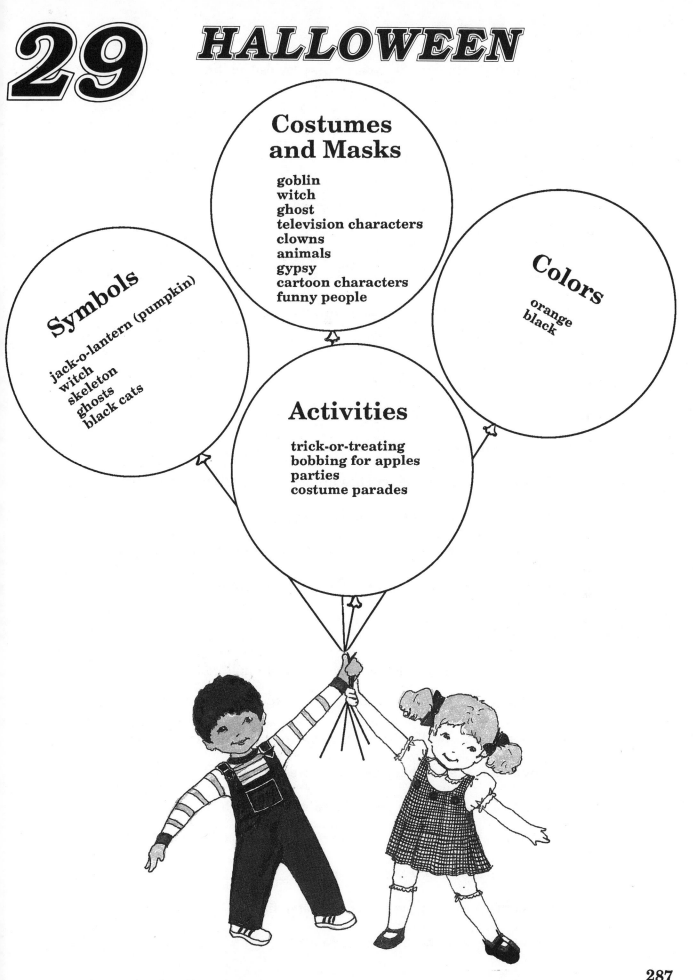

29 HALLOWEEN

Costumes and Masks

goblin
witch
ghost
television characters
clowns
animals
gypsy
cartoon characters
funny people

Symbols

jack-o-lantern (pumpkin)
witch
skeleton
ghosts
black cats

Colors

orange
black

Activities

trick-or-treating
bobbing for apples
parties
costume parades

Theme Goals:

Through participating in the experiences provided by this theme, the children may learn:

1. Halloween colors.

2. Halloween costumes and masks.

3. Halloween activities.

4. Halloween symbols.

Concepts for the Children to Learn:

1. Orange and black are Halloween colors.

2. Costumes and masks are worn on Halloween.

3. A costume is clothes for pretending.

4. A mask is a covering we put over our face.

5. A pumpkin can be cut to look like a face.

6. Ghosts, black cats and witches are symbols of Halloween.

7. People go trick-or-treating on Halloween.

8. A costume parade is a march with many children who are dressed up.

9. Bobbing for apples is an activity at Halloween parties.

Vocabulary:

1. **Halloween**—a day when children dress up and go trick-or-treating.

2. **jack-o-lantern**—a pumpkin cut to look like a face.

3. **trick-or-treat**—walking from house to house to ask for candy or treats.

4. **witch**—a make-believe person who wears black.

5. **ghost**—a make-believe person who wears all white.

6. **goblin**—a Halloween character.

7. **costume**—clothing worn to pretend.

8. **mask**—face covering worn when pretending.

9. **pretending**—acting like someone else.

Bulletin Board

The purpose of this bulletin board is to have the children practice visual discrimination skills. To prepare the bulletin board, construct pumpkins out of orange colored tagboard. The number will depend upon the developmental appropriateness of the group of children. An alternative would be to use white tagboard colored orange with paint or markers. Divide the pumpkins into pairs. Draw a different kind of face for each pair of pumpkins. Hang one pumpkin from each pair on the left side of the bulletin board as illustrated. Attach an orange string to each pumpkin. On the right side of the bulletin board, hang the matching pumpkins. See illustration. Attach a push pin to each of these pumpkins. The child can match the faces on the pumpkins by winding the correct string around the correct push pin.

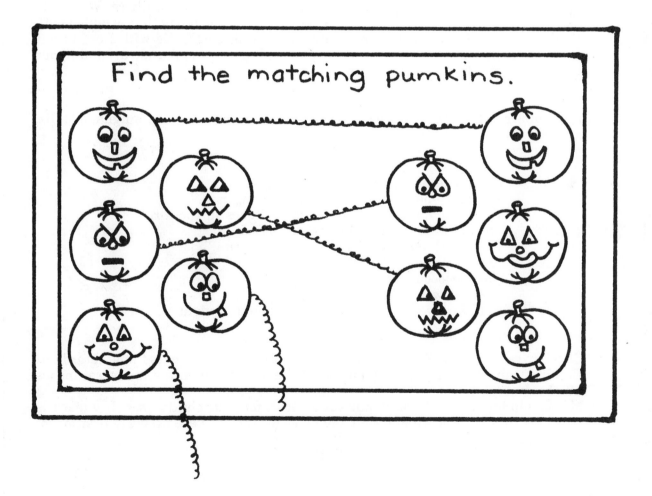

Parent Letter

Dear Parents,

The month of October has a special holiday for children—Halloween! Consequently, our theme this week will center on Halloween. Many learning experiences have been planned for this week to promote an awareness of colors that are associated with Halloween, as well as symbols that represent Halloween such as pumpkins, black cats, bats and witches.

This Week At School

Some of the Halloween activities planned for the week include:

* discussing Halloween safety procedures, especially while trick-or-treating.
* carving a jack-o-lantern for the classroom.
* roasting pumkin seeds and baking a pumpkin pie.
* trying on a variety of costumes in the dramatic play area.
* creating designs with pumpkin seeds and glue on paper.

Halloween Party!

We will be having a Halloween party on Friday. You are welcome to send a costume to school with your child that day. The costume can be simple. A funny hat, a pair of silly glasses, a wig or a little makeup would be fine Halloween attire. We would appreciate it if you could send the costume and accessories in a bag that is labled with your child's name. This will prevent a mix-up of belongings. We will dress in our costumes about 2:00 p.m. Then we will have a small party and parade around in our costumes. It should be a fun day. Join us!

At Home

To get into the spirit of Halloween and to help your child develop language skills, practice the following Halloween rhyme:

"Five Little Pumpkins"

Five little pumpkins sitting on a gate.
The first one said, "Oh my, it's getting late."
The second one said, "There are witches in the air."
The third one said, "But we don't care."
The fourth one said, "Let's run. Let's run."
The fifth one said, "It's Halloween fun!"
"Woooooooooo" went the wind,
And out went the lights.
And the five little pumpkins rolled out of sight.

To ensure a safe Halloween:

* Check to see if your child's costume is flame resistant or at least flame retardant.
* Children can easily trip in long garments. Be sure the hemline is several inches off the ground.
* Masks and hoods can slip and make it difficult for your child to see. If a mask is worn, be sure it is secure and that the holes for the eyes are properly positioned. An alternative to wearing a mask is to use make-up.
* Finally, check the batteries in the flashlight!

Have a safe and happy Halloween.

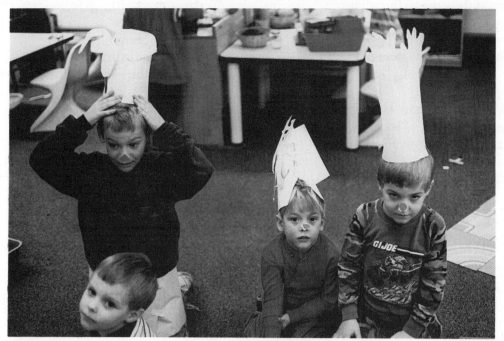

FIGURE 29 Costumes are the highlights of Halloween.

Music:

1. **"Flying Witches"**
   (Sing to the tune of "When the Saints Come Marching In")

   Oh, when the witches
   Come flying by.
   Oh, when the witches come flying by,
   It will be Halloween night,
   When the witches come flying by.

2. **"One Little, Two Little, Three Little Pumpkins"**
   (Sing to the tune of "One Little, Two Little, Three Little Indians")

   One little, two little, three little pumpkins,
   Four little, five little, six little pumpkins,
   Seven little, eight little, nine little pumpkins,
   Ready for Halloween night!

3. **"Have You Made a Jack-O-Lantern?"**
   (Sing to the tune of "Muffin Man")

   Have you made a jack-o-lantern,
   A jack-o-lantern, a jack-o-lantern?
   Have you made a jack-o-lantern
   For Halloween night?

Fingerplays:

JACK-O-LANTERN

I am a pumpkin, big and round.
  (show size with arms)
Once upon a time, I grew on the ground.
  (point to ground)
Now I have a mouth, two eyes, and a nose.
  (point to each)
What are they for do you suppose?
  (point to forehead & "think")
Why—I'll be a jack-o-lantern on Halloween night.

FIVE LITTLE WITCHES

Five little witches standing by the door.
  (hold up five fingers)
One flew out and then there were four.
  (flying motion with hand)
Four little witches standing by a tree.
  (four fingers)
One went to pick a pumpkin and then there were three.
  (picking motion then three fingers)
Three little witches stirring their brew.
  (stir)
One fell in and then there were two.
  (two fingers)

Two little witches went for a run.
  (run with fingers)
One got lost and then there was one.
  (one finger)
One little witch, yes, only one.
  (one finger)
She cast a spell and now there are none.
  (make motions as if to cast spell and
  then put hands in lap)

HALLOWEEN FUN

Goblins and witches in high pointed hats,
  (hands above head to form hat)
Riding on broom sticks and chasing black
cats.
  (ride broomstick)
Children in costumes might well give a
fright.
  (look frightened)
Get things in order for Halloween night.
We like our treats
  (nod head)
And we'll play no mean pranks.
  (shake head)
We'll do you no harm and we'll only say
"thanks!"

THE JACK-O-LANTERN

Three little pumpkins growing on a vine.
  (three fingers)
Sitting in the sunlight, looking just fine.
  (arms up like sun)
Along came a ghost who picked just one
  (one finger)
To take on home for some Halloween fun.
  (smile)
He gave him two eyes to see where he goes.
  (paint two eyes)
He gave him a mouth and a big handsome
nose.
  (point to mouth & nose)
Then he put a candle in.
  (pretend to put in candle)
Now see how he glows.
  (wiggle fingers from center of body out
  until arms are extended)

I'VE A JACK-O-LANTERN

I've a jack-o-lantern
  (make a ball with open fist, thumb at top)

With a great big grin.
  (grin)
I've got a jack-o-lantern
With a candle in.
  (insert other index finger up through
  bottom of first)

HALLOWEEN WITCHES

One little, two little, three little witches,
  (hold up one hand, nod fingers at each count)
Fly over the haystacks
  (fly hand in up-and-down motion)
Fly over ditches
Slide down moonbeams without any hitches
  (glide hand downward)
Heigh-ho! Halloween's here

THE FRIENDLY GHOST

I'm a friendly ghost—almost!
  (point to self)
And I chase you, too!
  (point to child)
I'll just cover me with a sheet
  (pretend to cover self ending with hands
  covering face)
And then call "scat" to you.
  (uncover face quickly and call out "scat")

WITCHES' CAT

I am the witches' cat.
  (make a fist with two fingers extended
  for cat)
Meoow, Meoow.
  (stroke fist with other hand)
My fur is black as darkest night.
My eyes are glaring green and bright.
  (circle eyes with thumb and forefingers)
I am the witches' cat.
  (make a fist again with two fingers
  extended and stroke fist with other hand)

MY PUMPKIN

See my pumpkin round and fat.
  (make circle with hands, fingers spread
  wide, touching)
See my pumpkin yellow.
  (make a smaller circle)
Watch him grin on Halloween.
  (point to mouth which is grinning wide)
He is a very funny fellow.

Science:

1. Carve Pumpkins

Purchase several pumpkins. Carve them and save the seeds for roasting. An alternative activity would be to use a black felt-tip marker to draw facial features on the pumpkin. Pumpkins can also have added accessories. For example, a large carrot can be used for a nose, parsley for hair, cut green peppers for ears, radishes for eyes and a small green onion can be placed in a cut mouth for teeth.

2. Roasting Pumpking Seeds

Wash and dry pumpkin seeds. Then spread the seeds out on a cookie sheet to dry. Bake the seeds in a preheated oven at 350 degrees until brown. Salt, cool and eat at snack time.

3. Plant Pumpkin Seeds

Purchase a packet of pumpkin seeds. Plant the pumpkin seeds in small paper cups. Set the paper cups with the pumpkin seeds in a sunny place. Water as needed. Observe to see if there is growth on a daily basis.

Dramatic Play:

Costume

Add Halloween costumes to the dramatic play area. (Some teachers purchase these at thrift stores or sales. From year to year they are stored in a Halloween prop box.)

Arts and Crafts:

1. Spooky Easel

Provide orange & black paint at the paint easels.

2. Pumpkin Seed Pictures

Dye pumpkin seeds many colors. Place the seeds with paste and paper on a table in the art area. The children then can create their own pictures.

3. Crayon Wash

On the art table, place paper, light colored crayons, tempera paint and brushes. The children can draw on paper with light colored crayons. After this, they can paint over the entire picture.

4. Masks

Yarn, paper plates, felt tip markers and any other accessories needed to make masks interesting can be placed on a table in the art area. If desired, yarn can be used as hair on the mask.

Sensory:

1. Measuring Seeds

Pumpkin seeds and measuring cups can be added to the sensory table. The children will enjoy feeling and pouring seeds.

2. Goop

Add dry cornstarch to the sensory table. Slowly add enough water to make it a "goopy" consistency. If desired, add coloring to make it black or orange.

Large Muscle:

Ghost, Ghost, Witch

This game is played like "Duck, Duck, Goose." Form a circle and kneel. Choose one child to walk around the outside of the circle chanting, "Ghost, ghost, ghost." When the child taps another child and says "witch," the child tapped chases the initiator around the circle, attempting to tag the child. If the child who is "it" returns to the tapped child's spot before the other, he can lose his turn. If not, the child continues walking around the circle, repeating the same procedure.

Field Trips/Resource People:

1. Pumpkin Patch

Visit a pumpkin patch. During the tour point out various sized pumpkins. Discuss how the pumpkins grow, as well as their shapes, sizes, etc.

2. Halloween Safety

A police officer can be invited to talk with the children about Halloween safety.

Math:

1. Counting Pumpkin Seeds

Cut circles from construction paper. The number needed will depend upon the developmental level of the children. Write a numeral on each paper circle and place each into a pie tin. The children may count pumpkin seeds into the tins matching the circles.

2. Weighing Pumpkin Seeds

In the math area, place a scale and pumpkin seeds. The children may elect to experiment by balancing the scale with the pumpkin seeds.

Group Time (games, language):

1. Thank You Note

Write a thank you note to any resource person. Encourage all of the children to participate by sharing what they liked or saw.

2. Costume Parade

On Halloween day, the children can dress up in costumes and march around the room and throughout the school to music. If available, a walk to a local nursing home may be enjoyed by the children as well as the elderly.

Cooking:

1. Pumpkin Pie

1 unbaked pie shell
2 cups (16-17 ounces) pumpkin
1 can sweetened condensed milk
1 egg
1/2 teaspoon salt
2 teaspoon pumpkin pie spice

Blend all of the ingredients in a large mixing bowl. Pour the mixture into the pie shell. Bake the pie in an oven preheated to 375 degrees for 50 to 55 minutes or until a sharp knife blade inserted near center of pie is clean when removed. Cool and refrigerate the pie for 1 hour before serving. Top with whipped cream if desired.

2. Pumpkin Patch Muffins

3 cups flour
1 cup sugar
4 teaspoons baking powder
1 teaspoon salt
1 teaspoon pumpkin pie spice
1 cup milk
1 cup canned pumpkin
1/2 cup (1 stick) butter or margarine, melted
2 eggs, beaten

Sift the flour, sugar, baking powder, salt and pumpkin pie spice into a large mixing bowl. Add the milk, pumpkin, melted butter and eggs. Mix with a wooden spoon just until flour is moist. (Batter will be lumpy.) Place paper liners in the muffin tins and fill 2/3 full with batter. Bake in a preheated 400-degree oven 20 minutes or until muffins are golden. Cool in muffin tins 10 minutes on a wire rack. Remove muffins from muffin tins and finish cooling on wire racks. Pile into serving baskets and serve warm for snack.

3. Witches' Brew

5 cups cranberry juice, unsweetened
5 cups apple cider, unsweetened
1 or 2 cinnamon sticks
1/4 teaspoon ground nutmeg

Place ingredients in a large saucepan. Cover, heat and simmer for 10 minutes. Serve warm.

4. Roasted Pumpkin Seeds

Soak pumpkin seeds for 24 hours in salt water (1/4 cup salt to 1 cup water). Spread on cloth-covered cookie sheet and roast at 100 degrees for 2 hours. Turn oven off and leave seeds overnight.

5. Non-bake Pumpkin Pie

1 can prepared pumpkin pie
1 package vanilla instant pudding
1 cup milk

Mix and pour into baked pie shell or graham cracker pie shell.

DECORATING A PUMPKIN

In carving or decorating a pumpkin with the children you can discuss:

* the physical properties of pumpkins—color, texture, size, shape (both outside and inside).
* what food category to which pumpkins belong.
* what other forms pumpkins can be made into after scooped out of the shell.
* where pumpkins grow (plant some of the seeds).

* what size and shape to make the features of the pumpkin, including eyes, nose, mouth and what kind of expression to make.

Accessories:

1 bunch parsley (hair)
1 carrot (nose)
2 string beans (eyebrows)
2 radishes (eyes)
1 green pepper (ears)

1 stalk celery (teeth)
1 large pumpkin (head)

Prepare the pumpkin in the usual manner; that is, cut off the cap and scoop out the seeds inside. Save the seeds for roasting. If desired, individual vegetable pieces may be attached by carving or inserting toothpicks.

Records:

The following records can be found in preschool educational catalogs:

1. **Holiday Songs and Rhythms.** Hap Palmer.

2. **Holiday Songs For All Occasions.** Kimbo Records.

3. **Holiday Action Songs.** Kimbo Records.

Books and Stories:

The following books and stories can be used to complement the theme:

1. **The Halloween Party.** Lonzo Anderson. (New York: Charles Scribner's Sons, 1974).

2. **The Terrible Trick-or-Treat.** Edith Battles. (New York: Young Scott Books, 1970).

3. **Clifford's Halloween.** Norman Bridwell. (New York: Four Winds Press, 1966).

4. **The Witch Next Door.** Norman Bridwell. (New York: Four Winds Press, 1965).

5. **Georgie's Halloween.** Robert Bright. (New York: Doubleday, 1958).

6. **The Trip.** Ezra Jack Keats. (New York: Greenwillow Books, 1978).

7. **The Attic Witch.** Sonia O. Lisker. (New York: Four Winds Press, 1973).

8. **That Terrible Halloween Night.** James Stevenson. (New York: Greenwillow Books, 1980).

9. **Pumpkin Moonshine.** Tasha Tudor. (New York: Henry Z. Walck, 1938).

10. **Halloween with Morris and Borris.** Bernard Wiseman. (New York: Dodd, Mead and Company, 1975).

11. **My First Halloween Book.** Colleen L. Reece. (Chicago: Childrens Press, 1984).

Puzzles:

The following puzzles can be found in preschool educational catalogs:

1. **"Halloween"** 22 pieces. Judy/Instructo.

2. **"Jack-o-Lantern"** 7 pieces. Puzzle People.

3. **"Halloween"** 7 pieces. Puzzle People.

30 HANUKKAH
(CHANUKAH)

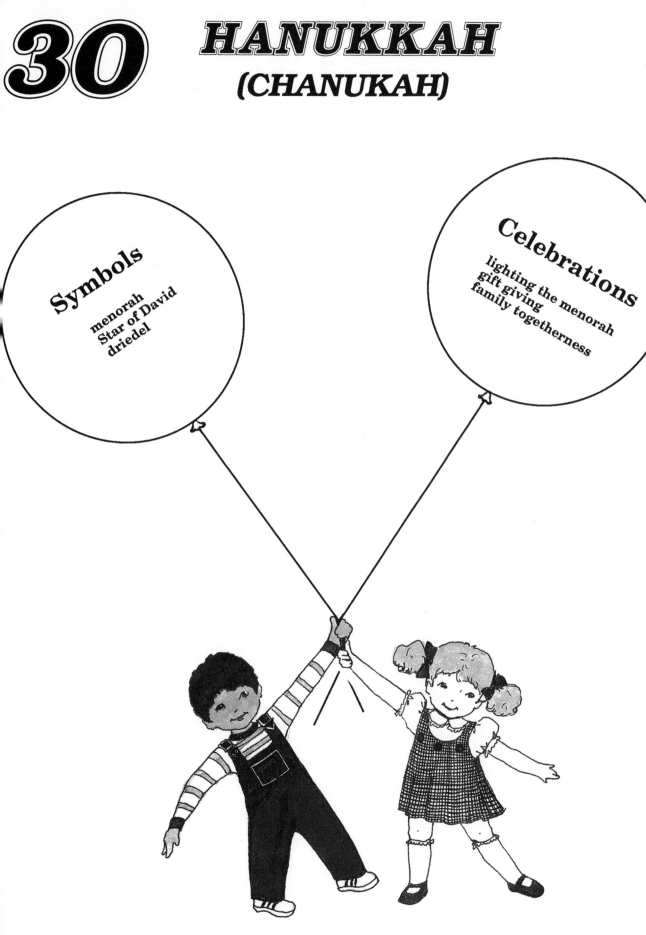

Symbols
menorah
Star of David
driedel

Celebrations
lighting the menorah
gift giving
family togetherness

Theme Goals:

Through participating in the experiences provided by this theme, the children may learn:

1. The story of Hanukkah.

2. Symbols of Hanukkah.

3. Hanukkah celebrations.

Concepts for the Children to Learn:

1. Hanukkah is a Jewish holiday.

2. Hanukkah is a time for giving and sharing with others.

3. The menorah, the dreidel and the Star of David are symbols of Hanukkah.

4. Hanukkah is celebrated for eight days.

Vocabulary:

1. **latkes**—potato pancakes eaten during Hanukkah.

2. **dreidel**—four-sided toy that spins like a top.

4. **Star of David**—star-shaped figure, symbol of Hanukkah.

4. **menorah**—eight-branched candlestick. The middle or ninth candle is taller than the other eight and is called the shammash.

5. **Hanukkah**—eight-day Jewish festival of lights. A celebration of the Jewish people's fight long ago to win the right to practice their religion. One candle is lighted on the menorah each day.

Bulletin Board

The purpose of this bulletin board is to develop an awareness of the passage of time as well as the math concept of sets. This bulletin board starts out with the base of the menorah. Each day of Hanukkah the children work together to construct a candle and a flame to add to the menorah. Candles and flames are most interesting when made using a wide variation of mediums: glitter, feathers, cut construction paper, yarn, etc.

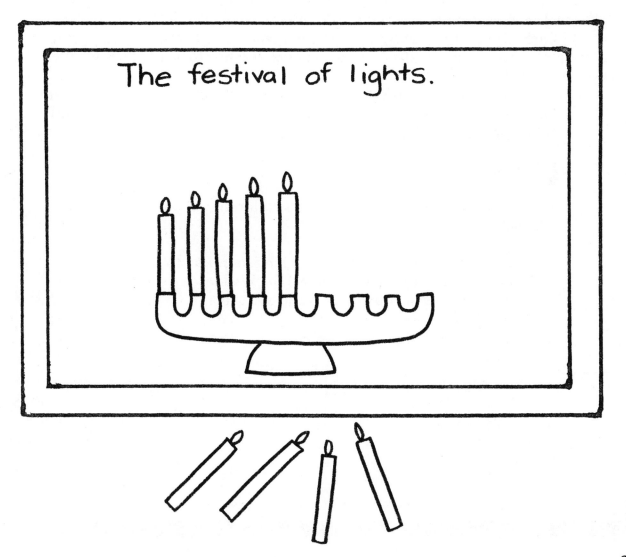

The festival of lights.

Parent Letter

Dear Parents,

For the next eight days, we will be celebrating Hanukkah. Hanukkah commemorates the victory of the Jews over the Syrians. Hanukkah, also known as the Festival of Lights, is celebrated for eight days in either November or December. In 175 B.C. a Syrian King, Anitochus, ordered the Jewish Temple destroyed. After the Syrians destroyed the Temple, Judah Maccabee formed a small but powerful army to defend the Jews. The Maccabees rebuilt the Temple and the legend states that when it was time to light the Temple lamp for rededication, there was only enough sacred oil to burn for one day. Miraculously, it burned for eight days!

Hanukkah is celebrated by the lighting of a special candelabra called a menorah. In the menorah there is one holder for each of the eight nights and one for the shammash. Shammash means servant in Hebrew; this is the candle that is used to light the others. The candles are lit beginning on the right side and moving to the left.

Each night, after the lighting of the menorah, the children are given small gifts. Traditionally this gift was gelt, money to be used while playing the dreidel game.

Hanukkah is one of the least solemn Jewish holidays. Unlike most Jewish holidays, work and schooling continues during the eight day celebration.

At School This Week

Some of the learning experiences the children will participate in this week include:

* playing a game with a dreidel, which is similar to a toy top.
* preparing latkes (potato pancakes) for Wednesday's snack.
* creating wax-resist drawings at the art table.

Have a good week!

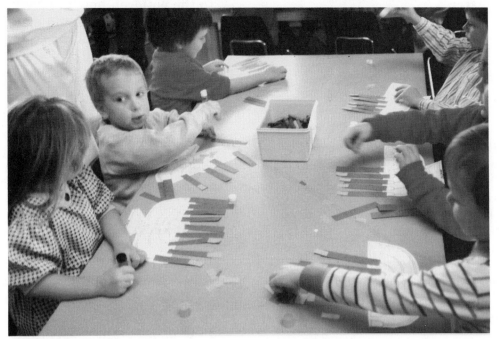

FIGURE 30 Hanukkah is time to light the menorah.

Music:

"Menorah Candles"
(Sing to the tune of "Twinkle, Twinkle, Little Star")

Twinkle, twinkle candles in the night,
Standing on the menorah bright,
Burning slow we all know,
Burning bright to give us light.
Twinkle, twinkle candles in the night,
Standing on the menorah bright.

Fingerplays:

THE MENORAH CANDLE

I'm a menorah candle
   (stand, point at self)
Growing shorter you can see
   (bend down slowly)
Melting all my wax
   (go down more)
Until there's nothing left to see.
   (sit down)

HANUKKAH LIGHTS

One light, two lights, three lights and four
   (hold up four fingers, one at a time)

Five lights, six lights, and three more,
   (hold up five fingers on other hand)
Twinkle, twinkle nine pretty lights,
   (move fingers)
In a golden menorah bright!
   (make cup with palm of hand)

MY DREIDEL

I have a little dreidel.
   (cup hands to form a square)
I made it out of clay.
   (move fingers in a molding motion)
And when it's dry and ready
   (flatten hands as if to hold in hand—
   palm up, pinkies together)
Then with it I will play.
   (pretent to spin dreidel on the floor)

Science:

1. **Potato Sprouts**

Provide each child with a clear plastic cup. Fill the plastic cup half way with water. Place a potato part way in the water supported by toothpicks to keep it from dropping into the jar. Put the end with tubers into the water. The other end should stick out of the water. Refill with fresh water as it evaporates and watch the roots begin to grow and leaves start to sprout.

301

2. Candle Snuffer

Demonstrate how a candle snuffer is used to put out a flame. (Check licensing regulations prior to the activity.)

3. Light

Light a candle. Discuss other sources of light. (Examples: sun, lamp, flashlight, traffic lights, etc.)

4. Sunlight Power

Fill two glasses half full of warm water. Stir some flour into one glass. In the other, dissolve a little yeast in the water, then add flour. Now set them both in a warm place for an hour and watch the results.

Dramatic Play:

1. Family Celebration

Collect materials for a special family meal. This may include dresses, hats, coats, plates, cups, plastic food, napkins, etc. The children can have a holiday meal.

2. Gift Wrapping Center

Collect various sized boxes, wrapping paper, tape and ribbon. The children can wrap presents for Hanukkah.

Sensory:

Sand Temples

Fill the sensory table with sand and moisten until the sand begins to adhere. The children may pack sand into cans to mold into desired shapes and build sand temples from the molded forms.

Arts and Crafts:

1. Star of David

Provide the children with triangles cut from blue construction paper. Demonstrate to the children how to invert one triangle over the other to form a star. The stars may be glued to construction paper.

2. Potato Art

Slice potatoes in half. The children may dip the potato halves in shallow pans containing various colors of tempera paint and then create designs on construction paper.

3. Hanukkah Handprints

Provide the chidlren with construction paper, brushes and tempera paint in shallow pans. Paint each of the children's hands with a brush that has been dipped in tempera paint. The children then may place their hands on the construction paper, creating handprints.

4. Dreidel Top

Collect and wash out 1/2-pint milk containers. Tape the top down so that the carton forms a square. Provide construction paper squares for the children to paste to the sides of the milk carton. The children may decorate with crayons or felt-tip markers. Upon completion, punch an unsharpened pencil through the milk container so that the children may spin it like a top.

5. Star of David Mobile

Provide each child with two drinking straws. Demonstrate to the children how to bend the straws so that they make triangles. Glue the straw triangles together, inverting one over the other to make a six-pointed star. Tie string to the star and hang from a window or ceiling.

Resource People:

Invite a rabbi or parent of the Jewish faith to come and talk about Hanukkah and how it is celebrated.

Large Muscle:

1. Dreidel Dance

The children can dance the dreidel dance by standing in a circle and spinning as they sing this song to the tune of "Row, Row, Row, Your Boat."

Dreidel, dreidel, dreidel,
A-spinning I will go.
Speed it up and slow it down,
And on the ground I'll go!

2. Frying Donuts—Dramatic Play

Children can act out frying donuts as they sing this song to the tune of "I Have a Little Turtle."

I have a little donut,
It is so nice and light,
And when it's all done cooking,
I'm going to take a bite!

Frying donuts usually pop up and out of the frying oil when they are finished cooking. The children can act out these motions. The oil used in frying the donuts is significant in the Hanukkah celebration. It signifies the oil burned in the Temple.

Math:

1. Sort the Stars

Provide children with various colored stars. The children can match the colors. A variation would be to have stars of various sizes. The children could sequence the stars from largest to smallest.

2. Hanukkah Puzzles

Mount pictures of a menorah and the Star of David on tagboard. Cut into pieces. Laminate. The number of pieces will depend upon the children's developmental age.

3. Candle Holder and Candle Match

Have a variety of candle holders set out with candles. The children will have to match the candles to the correct sized candle holder.

Group Time (games, language):

1. Hot Potato

Ask the children to sit in a circle. Provide one child with a real, a plastic or a potato constructed from tagboard. Play music. As the music is playing, the children pass the potato around the circle until the music stops. The one holding the potato is out of the circle. Game continues until one child is left or the children no longer wish to play.

2. Dreidel Game

Each player starts with 10 to 15 pennies, nuts, or raisins. Each player places an object in the center of the circle. The dreidel is spun by one of the players, while the following verse is chanted:

I have a little dreidel.
I made it out of clay.
And when it's dry and ready.
Then with it I will play.

Whether the spinning player wins or loses depends on which side of the dreidel lands upward when it falls. The following may be used as a guide:

Nun (N) means nothing: player receives nothing from the pot.
Gimmel (G) means all: player receives everything from the pot.
Hay (H) means half: player takes 1/2 of the pot.
Shin (S) means put in: player adds two objects to the pot.

When one player has won all of the objects the game is completed.

3. Gelt Hunt

Make a silver coin by cutting out a 4-inch round piece of cardboard and covering it with aluminum foil. Hide the coin (gelt) in the classroom and play a hide-and-seek game. For younger children hide the gelt in an obvious place.

(Gelt is the Hebrew word for money. Traditionally, small amounts of gelt are given to children each night of Hanukkah.)

Social Studies:

1. Menorah

Glue eight wooden or styrofoam spools of equal size to a piece of wood, leaving a space in the middle. Glue a larger spool in the middle, thus having four smaller spools on each side. Spray with gold or silver paint. The menorah can be lit during the eight days of Hanukkah during group time. Explain the meaning of the menorah to the group as well.

2. Hanukkah Celebration

Display pictures at the child's eye level of the Hanukkah celebration. Examples would include such pictures as lighting the menorah, a family meal, etc.

3. Human Menorah

The children can make a human menorah by positioning themselves to resemble a menorah. A menorah is a lamp with nine flames which is used to celebrate Hanukkah. Two children can lie head-to-toe on the floor to form the base. Have nine children stand behind the base to form the candles. The tallest child can stand in the middle and be the shammash. The shammash is the center candle that lights the other candles. The children can make flames out of construction paper for the candles to hold as they are lit.

Cooking:

1. Latkes

6 medium-sized potatoes washed, pared and grated
1 egg
3 tablespoons flour
1/2 teaspoon baking powder

In a large bowl, mix the egg and the grated potatoes. Add the flour and baking powder. Drop by spoonsful into hot cooking oil in a frying pan. Brown on both sides. Drain on paper towel. Latkes may be served with applesauce or sour cream.

2. Hanukkah Honey and Spice Cookies

1/2 cup (1 stick) margarine, softened
1/2 cup firmly packed dark brown sugar
1/2 cup honey
2 1/2 cups unsifted flour
2 teaspoons ground ginger
1 teaspoon baking soda
1 teaspoon ground cinnamon
1 teaspoon ground nutmeg
1/2 teaspoon salt
1/4 teaspoon ground cloves

In a large mixing bowl cream margarine and sugar. Beat in honey and egg until well combined. In a small bowl combine flour, ginger, baking soda, cinnamon, nutmeg, salt and cloves. Add to honey mixture. Beat on low speed until well blended. Cover dough and chill at least 1 hour or up to 3 days. Heat oven to 350 degrees. Grease cookie sheets. Set aside. Working quickly with 1/4 of the dough at a time, roll out on floured surface to 1/4-inch thickness. Cut into desired shapes, including a dreidel, menorah or star. Using a spatula, place cookies on prepared cookie sheets 1 inch apart. Reroll scraps. Bake for 7 minutes. Transfer to wire racks to cool. Makes about 4 dozen cookies.

3. Ka'achei Sumsum—Bagel Cookies

4 cups of flour
1 cup margarine
1 teaspoon salt
3 tablespoons cake-form yeast
1 egg
1 cup lukewarm water
1/4 teaspoon sugar

Place yeast and sugar in a bowl. Pour over lukewarm water. Put in a warm place for 10 minutes or until yeast rises. Prepare a dough from the flour, margarine, salt and dissolved yeast mixture. Cover dough with a towel, put in a warm place for 2 hours. When dough rises, take small pieces and roll into strips about 4 inches long. Join the ends to form a bagel. Brush each one with beaten egg and place on a greased baking sheet. Bake in a 350-degree oven for 20 to 30 minutes.

Source: *The Art of Israeli Cooking.* Aldo Nahoum (editor). (New York: Holt, Rinehart and Winston, 1970).

4. K'naidlach Soup

3 eggs
3 1/2 cups matzo meal
1/2 chicken bouillon cube
1 teaspoon celery leaves, chopped
nutmeg
juice of 1/2 lemon
salt
pepper

Beat eggs well. Add bouillon cube, salt, pepper and a pinch of nutmeg. Add lemon juice and celery leaves. Continue to beat. Slowly add matzo meal, using a wooden spoon to stir. When matzo meal thickens, knead by hand. After matzo meal has been thoroughly kneaded, form small balls (1 inch). Arrange in a deep dish and leave in refrigerator for at least 3 hours. Prepare a clear chicken soup and when it reaches boiling, drop in matzo balls. Let cook for 10 to 12 minutes. Serve 3 to 4 balls per bowl of soup. Add lemon juice to taste.

Source: *The Art of Israeli Cooking.* Aldo Nahoum (editor). (New York: Holt, Rinehart and Winston, 1970).

Records:

The following records can be found in preschool educational catalogs:

1. **Holiday Songs and Rhythms.** "Hanukkah" Hap Palmer.

2. **Holiday Songs for All Occasions.** "Hanukkah" Kimbo.

3. **Kindergarten Songs, Record 1.** "My Dreidel" Bowmar.

4. **Folk Songs of Israel.** "O Hanukkah" Bowmar.

5. **Israeli Children's Songs.** Ben-Ezra, Folkways.

6. **Songs to Share.** United Synagogue Book Service.

Books and Stories:

The following books and stories can be used to complement the theme:

1. **Hanukkah.** Norma Simon. (New York: Thomas Y. Crowell, 1966).

2. **Hanukkah in My House.** Norma Simon. (New York: United Synagogue Book Service, 1960).

3. **My First Hanukkah Book.** Aileen Fisher. (Chicago: Childrens Press, 1985).

4. **Potato Pancakes All Around.** Marilyn Hirsch. (Philadelphia: JPS, 1982).

5. **Hanukkah Money.** Shalom Aleichem.

6. **The Story of Chanukah for Children.** Beverly Rae Charette.

7. **A Picture Book of Jewish Holidays.** David Adler. (New York: Holiday House, 1982).

8. **Rainbow Candles.** Myra Shostak. (New York: Kar Ben, 1986).

9. **My Very Own Chanukah Book.** Judyth Robbins. (New York: Kar Ben, 1977).

10. **It's Chanukah.** Ellie Gellman. (New York: Kar Ben, 1985).

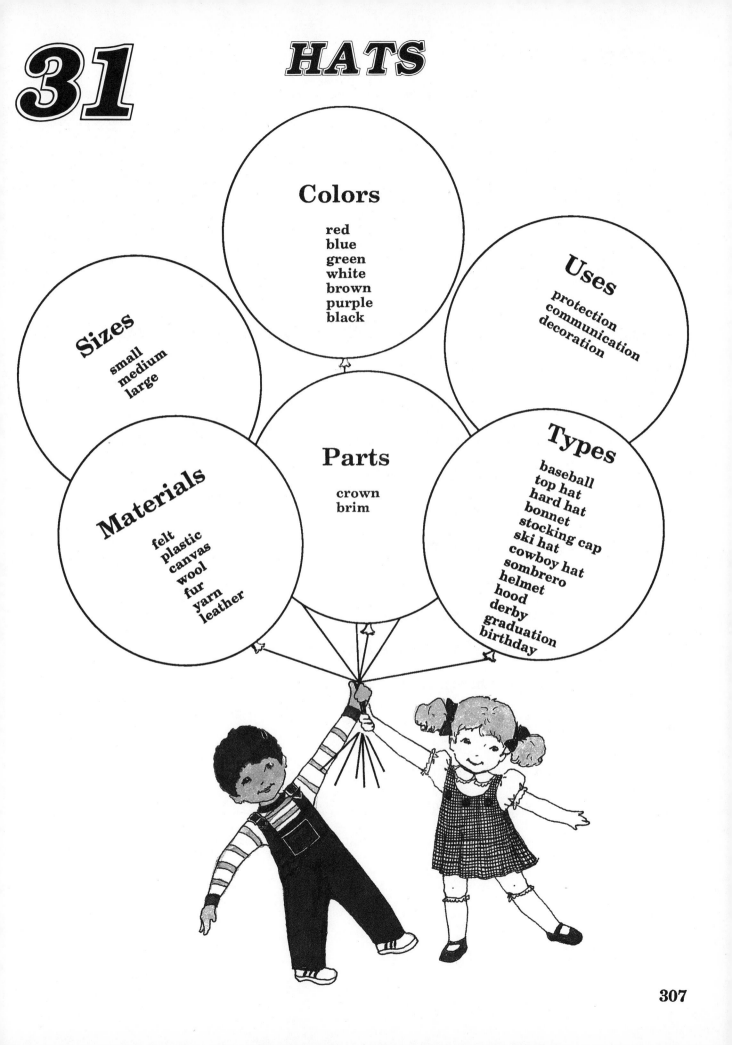

31

HATS

Colors

red
blue
green
white
brown
purple
black

Uses

protection
communication
decoration

Sizes

small
medium
large

Parts

crown
brim

Types

baseball
top hat
hard hat
bonnet
stocking cap
ski hat
cowboy hat
sombrero
helmet
hood
derby
graduation
birthday

Materials

felt
plastic
canvas
wool
fur
yarn
leather

Theme Goals:

Through participating in the experiences provided by this theme, the children may learn:

1. Types of hats.

2. Uses for hats.

3. Materials used to make hats.

4. Parts of a hat.

5. Colors and sizes of hats.

Concepts for the Children to Learn:

1. Hats are worn on our heads.

2. Some hats keep us warm.

3. Felt, plastic, cloth and yarn are all materials used to make hats.

4. Hats come in different sizes.

5. Hats come in different colors.

6. Some hats have special names.

7. Some hats can keep us cool.

8. Hats can be worn for fun.

9. Some people wear hats when they are working.

10. Most hats have a crown and a brim.

Vocabulary:

1. **hat**—a covering for the head.

2. **crown**—top part of the hat.

3. **brim**—the part of a hat that surrounds the crown.

Bulletin Board

The purpose of this bulletin board is to have the children match the colored pieces to their corresponding shadow, thereby developing visual discrimination skills. To construct the bulletin board, draw different types of hats on white tagboard. Color the hats with watercolor markers and cut out. Trace the cut out hats onto black construction paper to create shadows. Then cut the shadows out and attach to the bulletin board. A magnet piece or a push pin can be fastened to the shadow. A magnet piece or a hole can be applied to the colored hats.

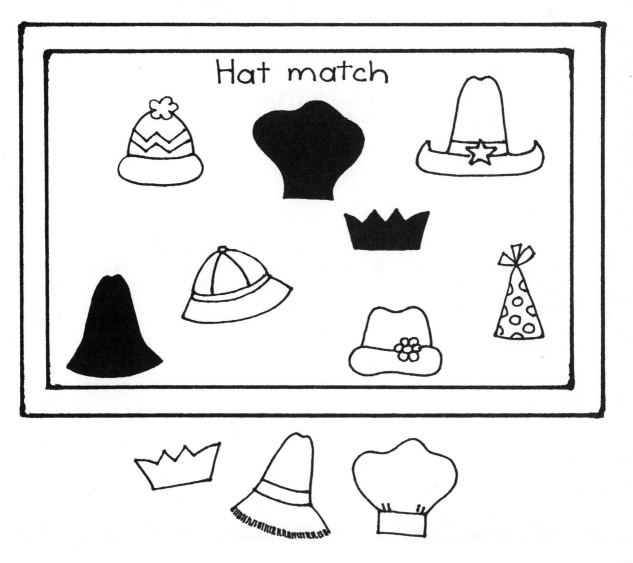

Parent Letter

Dear Parents,

This week the curriculum will focus on an article of clothing worn on our heads—hats! Through this unit the children will become familiar with occupations and sports for which hats are worn, materials used to make hats and purposes of hats such as for protection, decoration and identification.

At School This Week

Some of the learning activities planned for the week include:

* playing in the Hat Store located in the dramatic play area.
* making paper plate hats at the art table.
* listening to and dramatizing the story *Caps for Sale* by Esphyr Slobodkina.

Special Request!

On Friday we will have a Hat Day. The children will show and wear hats that they have brought from home. If your child wishes to share a special hat, please label it and send it to the center with your child in a paper bag. This will help us to keep track of which hat belongs to each child. Thank you for your help.

At Home

Ask your child to help you search the closets of your home for hats. To develop classification skills, discuss the colors and types of hats with your child. Are there more seasonal hats or sports hats? What are the hats made from? Why were those materials used?

Hats off to a good week!

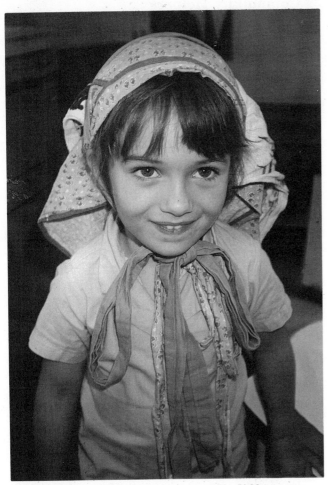

FIGURE 31 Hats come in all different styles.

Music:

1. "My Hat"
(traditional song)

My Hat it has three corners.
  (point to head, hold up three fingers)
Three corners has my hat.
  (hold up three fingers, point to head)
And had it not three corners
  (hold up three fingers)
It wouldn't be my hat.
  (shake head, point to head)

Variation: Make three cornered paper hats to wear while acting out this song.

Science:

What's It Made Of?

Hats representing a variety of styles and materials can be placed on the science table. Magnifying glasses can also be provided to allow the children to explore. They can look at, feel and smell the hats.

Dramatic Play:

1. Sports Hats

Provide football helmets and jerseys, baseball hats, batters' helmets and uniforms. Encourage the children to pretend they are football and baseball players.

2. Construction Site

Provide the children with toy tools, blocks, and construction hard hats.

3. Hat Store

Firefighter hats, bonnets, top hats, hard hats, bridesmaids' hats, baby hats, etc. can all be available in the hat store. Encourage the children to buy and sell hats using a cash register and play money.

Arts and Crafts:

1. Easel Ideas

* top hat shaped paper
* baseball cap shaped paper
* football helmet shaped paper
* graduation cap shaped paper

2. Paper Plate Hats

Decorate paper plates with many different kinds of scraps, glitter, construction paper and crepe paper. Punch a hole, using a paper punch, on each side of the hat. Attach strings so that the hat can be tied on and fastened under the chin.

Large Muscle:

Hat Bean Bag Toss

Lay several large hats on the floor. Encourage the children to stand about two feet from the hats and try to throw the beanbags into the hats.

Field Trips/Resource People:

1. Hat Store

Visit a hat store or hat department of a store. Examine the different kinds, sizes and colors of hats.

2. Sports Store

Visit a sporting goods store. Locate the hat section. Observe the types of hats used for different sports.

Math:

1. Hat Match

Construct pairs of hat puzzles out of tagboard. On each pair, draw a different pattern. Encourage the children to mix the hats up and sort them by design.

2. Hat Seriation

Collect a variety of hats. The children can arrange them from smallest to largest and largest to smallest. Also they can classify the hats by colors and uses.

Social Studies:

Many of these activities lend themselves to group time situations.

1. Weather or Not to Wear a Hat

Discuss the different kinds of hats that are worn in cold weather. Ask questions such as "What parts of our body does a hat keep warm?" "What kind of hats do we wear when it is warm outside?" "How does a hat help to keep us cool?"

2. Sports Hats

Make an arrangement of different sports hats. Place a mirror close by. The children can try on the hats.

3. Community Helpers

Many people in our community wear hats as part of their uniform. Collect several of these hats such as firefighter, police officer, mail carrier, baker, etc. and place in a bag for a small group activity. Identify one child at a time to pull a hat out of the bag. Once the hat is removed, the children can identify the worker. Older children may be able to describe the activities of the identified worker.

Group Time (games, language):

1. "My Favorite Hat Day"

Encourage the children to share their favorite hats with the class on a specific day. Talk about each hat and ask where it was bought or found. Colors, sizes and shapes can also be discussed.

2. Dramatization

Read the story *Caps for Sale*. After the children are familiar with the storyline, they may enjoy acting out the story.

Cooking:

The children may enjoy wearing baker's hats for the cooking experiences! Ask a bakery or fast-food restaurant to donate several for classroom use.

1. Cheese Crunchies

1/2 cup butter or margarine
1 cup all-purpose flour
1 cup shredded cheddar cheese
pinch of salt
1 cup rice cereal bits

Cut the butter into 6 or 8 slices and mix together with the flour, cheese and salt. Use fingers or fork to mix. Knead in the cereal bits; then roll the dough into small balls or snakes. Press them down flat and place onto an ungreased cookie sheet. Bake at 325 degrees for approximately 10 minutes. Cool and serve for snack.

2. Hamantaschen from Israel

Children in Israel eat hamantaschen on the holiday of Purim. A hamantaschen is a pastry that represents the hat worn by the evil Haman, who plotted against the ancient Jews. Today, Israeli children dress in costumes, parade in the streets and have parties on Purim.

7 tablespoons butter or margarine
1/3 cup sugar
2 eggs
2 1/2 cups flour
1/4 cup orange juice
1 teaspoon lemon juice
1 jar prune or plum jam

Cream the butter or margarine and sugar together in a large mixing bowl. Separate the eggs. Discard the whites. Add the yolk to the mixture and stir. Add the flour and juices to the mixture and mix to form dough. On a floured board, roll the dough to about 1/8-inch thickness. Use a cookie cutter to cut into 4-inch circles. Spoon a tablespoon of jam into the center of each circle and fold up 3 edges to create a triangle shape. Leave a small opening at the center. (Other fillings, such as poppy seeds or apricot jam, can be used.) Place the shaped dough on a cookie sheet and bake for 20 minutes in a 350-degree preheated oven. Serve for snack.

HATS

A variety of hats can be collected for use in the dramatic play area. Some examples are:

firefighter	motorcycle helmet	berets
police officer	cloche	top hat
visor	sports:	cowboy
sun bonnets	football	stocking cap
sombrero	baseball	mail carrier
straw hats	chef	bicycle helmet
mantilla	sailor	pillbox
party (birthday)	hard hats	scarves
nurse's cap	ski caps	headband
railroad engineer		

Books and Stories:

The following books and stories can be used to complement the theme:

1. **Caps for Sale.** Esphyr Slobodkina. (New York: Young Scott Books, 1947).

2. **The Hat.** Tomi Ungerer. (New York: Parents Magazine, 1970).

3. **The 500 Hats of Bartholomew Cubbins.** Dr. Seuss. (The Vanguard Press: 1938).

4. **Jennie's Hat.** Ezra Jack Keats. (New York: Harper and Row, 1966).

5. **Paddy's New Hat.** John S. Goodall. (New York: Atheneum, 1980).

6. **The Hat.** Faith and John Hubley. (New York: Harcourt, Brace and Jovanovich, 1974).

7. **The Cat in the Hat.** Dr. Seuss. (New York: Random House, 1957).

8. **Old Hat New Hat.** Jan and Stan Berenstein. (New York: Random House, 1970).

9. **I Want A Hat Like That.** Tom Cooke (ill.). (New York: Golden Press, 1987).

10. **A Three Hat Day.** Laura Geringer. (New York: Harper and Row, 1985).

11. **Fur.** Jan Mark. (New York: Harper and Row, 1986).

12. **Who Took Farmer's Hat?** (New York: Harper and Row, 1963).

13. **Santa's Hat.** Claire Schumacher. (New York: Prentice Hall Books, 1987).

Puzzles:

The following puzzles can be found in preschool educational catalogs:

1. **"Occupation Hats"** 6 pieces. Puzzle People.

2. **"Hats"** 5 pieces. Constructive Playthings.

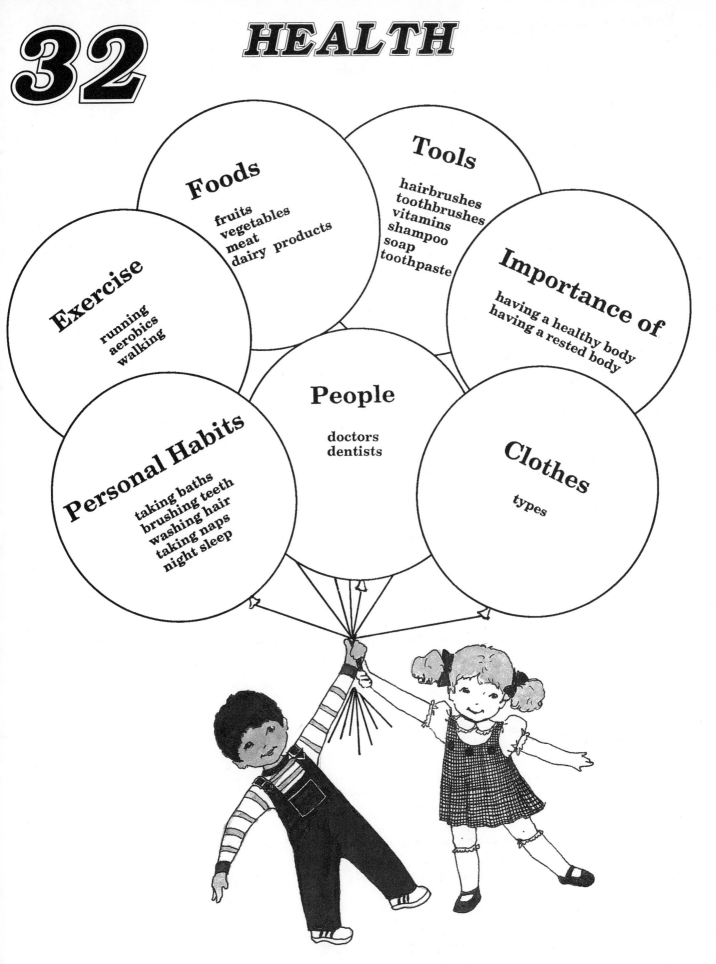

Foods
fruits
vegetables
meat
dairy products

Tools
hairbrushes
toothbrushes
vitamins
shampoo
soap
toothpaste

Exercise
running
aerobics
walking

Importance of
having a healthy body
having a rested body

People
doctors
dentists

Personal Habits
taking baths
brushing teeth
washing hair
taking naps
night sleep

Clothes
types

Theme Goals:

Through participating in the experiences provided by this theme, the children may learn:

1. Importance of good health.

2. Health foods.

3. Exercise clothes.

4. Tools used for health needs.

5. Exercises for health.

6. Health habits.

7. Health occupations.

Concepts for the Children to Learn:

1. We need to take good care of our bodies.

2. Vitamins, shampoo, soap and toothpaste are health aids.

3. Doctors and dentists provide health checkups.

4. Running, aerobics and walking are all forms of exercise.

5. Fruits, vegetables, dairy products and meat keep our bodies healthy.

6. Our bodies need rest.

7. Different types of clothing are worn during exercise.

8. Brushing teeth, washing hair and bathing are ways to keep our bodies clean.

9. Hairbrushes and toothbrushes are health tools.

Vocabulary:

1. **exercise**—moving body parts.

2. **health**—feeling good.

3. **nutrition**—eating foods that are good for our body.

4. **cleanliness**—keeping our body parts free from dirt.

5. **diet**—the food we eat.

6. **check-up**—a visit to a doctor to make sure you are healthy.

Bulletin Board

The purpose of this bulletin board is to have the children match the health aids to their corresponding shadow. Construct health aids from white tagboard such as a toothbrush, toothpaste, comb, brush and soap. Color the objects with colored felt-tip markers and laminate. Trace each of the health aids onto black construction paper to construct shadows as illustrated. Staple the shadow aids on the bulletin board by either affixing magnets or using push pins. Then punch a hole in the health aids for the children to hang them on the appropriate shadow.

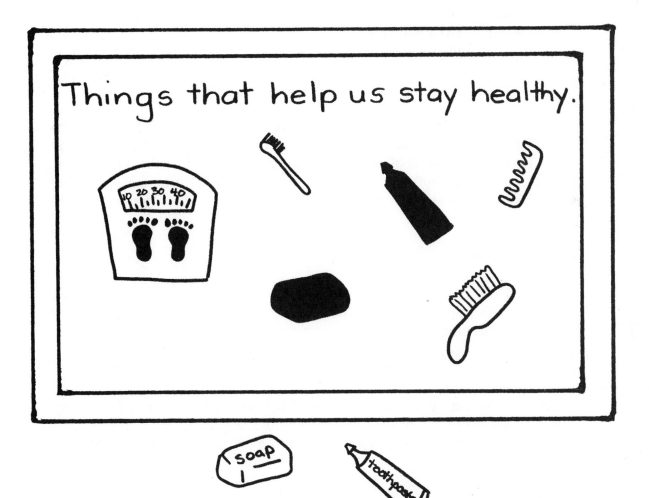

Parent Letter

Dear Parents,

This week at school we will be starting a unit on health. This unit will include many aspects of health. We will be discussing foods that are good for us, important personal habits and exercise. Through this unit the children will develop an awareness of how important it is to keep their bodies healthy.

At School This Week

Some of the learning experiences planned for the week include:

* tracing our bodies at the art center.
* visiting Dr. Thomas, the dentist, at his office.
* having a visit by an aerobics instructor.
* creating healthy snacks.
*weighing and measuring ourselves.

Field Trip

Arrangements have been made to visit Dr. Thomas's office on Th rs day of this week. Dr. Thomas will give us a tour of the dental clinic and show us various pieces of dental equipment. We will walk to his office, leaving school at 10:00 a.m. and return just in time for lunch. Please have your child at school by 10:00 am if he wishes to participate. Parents, please feel free to join us.

Just a Reminder

If your child's toothbrush at school is missing, please send another one. We teach the importance of dental hygiene by brushing our teeth after all meals and snacks at school.

At Home

Cotton swabs may be used instead of brushes for painting. They may also be used to dot paper with different colors. Painting is a valuable sensory experience for a child. It provides an opportunity to experiment with color.

Have a good week!

I scrub all my teeth for awhile.
I swish the water to rinse them and then
   (puff out cheeks to swish)
I look at myself and I smile.
   (smile at one another)

Science:

Soap Pieces

Add different kinds of soaps and a magnifying glass to the science area. Talk about what each one is used for.

Dramatic Play:

1. **Health Club**

Mats, fake weights (made from large tinker toys), headbands and music to represent a health club can be placed in the dramatic play area.

2. **Doctor's Office (Hospital)**

White clothing, stethoscopes, thermometers, magazines, bandages, cots, sheets and plastic syringes without needles can be placed in the dramatic play area to represent a hospital.

3. **Restaurant**

Tables, tablecloths, menus and tablets for taking orders can be placed in the dramatic play area. Paste pictures of food on the menus. A sign for the area could be "Eating for Health."

Arts and Crafts:

1. **Paper Plate Meals**

Magazines for the children to cut food pictures from the four food groups should be provided. The pictures can be pasted on a paper plate to represent a balanced meal.

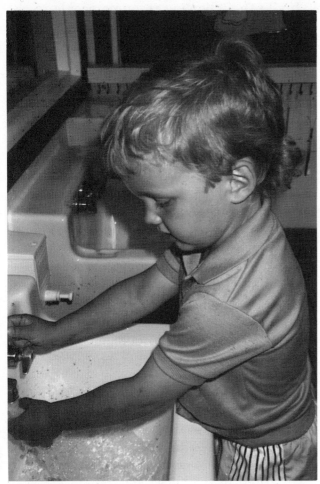

FIGURE 32 Washing hands before eating is important to healthy living.

Music:

1. **"Brush Your Teeth"** by Raffi.

2. **"My Body"**
(Sing to the tune of "Where is Thumbkin?")

This is my body.
This is my body.
It's the only one I've got.
It's the only one I've got.
I'm going to take good care of it.
I'm going to take good care of it.
Yes I am. Yes I am.

Fingerplays:

BRUSHING TEETH

I jiggle the toothbrush again and again.
   (pretend to brush teeth)

2. Body Tracing

Instruct each child to lay on a large piece of paper. Trace the child's body and let him take the tracing home and decorate it with his parents. After this, it can be returned to school for display. This activity should help the children become aware of individual uniqueness and fosters parent-child interaction.

Sensory:

Add shampoo or dish detergent to the sensory table.

Large Muscle:

1. Weight Awareness

The object of this activity is to become aware of weight and to feel the difference between heavy and light. To do this, the child should experiment with body force. Exercise in the following ways: lift arms slowly and gently, stomp on the floor, walk on tiptoes, kick out one leg as hard as possible, very smoothly and lightly slide one foot along the floor. Music can be added to imitate aerobics.

2. Mini-Olympics

Set up various areas for jumping jacks, jogging, relays and a "beanbag launch." For the "launch" put a beanbag on the top edge of a child's foot and launch it by kicking. Observe the distance each beanbag goes.

Field Trips/Resource People:

1. Take a field trip to:

* hospital
* health care facility
* doctor's office
* dentist's office
* beauty shop
* health club
* drug store

2. Invite the following resource people to visit the classroom:

* doctor
* nurse
* dentist
* dietician
* aerobics instructor
* beautician

Math:

1. Food Group Sorting

Create a food group display. To do this, encourage the children to bring empty food containers. The food containers can be sorted into food groups. This could be a small group activity or a choice during the self-selected play period.

2. Height and Weight Chart

Weigh and measure each of the children at various times throughout the year. Record the data on a chart. This chart can be posted in the classroom.

Group Time (games, language):

Tasting Party

Prepare for a tasting party. Collect a wide variety of foods. For example, the children could experiment with bananas by dipping them in wheat germ, peanut butter, honey, raisins, etc. To extend this activity, charts can be prepared listing the children's favorite foods.

Cooking:

Fruit Tree Salad

On a plate place a lettuce leaf. On the center of the lettuce, place a pineapple slice. In the hole of the pineapple, place two peeled bananas. Drain 1 small can of fruit cocktail. Spoon the fruit over the bananas.

Records:

The following records can be found in preschool educational catalogs:

1. **Aerobics for Kids.** Georgiana Liccione Stewart. Kimbo Educational Records.

2. **Fun Activities for Toddlers.** Laura Johnson. Kimbo Educational Records.

3. **Health-Cleanliness-Safety.** Irving Caesar. Songlets for Project Head Start. Cleanliness Bureau.

4. **Children's Body Awareness and Movement Exercises.** Stallman Records.

Books and Stories:

The following books and stories can be used to complement the theme:

1. **What It's Like to be a Doctor.** Arthur Shay. (New York: Reilly and Lee Books, 1971).

2. **Michael and the Dentist.** Bernard Wolf. (Locust Valley, NY: Four Winds Press, 1980).

3. **Time to Take a Bath, Shirley.** John Burningham. (New York: Crowell, 1978).

4. **Too Many Lollipops.** Robert M. Quackenbush. (New York: Parents Magazine Press, 1975).

5. **Sleepy People.** M.B. Goffstein. (New York: Farra, Straus and Geroux, 1966).

6. **Yoga for Children.** Eve Diskin. (New York: Arco Publishers, 1977).

7. **You Can't Move Without Muscles.** Paul Showers. (New York: Crowell, 1982).

8. **No Measles, No Mumps for Me.** Paul Showers. (New York: Crowell, 1980).

9. **Body Works, the Kid's Guide to Food and Fitness.** Carol and Bernick Bershad. (New York: Random House, 1979).

10. **Magic Monsters Learn about Health.** Jane Belk Moncure. (New York: Crowell, 1980).

11. **Nicky Goes to the Doctor.** Richard Scarry. (New York: Golden Book Press, 1972).

12. **Phoebe Dexter Has Harriet Peterson's Sniffles.** Laura J. Numeroff. (New York: Greenwillow, 1977).

13. **The Food We Eat.** Bobbie Kalman and Susan Hughes. (New York: Crabtree Publishing Company, 1986).

Puzzles:

The following puzzles can be found in preschool educational catalogs:

1. **"Fruit and Vegetable Puzzle"** 5 pieces. Judy/Instructo.

2. **"Body Parts Puzzle"** Judy/Instructo.

3. **"Brushing Teeth"** 4 pieces. Judy/Instructo.

4. **Nutrition puzzles** by LaYaled:

   "Breakfast" 13 pieces.

   "Lunch" 13 pieces.

   "Dinner" 13 pieces.

33 HOMES

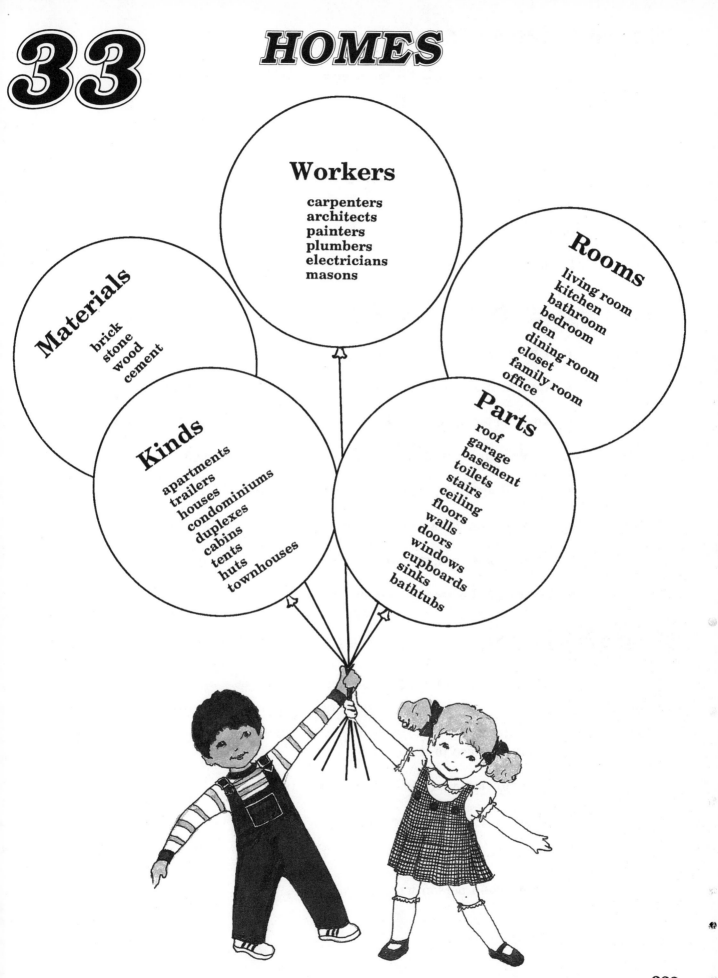

Workers
- carpenters
- architects
- painters
- plumbers
- electricians
- masons

Materials
- brick
- stone
- wood
- cement

Rooms
- living room
- kitchen
- bathroom
- bedroom
- den
- dining room
- closet
- family room
- office

Kinds
- apartments
- trailers
- houses
- condominiums
- duplexes
- cabins
- tents
- huts
- townhouses

Parts
- roof
- garage
- basement
- toilets
- stairs
- ceiling
- floors
- walls
- doors
- windows
- cupboards
- sinks
- bathtubs

Theme Goals:

Through participating in the experiences provided by this theme, the children may learn:

1. Home builders.

2. Parts of a home.

3. Rooms in a home.

4. Kinds of homes.

5. Building materials.

Concepts for the Children to Learn:

1. A home is a place to live.

2. Apartments, condominiums, trailers and houses are all kinds of homes.

3. Most homes have a kitchen, bedroom, bathroom and living room.

4. Homes can be built from brick, stone, wood or cement.

5. The ceiling, floor, roof and windows are parts of a home.

6. Construction workers build houses.

7. Homes come in many sizes.

8. Homes can be decorated many ways.

Vocabulary:

1. **apartment**—a building including many homes.

2. **duplex**—a house divided into two separate homes.

3. **house**—a place to live.

4. **construction worker**—a person who builds.

5. **kitchen**—a room for cooking.

6. **bedroom**—a sleeping room.

7. **architect**—a person who designs homes.

Bulletin Board

The purpose of this bulletin board is to develop classification skills. Draw an unfurnished model of a home on a large sheet of tagboard as illustrated. Include the basic rooms like kitchen, bedroom and living room. Draw and cut furnishings to add to the home. Laminate home and furnishings. The children can place the furnishings in the proper room by using "fun tack" or magnetic strips on the furnishings.

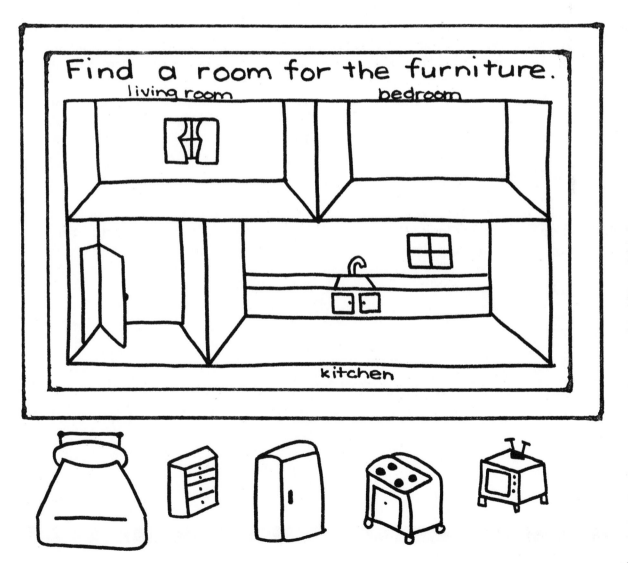

Parent Letter

Dear Parents,

This week our unit will focus on our homes. Since everyone's home is unique we will be discussing how homes differ. We will also be discussing activities we do in our home and the rooms in our homes.

At School This Week

Some of our activities this week will include:

* constructing homes out of cardboard boxes and paper in the art area.
* acting out the story of *The Three Little Pigs* in the dramatic play area.
* building at the workbench.

A special activity this week will include making placemats, but we need your help. For our placemats we will need a few pictures of your family, home, or both. These will be glued to construction paper and laminated during our project. They will not be returned in their original form. Thank you!

This week we will also be taking a neighborhood tour to observe the various types of homes in the area. We will be taking our walk at 10:00 a.m. on Thursday. Please feel free to join us!

At Home

To develop observation skills, take your child on a walk of your neighborhood to look at the houses in your area. Talk about the different colors and sizes of dwellings. Enjoy your special time with your child!

Enjoy your week!

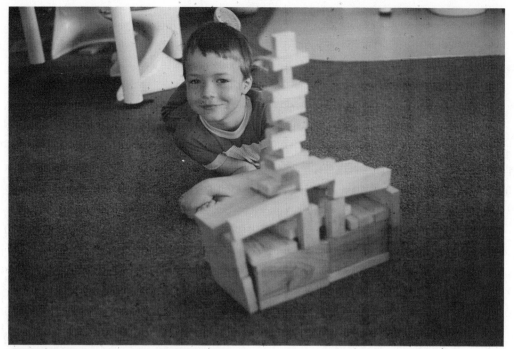
FIGURE 33 Proud of his home.

Music:

"This is the Way We Build Our House"
(Sing to the tune of "Here We Go 'Round the Mulberry Bush")

This is the way we build our house
So early in the morning.

Other suggestions:
This is the way we paint the house.
This is the way we wash the car.
This is the way we rake the leaves.

Fingerplays:

MY HOUSE

I'm going to build a little house
  (fingers make roof)
With windows big and bright
  (stand with arms in air)
Drifting out of sight.
In winter when the snowflakes fall
  (hands flutter down)
Or when I hear a storm
  (hand cupped to ear)
I'll go sit in my little house
  (sit down)
Where I'll be snug and warm.
  (cross arms over chest)

WHERE SHOULD I LIVE?

Where should I live?
In a castle with towers and a moat?
  (make a point with arms over head)
Or on a river in a houseboat?
  (make wave like motions)
A winter igloo made of ice may be just the thing
  (pretend to pack snow)
But what would happen when it turned to spring?
  (pretend to think)
I like tall apartments and houses made of stone,
  (stretch up tall)
But I'd also like to live in a blue mobile home.
  (shorten up)
A cave or cabin in the woods would give me lots of space
  (stretch out wide)
But I guess my home is the best place!
  (point to self)

KNOCKING

Look at _____ knocking on our door.
  (knock)
Look at _____ knocking on our door.
  (knock)

Come on in out of the cold
   (shiver)
Into our nice, warm home.
   (rub hands together to be warm)

MY CHORES

In my home, I wash the dishes
   (pretend to wash)
Vacuum the floor
   (push vacuum)
And dust the furniture.
   (dust)
Outside my home, I rake the leaves
   (rake)
Plant the flowers
   (plant)
And play hard all day.
   (wipe sweat from forehead)
When the day is over
I eat my supper,
   (eat)
Read a story
   (read)
And go to sleep.
   (put head on hands)

Science:

Building Materials

Building materials with magnifying glasses should be placed in the science area. The children may observe and examine materials. Included may be wood, brick, canvas, tar paper, shingles, etc.

Dramatic Play:

1. Tent Living

A small tent can be set up indoors or outdoors depending upon weather and space. Accessories such as sleeping bags, flashlights, rope, cooking utensils and backpacks should also be provided if available.

2. Cardboard Houses

Collect large cardboard boxes. Place outdoors or in an open classroom area. The children may build and construct their own homes. If desired tempera paint can be used for painting the homes. Wallpaper may also be provided.

3. Cleaning House

Housecleaning tools such as a vacuum cleaner, dusting cloth, sponges, mops and brooms can be placed in the dramatic play area. During the self-selected play periods the children may choose to participate in cleaning.

Arts and Crafts:

1. Shape Homes

An assortment of construction paper shapes such as squares, triangles, rectangles and circles should be placed on a table in the art area. Glue and large piece of paper should also be provided.

2. Tile Painting

Ask building companies to donate cracked, chipped or discontinued tiles. The children can paint tiles.

3. Homes I Like

The children can cut pictures of homes, rooms, appliances and furniture from magazines. They can glue these pieces on large construction paper pieces. The construction paper can be stapled. A cover can also be added and labeled "Things In My Home."

4. Household Tracings

Several household items such as a spatula, wooden spoon, pizza cutter or cookie cutter can be placed on the art table. Also include paper, scissors and crayons. These items can be traced. Some of the older children may color and cut their tracings.

Sensory:

1. Identifying Sounds

Record several sounds found in the home such as a vacuum cleaner, television, water running and a toilet flushing. Encourage children to name sounds. For older children, this could also be played as a lotto game. Make cards containing pictures of sounds, vary pictures from card to card. When a sound is heard, cover the corresponding picture with a chip.

2. Sand Castles

Add wet sand to the sensory table. Provide forms to create buildings, homes, etc. Examples may include empty cans, milk cartons, plastic containers, etc.

Large Muscle:

Pounding Nails

Collect building materials such as soft pine scraps and styrofoam for the workbench. Adult supervision is always required with this activity.

Field Trips/Resource People:

1. Neighborhood Walk

Walk around the neighborhood. Observe the construction workers' actions and tools.

2. Construction Site

If available visit a local construction sight. Discuss the role of the construction worker.

3. Resource People

The following resource people could be invited to the classroom:

* builder
* architect
* plumber
* painter
* electrician

Math:

My House

Construct a "My House" book for each child. On the pages write things like

"My home has _____ steps."
My home is the color _____.
My home has _____ windows.
There are _____ doors in my home.
My home has _____ keyholes.

Other ideas could include the number of beds, people, pets, etc. Send this home with the child to complete with parents.

Social Studies:

Room Match

Collect several boxes. On one box print kitchen; on another print bathroom; on another print living room; and on another print bedroom. Then cut objects related to each of these rooms from catalogs. The children may sort objects by placing them in the appropriate boxes. To illustrate, dishes, silverware and a coffee pot would be placed in the box labeled kitchen.

Group Time (games, language):

Construct a "My home is special because. . ." chart. Encourage each child to name a special thing about their home. Display the chart at the children's eye level in the classroom for the week.

Cooking:

Individual Pizza

English muffins
pizza sauce
grated mozzarella cheese

Spread a tablespoon of sauce on each muffin half. Sprinkle the top with grated cheese. Bake in a preheated oven at 375 degrees until cheese melts.

Records:

The following records can be found in preschool educational catalogs:

1. **American Folk Songs For Children.** Pete Seegar. Folkway Records.

2. **A Place of Our Own.** Fred Rogers. Dickwick International, Inc.

3. **My Street Begins At My House.** Ella Jenkins.

Books and Stories:

The following books and stories can be used to complement the theme:

1. **Rabbit's New Rug.** Judy Delton. (New York: Parents Magazine Press, 1979)

2. **Adam's World—San Francisco.** Kathleen Fraser and Miriam Levy. (Chicago: Albert Whitman and Company, 1971).

3. **The Biggest House.** Ruth Jaynes. (Los Angeles: Bowmar Publishing Company, 1968).

4. **Read and Tell!** Elin McCoy. (New York: Macmillan Publishing Company, Inc., 1975).

5. **Peter and Mr. Brandon.** Eleanor Schnick. (New York: Macmillan Publishing Company, Inc., 1973).

6. **We Were Tired of Living In a House.** Liesel Moak. (New York: Franklin Watts, Inc., 1962).

7. **Mary Jo's Grandmother.** Janice May Udry. (Chicago: Albert Whitman and Company, 1970).

8. **Tommy Builds a House.** Gunilla Wolde. (Boston: Houghton Mifflin Company, 1969).

9. **The House That Jack Built.** Paul Galdone. (New York: McGraw Hill, 1961).

10. **The Three Little Pigs.** Paul Galdone. (New York: Seabury Press, 1970).

11. **Alec's Sand Castle.** (New York: Harper and Row, 1972).

12. **My Home.** Renee Bartkowski. (Racine, WI: Western Publishing Company, Inc., 1976).

13. **The House Book.** Carol North. (Racine, WI: Western Publishing Company, Inc., 1985).

14. **Who Lives Here?** Sara Jeffrey. (New York: Dandelion Press, 1979).

15. **Apartment 3.** Ezra Jack Keats. (New York: Macmillan Publishing Company, Inc., 1971).

16. **Around the House.** Robert Durham. (Chicago: Childrens Press, 1987).

17. **Animal Homes.** Brian Wildsmith. (New York: Oxford University, 1980).

Puzzles:

The following puzzles can be found in preschool educational catalogs:

1. **"Mini Mall"** 19 pieces. Playskool.

2. **"Living Room"** 16 pieces. Playskool.

3. **"Bathroom"** 15 pieces. Playskool.

4. **"Kitchen"** 8 pieces. Playskool.

5. **"The City"** 20 pieces, Judy Floor Puzzles.

6. **"The Farm"** 20 pieces. Judy Floor Puzzles.

7. **"House"** 17 pieces. Childcraft.

8. **"Houses Beginner Inlay"** Childcraft.

9. **"Buildings We See"** 4 pieces. Childcraft.

10. **"City"** 20 pieces. Childcraft.

11. **"Carpenter"** 13 pieces. Judy/Instructo.

34 INSECTS AND SPIDERS

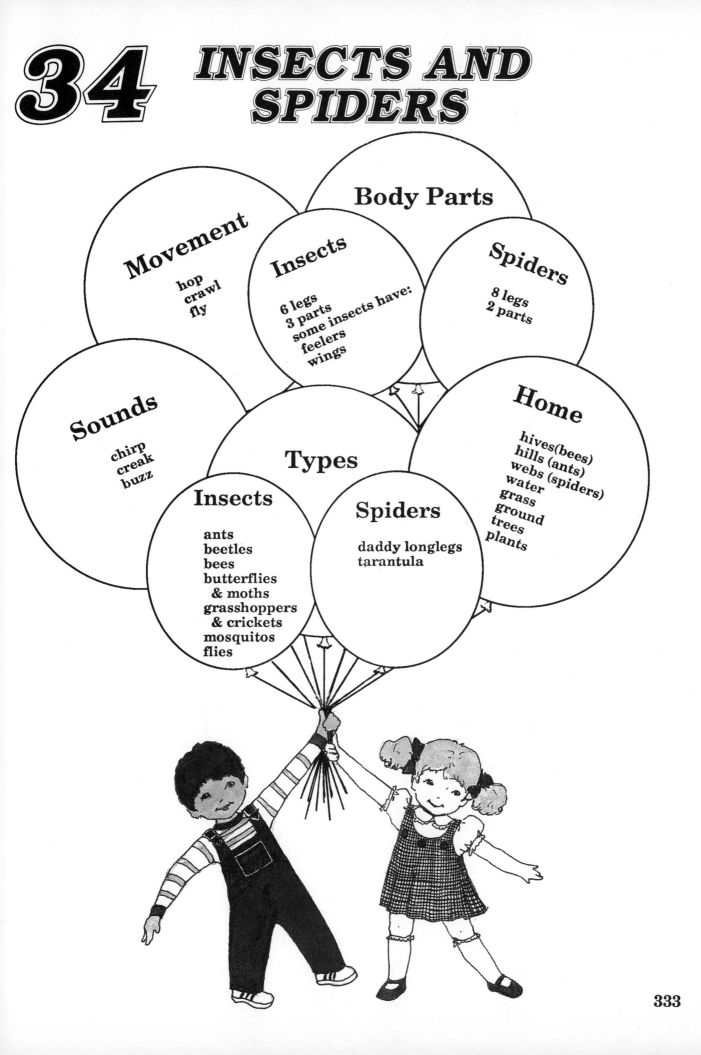

Movement

hop
crawl
fly

Body Parts

Insects

6 legs
3 parts
some insects have:
feelers
wings

Spiders

8 legs
2 parts

Sounds

chirp
creak
buzz

Types

Insects

ants
beetles
bees
butterflies
 & moths
grasshoppers
 & crickets
mosquitos
flies

Spiders

daddy longlegs
tarantula

Home

hives(bees)
hills (ants)
webs (spiders)
water
grass
ground
trees
plants

Theme Goals:

Through participating in the experiences provided by this theme, the children may learn:

1. Ways to identify different insects and spiders.

2. Ways insects help us.

3. Ways spiders help us.

4. Places where spiders and insects live.

5. Ways that spiders and insects move from place to place.

Concepts for the Children to Learn:

1. There are many kinds of insects.

2. Insects are different in many ways: size, shape, color, eyes, mouths and number of wings.

3. Insects have six legs (three pairs) and if winged, four wings.

4. Spiders have eight legs (four pairs) and no wings.

5. Insects and spiders come from eggs.

6. Insects can help us by making honey and pollinating fruits and flowers.

7. Spiders can help us by eating insect pests.

8. Most spiders spin a web.

9. Some insects fly, others walk.

10. Spiders spin a web to catch other insects to eat.

Vocabulary:

1. **insect**—small animal with three pairs of jointed legs.

2. **spider**—small animal with four pairs of legs.

3. **caterpillar**—the wormlike larvae of a butterfly or moth.

4. **pollinate**—the way insects help flowers to grow.

5. **spiderling**—a baby spider.

6. **antennae**—feelers on an insect that stick out from the head.

7. **pupa**—intermediate stage of an insect; chrysalis.

8. **moth**—night flying insect with four wings related to the butterfly.

9. **wasp**—winged insect with a poisonous sting.

10. **cricket**—small leaping insect known for its chirping.

Bulletin Board

The purpose of this bulletin board is to develop visual discrimination skills. Construct several butterflies, each of a different shape, out of tagboard. Trace on black construction paper for shadows. Laminate. Staple shadow butterflies to bulletin board. Punch holes in colored butterflies for children to hang on the push pin of the corresponding shadow butterfly.

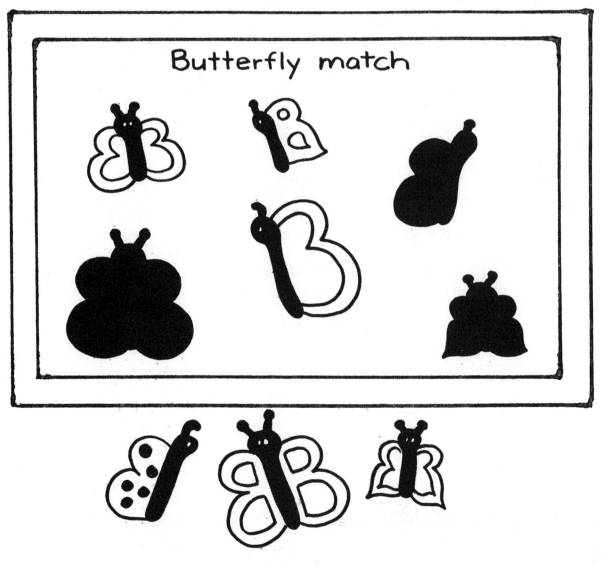

Parent Letter

Dear Parents,

We are continuing our study of animals. This week we move to a new category—insects and spiders. The children will become aware of the difference between insects and spiders and the ways that those creatures are helpful. Do you know the difference between insects and spiders? Most insects have three body parts and six legs. Spiders have two body parts and eight legs.

At School This Week

Some of the learning experiences scheduled for this week include:

* singing and acting out the song "One Elephant Went Out to Play." It's about an elephant that plays on a spider web!
* listening to a flannel board version of the story *The Very Hungry Caterpillar* by Eric Carle.
* watching and observing an ant farm set up in the science area.
* creating spiders and insects out of a variety of materials in the art area.

At Home

There are many ways to bring this unit into your home. Take a walk with your child and see how many spiders and insects you can find. Avoid touching unknown types of insects or spiders with your fingers. Instead, use a clear jar with a lid to observe the creature close up. Release the insect or spider after the observation.

We will be having a snack this week called ants on a log. Let your child make some for you! Spread peanut butter on pieces of celery. Top with raisins. Enjoy!

Have a great week!

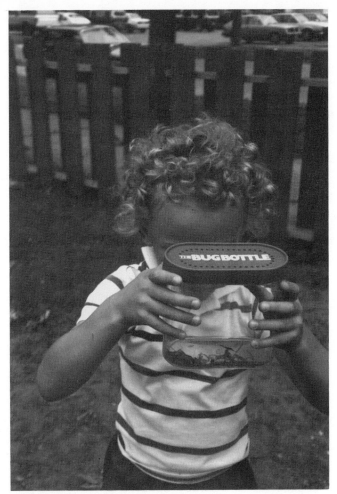

FIGURE 34 Watching many varieties of insects and spiders.

Music:

1. **"Bugs"**
(Sing to tune of "Frere Jacques")

Big bugs, small bugs, big bugs, small bugs,
See them crawl, see them crawl.
Creepy, creepy, crawling, never, never falling
Bugs, bugs, bugs. Bugs, bugs, bugs.

Thin bugs, fat bugs, thin bugs, fat bugs
See them crawl, on the wall.
Creepy, creepy, crawling, never, never falling
Bugs, bugs, bugs. Bugs, bugs, bugs.

Source: *Resources for Creative Teaching in Early Childhood Education.* Fleming, Hamilton and Hicks. (Chicago: Harcourt, Brace Jovanovich, Inc., 1977).

2. **"The Eensie Weensie Spider"**
(traditional)

The eensie weensie spider crawled up the water spout.
(walk fingers up other hand)
Down came the rain and washed the spider out.
(lower hands to make rain, wash out spider by placing hands together in front and extending out to either side)
Out came the sun and dried up all the rain
(form sun with arms in circle over head)
And the eensie weensie spider went up the spout again.
(walk fingers up other arm)

3. **"The Elephant Song"**

One elephant went out to play
On a spider's web one day.
He had such enormous fun,
That he called for another elephant to come.

Elephant! Elephant! Come out to play!
Elephant! Elephant! Come out to play!

Two elephants. . .

4. **"The Insects and Spiders"**
(Sing to the tune of "The Wheels on the Bus")

The bugs in the air fly up and down,
up and down, up and down.
The bugs in the air fly up and down
all through the day.

The spiders on the bush spin a web.
The crickets in the field hop up and down.
The bees in their hive go buzz, buzz, buzz.

Fingerplays:

ANTS

Once I saw an ant hill, with no ants about.
So I said "Little ants, won't you please come out?"
Then as if they heard my call, one, two, three, four, five came out.
And that was all!

BUMBLEBEE

Brightly colored bumblebee
Looking for some honey.
Flap your wings and fly away
While it still is sunny.

THE CATERPILLAR

A caterpillar crawled to the top of a tree.
  (index finger of left hand moves up right
  arm)
"I think I'll take a nap", said he.
So under a leaf, he began to creep
  (wrap right hand over left fist)
To spin his chrysalis and he fell asleep.
All winter long he slept in his chrysalis bed,
  (keep right hand over left fist)
Till spring came along one day, and said,
"Wake up, wake up little sleepy head."
  (shake left fist with right hand).
"Wake up, it's time to get out of bed!"
So, he opened his eyes that sun shiny day
  (shake fingers and look into hand)
Lo—he was a butterfly and flew away!
  (move hand into flying motion)

LITTLE MISS MUFFET

Little Miss Muffet
Sat on a tuffet
Eating her curds and whey.
Along came a spider
And sat down beside her
And frightened Miss Muffet away!

Spiders can be prepared in the art area.

Science:

1. Observe an ant farm

   The children can watch the ants dig tunnels,
   build roads and tunnels, build roads and
   rooms, eat and store food, etc. (Ant farms are
   available in some commercial play catalogs.)
2. Go outside and observe ant hills in the
   playground area.
3. Observe deceased flies and ants under a
   microscope.
4. Observe insects and spiders in a caged bug
   keeper or jars with holes in the lids.

5. Listen to a cricket during quiet time.
6. Capture a caterpillar and watch it spin a
   chrysalis and turn into a butterfly.

Dramatic Play:

1. **Scientist**

   The children can dress up in white lab
   coats and observe spiders and insects with
   magnifying glasses.

2. **Spider Web**

   Tie together a big piece of rope to resemble a spider web. Have children pretend
   they are spiders playing on their web.

3. **Spider Sac**

   Tape together a 10 foot by 25 foot piece of
   plastic on the sides. Blow it up with a fan
   to make a big bubble. Make a slit in the
   plastic for the entrance. The children can
   pretend to be baby spiders coming out of
   the spider sac when they are hatching.

4. The children can act out "Little Miss Muffet."

Arts and Crafts:

1. Cut easel paper in the shape of a
   butterfly.
2. Fingerpaint creepy crawly pictures.
3. Make insects and spiders out of clay. Use
   toothpicks, straws and pipe cleaner
   segments for the appendages.
4. Make insects and spiders with thumb
   prints. Children can draw crayon legs to
   make prints look like insects and spiders.
5. Egg carton caterpillars. Cut egg cartons
   in half, lengthwise. Each child paints a
   carton half. When dry, children can make
   a face on the end of the carton and insert
   pipe cleaners or straws for feelers.
6. Have children make spiders from black
   construction paper—one large black circle
   for a body and eight strips for legs.

338

Children can paste on two yellow circles for eyes. Hang by a string around the room.

7. Make ladybug shapes out of red and orange construction paper. Have children sponge paint dots and legs on the bugs.
8. Make butterfly templates.
9. Use butterfly templates and place crayon shavings between two pieces of waxed paper and iron. Put a butterfly template over the wax paper and glue it on. A pretty butterfly will be the final product!
10. Tissue paper butterflies. Have children lightly paint white tissue paper or use colored tissue paper. Fasten a pipe cleaner around the middle. Add circles on the ends for antennaes.
11. Balloon bugs. Blow up several long balloons. Cover them with strips of paper dipped in wallpaper paste. Put on three to four layers of this sticky paper. Let dry for two to three days. Then paint your own giant bug!
12. Have insect and spider stencils set out for the children to draw and trace.

Sensory:

Add soil and plastic insects to the sensory table.

Large Muscle:

Have children pretend to walk as different insects when in transition from one activity to another.

Field Trips/Resource People:

1. Go on a walk to a nearby park to find bugs. Look under rocks, in cracks, in sidewalks, in bushes, etc.
2. Have someone who has a butterfly collection come in.
3. Visit a pet store. Ask them to show you what kind of insects they feed to the animals in the store. Do they sell any insects?
4. Invite a zoologist to come in and talk about insects and how important they are.

5. Invite an individual who raises bees to talk to the children. Ask him to bring in a honey comb for the children to taste.

Math:

1. **Butterfly Match**

   Make several triangles of different colors. On one triangle put the numbers 1 to 10; on the other make dots from 1 to 10. Have the children match the dots to the numbers and clip them together with a clothespin to form a butterfly.

2. **Lady Bug Houses**

   Paint several 1/2 pint milk cartons red. Write the numerals 1 to 10 on each. Make 50 small ladybugs dotting 5 sets of 1 to 10. Have children put ladybugs in their correct houses by matching dots to numerals.

3. **Numeral Caterpillar**

   Make a caterpillar with 10 body segments and a head. Have the children put the numbers in order to complete the caterpillar's body.

4. Sing the song "The Ants Go Marching One by One" and have the children act out the song using their fingers as numbers.

5. Make an insect and spider lotto or concentration game with stickers for children to play.

Social Studies:

1. Take the children on an insect hunt near your school. When children are finished, have everyone show the rest of the class what they found. Talk about where they found the insects (on a tree, under a log, etc.).
2. Have children make homes for all the insects they found. They can put dirt, grass, twigs and small rocks in jars and cans.

3. Discuss what it is like to be a member of a family. Ask the children if each member of their family has a certain job. Then focus on ant colonies or families. Ants live together much like people do, except ants live in a larger community. Each ant has a certain task within the community. Some of the jobs are:
* nurse: to look after the young
* soldier: defend colony and attack the enemies
* others: search for food; enlarge and clean the nest (house)

Group Time (games, language):

1. Matching Insects

Divide children into two groups. Hand out pictures of different spiders and insects, one to each group that matches one in the other group. Point to a child from one group and have that child act out the insect they have in some way (movement or noises). The child that has the same insect from the other group must go and meet the child in the middle and act out the insect also.

2. Have many pictures of insects and spiders on display. Talk about a new one every day. Where it lives, how it walks, what it might eat, etc.

Cooking:

1. Honey Bees

1/2 cup peanut butter
1 tablespoon honey
1/3 cup nonfat dry milk
2 tablespoons toasted wheat germ
unsweetened cocoa powder
sliced almonds

In a mixing bowl, mix peanut butter and honey. Stir in dry milk and wheat germ until well mixed. Lay waxed paper on a baking sheet. Using 1 tablespoon at a time, shape peanut butter mixture into ovals to look like bees. Put on baking sheet. Dip a toothpick in cocoa powder and press lightly across the top of the bees to make stripes. Stick on almonds for wings. Chill for 30 minutes.

Source: *Better Homes and Gardens Kids Snacks* (Iowa: Meredith Corporation, 1979).

2. Ants on a Log (traditional)

Cut celery pieces into 3-inch strips. Fill the cavity of the celery stick with peanut butter. Garnish with raisins. (As with all recipes calling for celery, this might be more appropriate for older children.)

Record:

The following record can be found in preschool educational catalogs:

Birds, Beasts, Bugs and Little Fishies. Pete Seeger.

Books and Stories:

The following books and stories can be used to complement the theme:

1. **Lucky Ladybugs.** Gladys Conklin. (New York: Holiday House, Inc., 1968).

2. **The Web in the Grass.** Bernie Freschet. (New York: Charles Scribner's Sons, 1972).

3. **Be Nice to Spiders.** Margaret B. Graham. (New York: Harper and Row, 1969).

4. **The Very Hungry Caterpillar.** Eric Carle. (New York: Scholastic Book Services, 1971).

5. **"I Can't," Said the Ant.** Polly Cameron. (New York: Coward McCann and Geoghegan, Inc., 1961).

6. **Ants and Bees.** Ronald Grood. (New York: Dunlap Company, 1979).

7. **The Spider's Web.** Julie Brinckloe. (New York: Doubleday Company, 1974).

8. **The Blue Bug and the Bullies.** Virginia Poulet. (Chicago: Childrens Press, 1971).

9. **My Lady Bug.** Herbert Wong and Matthew Vessel. (Reading, MA: Addison-Wesley Publishing Company, 1969).

10. **One, Two, Three with Ant and Bee: A Counting Story.** Angela Bonner. (New York: Watts Company, 1958).

11. **Insects.** Jeanne Brouillette. (Chicago: Follett Publishing Company, 1963).

12. **We Like Bugs.** Gladys Conklin. (New York: Holiday House, 1962).

13. **Buzz, Buzz, Buzzing Bees.** Gene Fulks. New York: Harper and Row, 1967).

14. **Only One Ant.** Lenore Klein. (New York: Dunlap Company, 1979).

15. **Spiders.** Lillian Bason. (Washington, DC: National Geographic Society, 1974).

16. **The Spider.** Margaret Lane. (New York: Dial Press, 1982).

17. **The Caterpillar.** Peter Curry. (New York: Scholastic, 1983).

18. **The Very Busy Spider.** Eric Carle. (New York: Philomel Books, 1985).

19. **See the Fly Fly.** Catherine Chase. (New York: Dandelion Press, 1979).

20. **How to Hide a Butterfly and Other Insects.** Ruth Heller. (New York: Grosset and Dunlap, 1985).

21. **Insects.** Illa Podendorf. (Chicago: Childrens Press, 1981).

22. **What Is A Butterfly?** Chris Arvetis. (Chicago: Childrens Press, 1987).

23. **From Egg to Butterfly.** Marlene Reidel. (Minneapolis, MN: Carolrhoda, 1981).

Puzzles:

The following puzzles can be found in preschool educational catalogs:

1. **"Butterfly"** 5 pieces. Judy/Instructo.

2. **"Lady Bug"** 5 pieces. Judy/Instructo.

3. **"Caterpillar and Butterfly"** Judy/Instructo.

4. **Giant Insect Puzzles**—Jumbo Jigsaw Puzzle.
   "Flea"
   "Grasshopper"
   "Mosquito"
   "Lightening Bug"

5. **Rubber Puzzles**—Lauri.
   "Bug" 15 pieces.
   "Butterfly" 12 pieces.

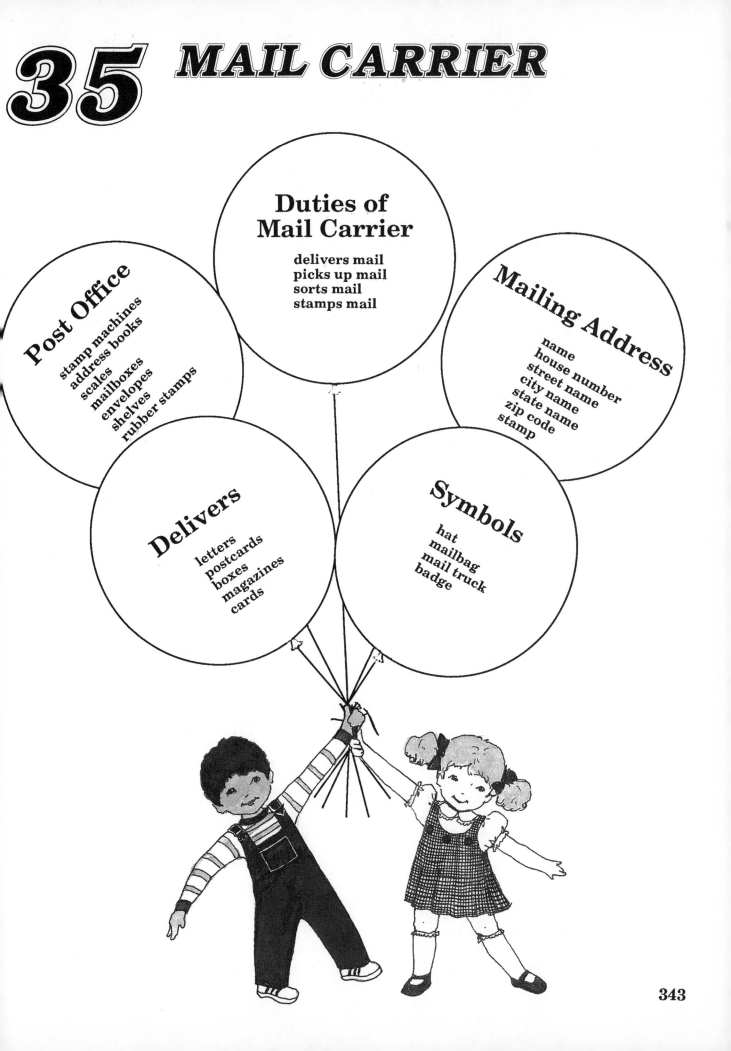

Duties of Mail Carrier

delivers mail
picks up mail
sorts mail
stamps mail

Post Office

stamp machines
address books
scales
mailboxes
envelopes
shelves
rubber stamps

Mailing Address

name
house number
street name
city name
state name
zip code
stamp

Delivers

letters
postcards
boxes
magazines
cards

Symbols

hat
mailbag
mail truck
badge

Theme Goals:

Through participating in the experiences provided by this theme, the children may learn:

1. Duties of a mail carrier.

2. Symbols identifying a mail carrier.

3. Objects found in a post office.

4. Parts of a mailing address.

5. Types of postal deliveries.

Concepts for the Children to Learn:

1. Mail carriers deliver mail.

2. The mail carrier usually wears a badge and a hat.

3. A mail carrier sometimes drives a truck.

4. Mail carriers deliver cards, letters, postcards, boxes and magazines.

5. Stamps are used for mailing.

6. Names, house numbers, street names, city names, state names and zip codes are on mailing labels.

7. A post office has stamp machines, address books, mailboxes and envelopes.

8. Scales are used to weigh mail.

Vocabulary:

1. **post office**—place where mail is sorted.

2. **letter**—a printed message.

3. **zip code**—the last numbers on a mailing address.

4. **address**—directions for the mail carrier.

5. **mail**—letters, cards, postcards, and packages.

6. **envelope**—a cover for a letter.

7. **stamp**—a sticker put on mail.

8. **mail carrier**—person who delivers mail.

9. **mail bag**—bag that holds letters and postcards.

Bulletin Board

The purpose of this bulletin board is to reinforce the mathematical skill of matching a set to its written numeral. Construct mailboxes out of tagboard. Each mailbox should include a flag, which is red colored and contains a numeral. The number will depend upon the maturity of the children. A set of dots, corresponding to the numeral on the flag, should be placed on the mailbox. Hang the mailboxes on the bulletin board. Next, construct letters by using small cards with sets of dots on them. The children can match the dots on the cards with the dots and numerals on the mailboxes. If desired, magnet pieces can be attached to both the mailboxes and the cards.

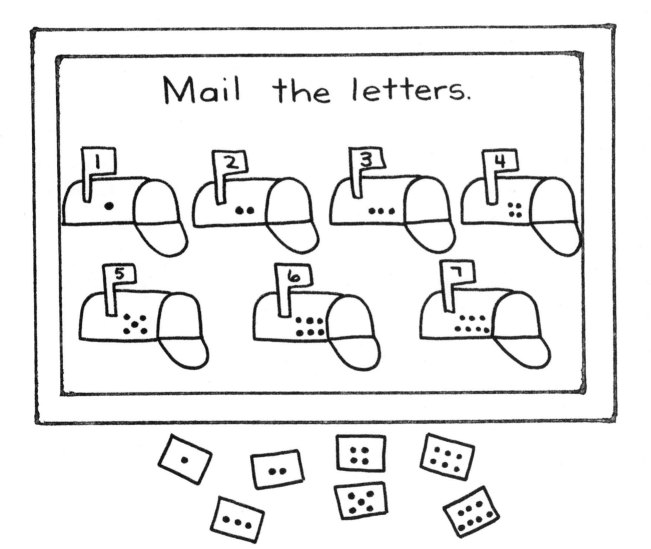

Parent Letter

Dear Parents,

We have been busy discussing the roles of a variety of community helpers these past weeks. This week we will focus on the mail carrier. The children will be learning about letters, stamps and addresses, and will be able to identify objects found in a post office. They will also become aware of how mail is delivered and what needs to be on a letter or package before it is delivered.

At School This Week

Some of the many learning activities scheduled for this week include:

* listening to the story *Adventures of a Letter* by Warren G. Schloat.
* playing in a post office set up in the classroom.
* making mailboxes and postcards.
* weighing letters and packages.
* delivering mail to our friends in our room.

At Home

Let your children help or watch you open the mail. Give your child the "junk mail" to play with. Show your child where your address is on your house and mailbox. You may also enjoy having your children dictate a letter to a grandparent, favorite aunt or cousin. As you write the letter, show your child the printed alphabet letters to develop an awareness of alphabet letters. After you finish the letter, address an envelope. Let your child lick the stamp and show the proper placement. Then it's off to the post office!

Have a great week!

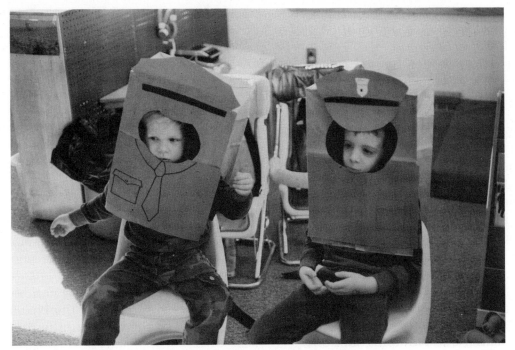

FIGURE 35 Delivering mail is a lot of work!

Music:

1. "Mailing Letters"
(Sing to the tune of "The Mulberry Bush")

This is the way we mail a letter,
Mail a letter, mail a letter.
This is the way we mail a letter,
So early in the morning.

2. "Let's Pretend"
(Sing to the tune of "Here We Are Together"
and "Did You Ever See a Lassie")

Let's pretend that we are mail carriers,
Are mail carriers, are mail carriers.
Let's pretend that we are mail carriers,
We'll have so much fun.
We'll carry the letters and put them in
boxes.
Let's pretend that we are mail carriers,
We'll have so much fun.

Fingerplays:

LITTLE MAIL CARRIER

I am a little mail carrier
  (point to self)
That can do nothing better.

I walk.
  (walk in place)
I run.
  (run in place)
I hop to your house.
  (hop in place)
To deliver your letter.

FIVE LITTLE LETTERS

Five little letters lying on a tray.
  (extend fingers of right hand)
Mommy came and took the first one away.
  (bend down thumb)
Daddy said, "This one's for me!"
I counted them twice, now there are three.
  (bend down pointer finger)
Brother Bill asked "Did I get any mail?"
He found one and cried "A letter from Gail."
  (bend down middle finger)
My sister Jane took the next to the last
And ran upstairs to open it fast.
  (bend down ring finger)
As I can't read, I am not able to see,
Whom the last one is for, but I hope it's for me!
  (wiggle last finger, clap hands)

THE POSTMAN

I come from the post office
  (walk from post office)

My mail sack on my back.
  (pretend to carry sack on back)
I go to all the houses
  (pretend to go up to a house)
Leaving letters from my pack.
  (pretend to drop letters into mailbox)
One, two, three, four
  (hold up fingers as you count)
What are these letters for?
  (pretend to hold letters as you count)
One for John. One for Lou.
  (pretend to hand out letters)
One for Tom and one for you!
  (pretend to hand out letters to others)

LETTER TO GRANDMA

Lick them, stamp them
  (make licking and stamping motions)
Put them in a box.
  (extend arms outward)
Hope that Grandma
Loves them alot!
  (hug self)

Dramatic Play:

1. Post Office

Develop the dramatic play area into a post office. Provide a mailbox, mail carrier hats, mailbag, stamps, cash register, rubber date stamps and a letter scale. The children may enjoy acting out the role of a mail carrier or a post office worker.

2. Letters

Provide a variety of writing materials. Include different colors of paper, writing tools and envelopes. The children can dictate a letter to a friend or a family member. After all interested children have completed dictation, apply stamps and walk to the nearest mailbox or post office. (Contact a local printer, office supply store or card shop and ask for discontinued samples or misprinted envelopes.)

Science:

1. Dress the Mail Carrier

Place flannel board pieces representing the seasonal clothing for a mail carrier. Let the children select the appropriate clothing for the weather. This may be an interesting activity to introduce daily during group time.

2. Weighing Mail

A variety of letters, boxes, stamps and a scale can be placed in the science area. The children can weigh letters and packages. This activity can be extended by placing materials in the boxes and weighing them noting the difference.

3. How Does the Mail Feel?

Place different types of envelopes and stationery on the sensory table for the children to explore. Include airmail paper, onion skin paper, bond paper, typing paper and different kinds of stationery. Also, provide a magnifying glass.

Field Trips/Resource People:

1. Post Office

Plan a field trip to the local post office. Observe the mailboxes, stamp machines, address books, scales and rubber stamps with the children. Mail a postcard back to the center. Count the number of days it takes to arrive.

2. Mail Carrier

Invite the mail carrier who delivers mail to your center or school to visit in the classroom. Ask the mail carrier to share their mailbag, hat, etc. with the children.

Social Studies:

Mailboxes

Plan a walk around the neighborhood. Observe the different types of mailboxes and addresses.

Math:

The number of items and numerals used in these activities need to be adjusted to reflect the developmental appropriateness of the children.

1. Dominoes

Create dominoes out of envelopes. Have the children match the numbers and dots.

2. How Many Stamps?

Write an individual numeral on an envelope. Make or collect many stamps. The children can place the correct number of stamps in the envelope with the corresponding numeral. A variation of this activity is to make mailboxes from shoeboxes. Again, write a numeral on each box. Make or collect many different envelopes. The children can put the correct number of letters in the corresponding mailboxes.

3. Package Seriation

Prepare several packages and letters of different sizes. The children can place the letters and packages in order from largest to smallest or smallest to largest.

Arts and Crafts:

1. Easel Ideas

Cut easel paper in the shape of envelopes, letters, stamps or mailbags.

2. Postcards

Have children make postcards at school to send to family and friends. Provide index cards. Let the children design the postcards.

Books and Stories:

3. Mailboxes

Make mailboxes out of old shoeboxes. Each child can decorate their own box. Names can be added by the child or teacher. Include a home address for older children.

4. Mail Truck

Construct a mail truck out of a large cardboard box. Provide paint for the children to decorate it. When dried, place chairs and, if available, a steering wheel inside for the children to drive.

5. Stamps

Collect assorted stamps or stickers. Cancelled stamps can be reglued. The children can make a stamp collage.

Group Time (games, language):

Thank You

Write a thank you note to the post master or mail carrier after visiting.

Cooking:

Zip Code Special

1 1/2 cups nonfat dry milk
2 cups fresh or frozen berries
1 teaspoon vanilla
1 cup water
1 tray ice cubes

Blend all ingredients in a blender. Serve and enjoy.

The following books and stories can be used to complement the theme:

1. **I Know a Postman.** Lorraine Hendroid. (New York: Putnam Company, 1967).

2. **Postal Service.** Johanna Petersen. (Minnesota: Lerner Publications, 1975).

3. **Let's Go to A Post Office.** Naomi Buchheimer. (New York: G. P. Putnam's Sons, 1970).

4. **Adventures of a Letter.** Warren G. Schloat. (New York: Charles Scribner's Sons, 1964).

5. **Let's Visit the Post Office.** Billy N. Pope. (Dallas: Taylor Publishing Company, 1967).

6. **A Letter to Amy.** Ezra Jack Keats. (New York: Harper and Row, Inc., 1968).

7. **Seven Little Postmen.** Margaret Wise Brown. (New York: The Golden Press, 1971).

8. **A Letter to Anywhere.** Al Hine. (New York: Harcourt, Brace and World, Inc., 1965).

9. **Read about the Postman.** Louis Slobodkin. (New York: Watts Company, 1966).

10. **My Mother the Mail Carrier.** Inez Maury. (New York: Feminist Press, 1967).

11. **Communication.** Julie Batchelor. (New York: Harcourt, Brace and World, Inc., 1953).

12. **The Post Office Book.** Gail Gibbons. (New York: Thomas Y. Crowell, 1982).

Puzzles

The following puzzles can be found in preschool educational catalogs:

1. **"Mail Carrier"** 6 pieces. Multi-Ethnic Career Puzzles. Judy/Instructo.

2. **"Mail Carrier"** 14 pieces. Constructive Playthings.

3. **"Mail Carrier"** 11 pieces. Judy/Instructo.

MUSIC

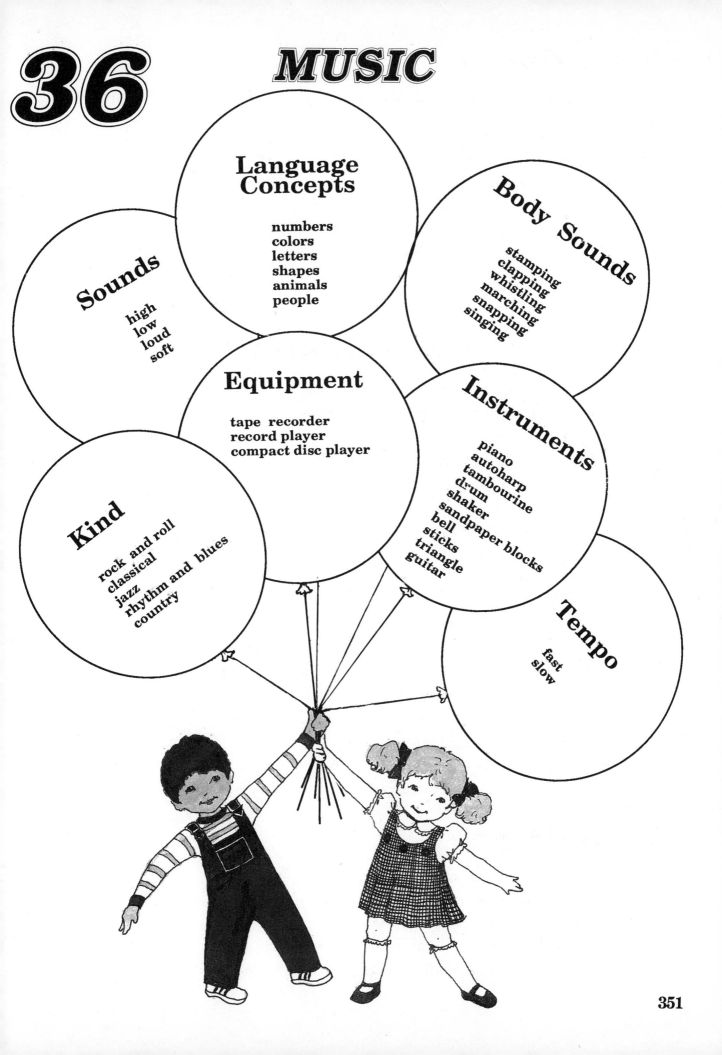

Language Concepts

numbers
colors
letters
shapes
animals
people

Body Sounds

stamping
clapping
whistling
marching
snapping
singing

Sounds

high
low
loud
soft

Equipment

tape recorder
record player
compact disc player

Instruments

piano
autoharp
tambourine
drum
shaker
sandpaper blocks
bell
sticks
triangle
guitar

Kind

rock and roll
classical
jazz
rhythm and blues
country

Tempo

fast
slow

Theme Goals:

Through participating in the experiences provided by this theme, the children may learn:

1. Music is a language.
2. Kinds of music.
3. Music tempos.
4. Language concepts.
5. Different sounds.
6. Names of many musical instruments.
7. Body sounds.
8. Equipment used for playing and recording music.

Concepts for the Children to Learn:

1. There are many types of instruments.
2. Each instrument has its own sound.
3. Music sounds can be high, low, loud and soft.
4. Music can express different moods.
5. Music can be played in different rhythms.
6. Songs can tell stories.
7. Our bodies are musical instruments.
8. Our hands can clap.
9. Our feet can stamp and march.
10. Our fingers can snap.
11. Our mouths can whistle and sing.
12. The piano, autoharp and guitar are played with our fingers.
13. Sticks are used on the triangle, drum, xylophone and bells.
14. We shake bells, shakers and tambourines.
15. We rub sandpaper blocks.
16. There are many kinds of music.
17. We can tape music with a recorder.
18. A record, tape or compact disc player can play music.

Vocabulary:

1. **music**—a way of expressing ideas and feelings.
2. **instrument**—makes musical sounds.
3. **tempo**—the speed of music.
4. **body sounds**—sounds made by moving one or more body parts.
5. **mallets**—special sticks used to play the xylophone and bells.

Bulletin Board

The purpose of this bulletin board is to develop visual discrimination skills. Create a musical bulletin board by drawing musical instruments on tagboard as illustrated. Color the instruments with markers, cut out and laminate. Trace these pieces onto black construction paper. Cut out the pieces and attach to the bulletin board. A magnet should be attached to both the colored pieces and the black shadow pieces. The children can match the appropriately shaped instrument piece to its shadow on the bulletin board.

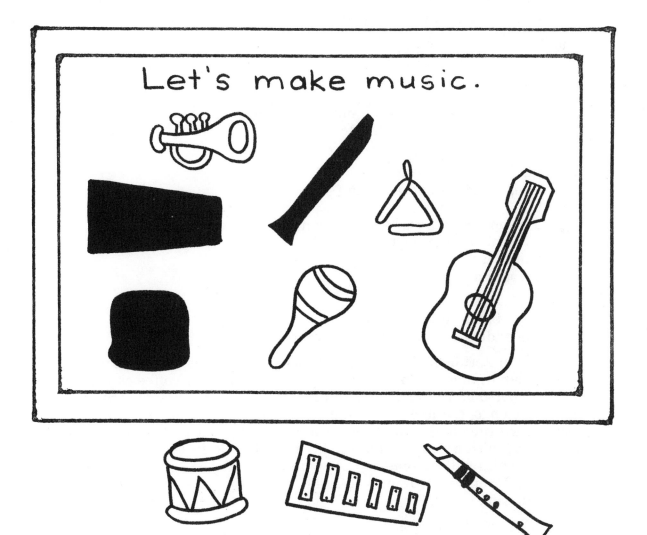

Parent Letter

Dear Parents,

We will be singing and playing instruments all week during our unit on music. Music is a way of communication and expressing oneself. For young children, singing is not that much different from talking—as I'm sure you've noticed from observing the children! Throughout the week the children will be making discoveries about the many sounds that we can make with our voices, body parts, and musical instruments.

At School This Week

A few highlights of our scheduled musical learning activities for the week include:

* making musical instruments.
* painting at the easel while listening to music with headphones.
* trying on band uniforms (courtesy of Mead School) in the dramatic play area.
* forming a rhythm band outside in the play yard.

At Home

To stimulate creativity and language, create verses with your child for this song to the tune of "Old McDonald Had A Farm:"

Mr. Roberts had a band,
E-I-E-I-O
And in his band he had a drum
E-I-E-I-O
With a boom, boom here, And a boom, boom, there,
Here a boom, there a boom,
Everywhere a boom, boom.
Mr. Roberts had a band,
E-I-E-I-O.

And in his band he had a horn...
Continue adding instruments that your child can think of.

Provide materials for your child to make simple musical instruments. A drum can be made using an empty oatmeal carton or coffee can. Your child can personalize the instrument by decorating the outside of the container with paper, crayons and markers. A kazoo can also be made with a cardboard tube and a small piece of waxed paper attached to the end of the tube with a rubber band. Poke a small hole in the waxed paper and your child will be ready to blow up a storm! The sounds produced by the different instruments can be compared to develop auditory discrimination skills.

Keep a song in your heart!

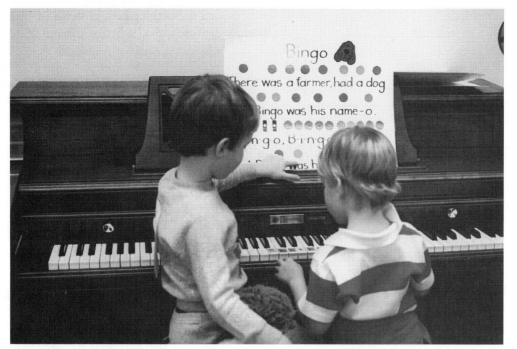

FIGURE 36 Music is a way to express yourself.

Music:

Music for this unit should consist of the children's favorite and well-known songs. The children will enjoy singing these songs, and you will be able to focus on the sound of the music. Here are some suggestions of traditional songs that most children enjoy:

1. "Old MacDonald Had a Farm"

2. "Five Green Speckled Frogs"

3. "The Farmer in the Dell"

4. "Row, Row, Row Your Boat"

5. "Mary Had a Little Lamb"

6. "Hickory Dickory Dock"

7. "If You're Happy and You Know It"

8. "ABC Song"

9. "The Little White Duck"

10. "Six Little Ducks"

Fingerplays:

I WANT TO LEAD A BAND

I want to lead a band
With a baton in my hand.
  (wave baton in air)
I want to make sweet music high and low.
Now first I'll beat the drum
  (drum beating motion)
With a rhythmic tum-tum-tum,
And then I'll play the bells
A-ting-a-ling-a ling,
  (bell playing motion)
And next I'll blow the flute
With a cheery toot-a-toot.
  (flute playing motion)
Then I'll make the violin sweetly sing.
  (violin playing motion)
Now I'm leading a band
With a baton in my hand.
  (wave baton in air again.)

IF I COULD PLAY

If I could play the piano
This is the way I would play.
  (move fingers like playing a piano)

If I had a guitar
I would strum the strings this way.
  (hold guitar and strum)

If I had a trumpet
I'd toot to make a tune.
  (play trumpet)

But if I had a drum
I'd go boom, boom, boom.
  (pretend to play a drum)

MUSICAL INSTRUMENTS

This is how a horn sounds
Toot! Toot! Toot!
  (play imaginary horn)

This is how guitars sound
Vrrroom, Vrrroom, Vrrroom
  (strum imaginary guitar)

This is how the piano sounds
Tinkle, grumble, brring.
  (run fingers over imaginary keyboard)

This is how the drum sounds
Rat-a-tat, grumble, brring.
  (strike drum, include cymbal)

JACK-IN-THE-BOX

Jack-in-the-box all shut up tight
  (fingers wrapped around thumb)
Not a breath of air, not a ray of light.
  (other hand covers fist)
How tired he must be all down in a heap.
  (lift off)
I'll open the lid and up he will leap!
  (thumbs pop out)

Science:

1. Water Music

Fill four identically sized crystal glasses
each with a different amount of water.
The children can trace their wet finger
around the rim of each glass. Each glass
will have a different tune. Older children
may enjoy reordering the glasses from the
highest to the lowest tone.

2. Pop Bottle Music

Fill six 12-ounce pop bottles, each with a
different amount of water. For effect, in

each bottle place a drop of food coloring,
providing six different colors. Younger
children can tap the bottles with a spoon
as they listen for the sound. Older
children may try blowing directly into the
opening for sound production.

3. Throats

Show the children how to place their
hands across their throat. Then have them
whisper, talk, shout and sing feeling the
differences in vibration.

4. Jumping Seeds

Set seeds or something small on top of a
drum. Then beat the drum. What happens?
Why? This activity can be extended by
having the childen jump to the drum beat.

5. Identifying Instruments

Prepare a tape recording of classroom
musical instruments. Play the tape, encouraging the children to identify the correct instrument related to each sound.

6. Matching Sounds

Collect 12 containers, such as film
canisters, milk cartons, or covered baby
food jars, that would be safe to use with
the children. Fill 2 containers with rice, 2
cans with beans, 2 cans with pebbles, 2
cans with water and the remaining cans
with dry pasta. Coins, such as pennies,
could be substituted. Color code each pair
of containers on the bottom. Let the
children shake the containers, listening to
the sounds, in an attempt to find the
matching pairs.

Dramatic Play:

1. Band

Collect materials for a band prop box
which may include band uniforms, a
baton, music stand, cassette player and
tapes with marching music. The children
can experiment with instruments.

2. Dramatizing

Add a cassette recorder and a small microphone to the dramatic play area. The children may enjoy using it for singing and recording their voices.

3. Disc Jockey

In the music area, provide a tape recorder and cassettes for the children.

Arts and Crafts:

1. Drums

Create drums out of empty coffee cans with plastic lids, plastic ice cream pails or oatmeal boxes. The children can decorate as desired with paper, paint, felt-tip markers or crayons.

2. Shakers

Collect a variety of egg-shaped panty hose containers. Fill each egg with varying amounts of sand, peas or rice, and securely tape or glue them shut. To compare sounds, empty film containers can also be filled.

3. Cymbals

Make cymbals out of old tin foil pans. Attach a string for the handles.

4. Tambourines

Two paper plates can be made into a tambourine. Begin by placing pop bottle caps or small stones between the plates. Staple the paper plates together. Shake to produce sound.

5. Easel Ideas

Cut easel paper into the shape of different instruments such as a drum, guitar or tambourine.

6. Musical Painting

On a table in the art area, place a tape recorder with headphones. The children can listen to music as they paint.

7. Kazoos

Kazoos can be made with empty paper towel rolls and waxed paper. The children can decorate the outside of the kazoos with colored felt-tip markers. After this, place a piece of waxed paper over one end of the roll and secure it with a rubber band. Poke two or three small holes into the waxed paper allowing sound to be produced.

8. Rhythm Sticks

Two wooden dowels should be given to each interested child. The sticks can be decorated with paint or colored felt-tip markers.

Large Muscle:

1. Body Movement Rhythms

Introduce a simple body movement. Then have the children repeat it until they develop a rhythm. Examples include:

* stamp foot, clap hands, stamp foot, clap hands
* clap, clap, stamp, stamp
* clap, stamp, clap, stamp
* clap, clap, snap fingers
* clap, snap, stamp, clap, snap, stamp
* clap, clap, stamp, clap clap, stamp

2. Body Percussion

Instruct the children to stand in a circle. Repeat the following rhythmic speech:

We walk and we walk and we stop (rest)
We walk and we walk and we stop (rest)
We walk and we walk and we walk and we walk
We walk and we walk and we stop. (stop)

3. March

Play different rhythm beats on a piano or another instrument. Examples include hopping, skipping, gliding, walking, running, tip-toeing, galloping, etc. The children can move to the rhythm.

Field Trips/Resource People:

1. Band Director

Visit a school band director. Observe the different instruments available to students. Listen to their sounds.

2. Who Can Play?

Invite parents, grandparents, brothers, sisters, relatives, friends, etc. to visit the classroom and demonstrate their talent.

3. Radio Station

Visit a local radio station.

4. Taping

Videotape the children singing and using rhythm instruments. Replay the video for the children. Save this for a future open house, parent meeting or holiday celebration.

Math:

1. Colors, Shapes and Numbers

Sing the song, "Colors, Shapes and Numbers" mentioned in the shapes unit or make up a song about shapes. Hold up different colors, shapes and numbers while you sing the song for the children to identify.

2. Number Rhyme

Say the following song to reinforce numbers:

One, two, three, four
Come right in and shut the door.
Five, six, seven, eight
Come right in it's getting late.
Nine, ten, eleven, twelve
Put your books upon the shelves.
Will you count along with me?
It's as easy as can be!

3. Ten in the Bed

Chant the following words to reinforce numbers:

There were 10 in the bed and the little one said,
"Roll over, roll over."
So they all rolled over and one fell out.

There were 9 in the bed and the little one said,
"Roll over, roll over."
So they all rolled over and one fell out.

Continue until there is only one left. The last line will be "...and the little one said, "Good Night!"

4. Music Calendar

Design a calendar for the month of your music unit. The different days of the week can be made out of musical notes and different instruments.

Social Studies:

1. Our Own Songs

Encourage the children to help you write a song about a common class experience. Substitute the words into a melody that everyone knows. ("Twinkle, Twinkle, Little Star" or "The Mulberry Bush").

2. Pictures

Add pictures of instruments and band players in the room to add interest and stimulate discussion.

3. Sound Tapes

Make a special tape of sounds heard in a home. Homes are full of different sounds. Included may be:

* people knocking on doors
* wind chimes
* telephone ringing
* tea kettle whistling
* clock ticking
* toilet flushing
* popcorn popping
* vacuum cleaner
* doorbell
* running water
* car horn

Play the tape and have the children listen carefully to identify the sounds.

Group Time (games, language):

1. Name Game

Say the following rhythmic chant as the whole class claps.

"Names, Names we all have names
Play a game as we say our names
Scott (class echoes) Scott
Melanie (class echoes) Melanie
Tommy (class echoes) Tommy."

Repeat until all the children have had their name repeated.

Source: *The Kinder-Music House.* (Fairfax County Public Schools, 1982).

2. Are You Here?

Sing the following song to the tune of "Twinkle, Twinkle, Little Star."

Hello children here we are,
At our school from near and far.
Today we are going to play a game,
Please stand when I call your name.

Source: *Channels to Children.* Beckman, Simmons, and Thomas. (Colorado: Channels to Children Publishing Company, Colorado, 1982).

Miscellaneous:

Instrument of the Day

Focus on a different instrument each day. Talk about the construction and demonstrate the instrument's sound.

Cooking:

Popcorn

Make popcorn and have the children listen to the sounds of the oil as well as the corn popping. Supervise this activity closely since the corn popper will become hot. This activity is most appropriate for older children—younger children may choke on popcorn.

Records:

The following records can be found in preschool educational catalogs:

1. **Simplified Lummi Stick Activities.** Kimbo.

2. **Getting to Know Myself.** Hap Palmer.

3. **Color Me a Rainbow.** Melody House.

4. **Music Skills.** Melody House.

5. **On The Move With Greg and Steve.** "Scat Like That" Youngheart Records.

6. **We All Live Together Series—Volume 3.** "Sing A Happy Song" Youngheart Records.

7. **Rhythm Band Time.** Melody House Records.

Books and Stories:

The following books and stories can be used to complement the theme:

1. **I Want to be a Musician.** Carla Green. (Chicago: Childrens Press, 1962).

2. **Music and Instruments for Children to Make.** John Hawkinson. (Niles, IL: Albert Whitman and Company, 1969).

3. **Picture Book of Musical Instruments.** Marion Lacey. (New York: Lothrop, Lee and Shepard Company, Inc., 1942).

4. **Hush Little Baby.** Aliki Brandenburg. (Englewood Cliffs, New Jersey: Prentice Hall, Inc., 1963).

5. **London Bridge is Falling Down.** Carla Greece. (Chicago: Childrens Press, 1962).

6. **The Cat in the Hat Song Book.** Dr. Seuss. (New York: Random House, 1967).

7. **Sing Mother Goose.** Opal Wheeler. (New York: E.P. Dutton and Company, Inc., 1945).

8. **Spring Song.** Jacqueline Jackson. (The Kent State University Press, 1969).

9. **Things That Go Bang.** Lisa Weil. (New York: McGraw Hill Book Company, 1969).

10. **What Makes an Orchestra?** Jan Balet. (New York: Henry Z. Walck Inc., 1951).

11. **The Magic Flute.** Stephen Spender. (New York: G.P. Putnam's Sons, 1966).

12. **Stories that Sing.** Ethel Crowninshield. (Boston: Boston Music Company, 1947).

13. **Bottom's Dream.** John Updike. (New York: Alfred A. Knopf, Inc., 1969).

14. **Really Rosie.** Maurice Sendak. (New York: Harper and Row, 1975).

15. **Over in the Meadow.** John Langstaff. (New York: Harcourt, Brace, and Company, 1957).

16. **Geraldine the Music Mouse.** Leo Lionni. (New York: Pantheon Books, 1979).

17. **Umbrella.** Taro Yashima. (New York: The Viking Press, 1958).

18. **The Boy With a Drum.** Eloise Wilkin. (New York: Golden Press, 1969).

19. **Old MacDonald Had a Farm.** Pam Adams (ill.). (Restrop Manor, England: Child's Play, 1975).

20. **This Old Man.** Pam Admas (ill.). (New York: Grosset and Dunlap, 1974).

21. **Percussion.** Dee Lillegard. (Chicago: Childrens Press, 1987).

22. **Woodwinds.** Dee Lillegard. (Chicago: Childrens Press, 1987).

23. **Down By the Bay.** Raffi. (New York: Crown Publishers, Inc., 1987).

24. **The Philharmonic Gets Dressed.** Karla Kuskin. (New York: Harper and Row, 1982).

25. **There Was An Old Lady Who Swallowed A Fly.** Pam Adams (ill.). (New York: Grosset and Dunlap, 1973).

26. **I See a Song.** Eric Carle. (New York: Thomas Y. Crowell Company, 1973).

Puzzles:

The following puzzles can be found in preschool educational catalogs:

1. **"Holiday Parade"** 20 pieces, Judy/Instructo.

2. **"Children of the Orchestra"** 9 pieces. Constructive Playthings.

37 NUMBERS

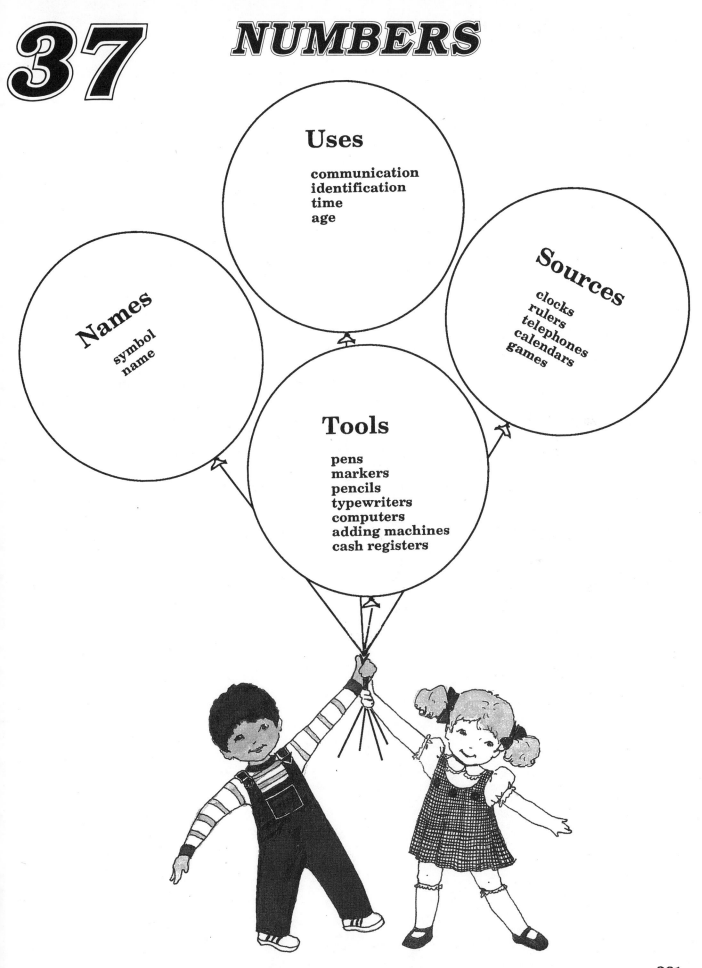

Uses
communication
identification
time
age

Names
symbol
name

Sources
clocks
rulers
telephones
calendars
games

Tools
pens
markers
pencils
typewriters
computers
adding machines
cash registers

361

Theme Goals:

Through participating in the experiences provided by this theme, the children may learn:

1. Uses of numbers.

2. Sources of numbers.

3. Number names.

4. Tools for recording numbers.

Concepts for the Children to Learn:

1. A number is a symbol.

2. Each number symbol has a name.

3. Pencils, typewriters and computers are tools used to make numbers.

4. Numbers can be found on clocks, rulers, telephones and calendars.

5. Communication, identification, time and age are uses for numbers.

6. Adding machines and cash registers have numerals.

Vocabulary:

1. **numeral**—a symbol that represents a number.

2. **number**—a symbol used to represent an amount.

Bulletin Board

The objective of this bulletin board is for the children to match the numeral to the set by winding the string around the other push pin. Construct the numerals out of tagboard. Construct objects familiar to the child to correspond to one type of object to each numeral. The number of objects and numerals should be developmentally appropriate for the group of children. Laminate. Staple 1, 2, 3, 4 and 5 down the left side of bulletin board. Staple the sets of objects in random order (3, 5, 1, 2, 4) down the right side of the bulletin board as illustrated. Affix a push pin with an attached long string by each numeral. Affix a push pin in front of each set row.

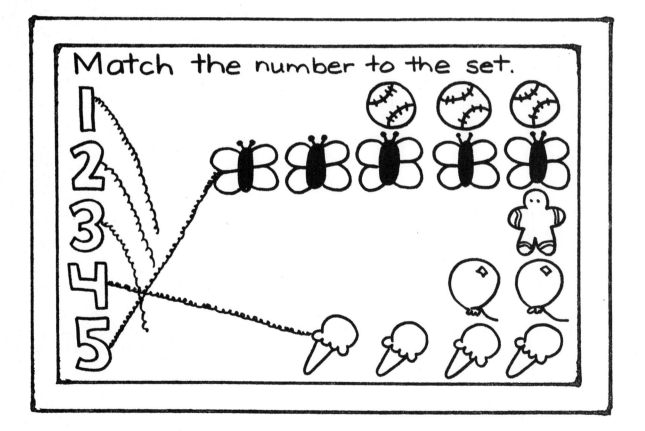

Parent Letter

Dear Parents,

This week at school we will be starting a unit on numbers. The children will be exposed to concepts of pairs, sets and halves and wholes. They will also be participating in activities that include the concepts of heavy/light, bigger/smaller and more/less.

At School This Week

Some of the play related activities for this week include:

* measuring with scales and rulers at the science table.
* charting our weight and height.
* listening to the book entitled *I Can Count* by Lynn Grundy.
* using number cookie cutters with playdough.
* bowling with numbered pins.

The personnel from the telephone company will be visiting us Tuesday. They will show us a variety of phones. They will also stress the importance of knowing our telephone number. Feel free to join us for this activity.

At Home

Cooking provides a concrete foundation for mathematical concepts. It involves amounts, fractions and measures. While you are cooking, have your child help. Count how many spoonsful it takes to fill a one cup measurer.

Your child can help you make this simple no-bake recipe for peanut butter treats.

Peanut Butter Treats

1/4 cup margarine
1/4 cup peanut butter
1 cup raisins
40 regular-sized marshmallows
5 cups rice cereal

Melt margarine over low heat. Add marshmallows and melt. Add the peanut butter and stir. Add the rice cereal and raisins, stir until everything is mixed well. Spread the mixture into a buttered pan and press into a firm layer. Cool and cut into squares.

Enjoy your week!

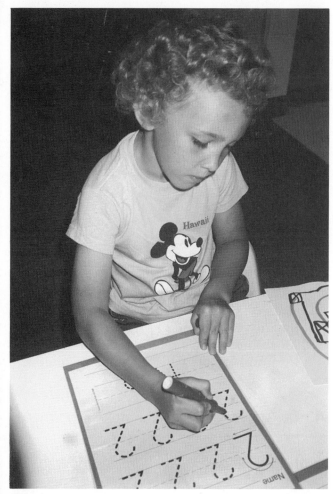

FIGURE 37 It takes time and practice to learn numbers.

Music:

1. **"Hickory Dickory Dock"**
   (traditional)

   Hickory dickory dock
   The mouse ran up the clock.
   The clock struck one,
   The mouse ran down.
   Hickory dickory dock.

2. **"Two Little Blackbirds"**
   (traditional)

   Two little blackbirds sitting on a hill
   One named Jack,
   One named Jill.
   Fly away Jack,
   Fly away Jill.
   Come back Jack,
   Come back Jill.
   Two little blackbirds sitting on a hill

One named Jack,
One named Jill.

Fingerplays:

I CAN EVEN COUNT SOME MORE

One, two, three, four
I can even count some more.
Five, six, seven, eight
All my fingers stand up straight
Nine, ten are my thumb men.

FIVE LITTLE MONKEYS SWINGING FROM A TREE

Five little monkeys swinging from the tree
Teasing Mr. Alligator, "You can't catch me."
Along comes Mr. Alligator as sneaky as can be
SNAP
4 little monkeys swinging from the tree.
3 little monkeys swinging from the tree.
2 little monkeys swinging from the tree.
1 little monkey swinging from the tree.
No more monkeys swinging from the tree!

ONE, TWO, THREE

1, 2, How do you do?
1, 2, 3 Clap with me.
1, 2, 3, 4 Jump on the floor.
1, 2, 3, 4, 5 Look bright and alive!
1, 2, 3, 4, 5, 6 Pick up your sticks.
1, 2, 3, 4, 5, 6, 7 We can count up to eleven.
1, 2, 3, 4, 5, 6, 7, 8 Draw a circle around your plate.
1, 2, 3, 4, 5, 6, 7, 8, 9 Get the trunks in the line.
1, 2, 3, 4, 5, 6, 7, 8, 9, 10 Let's do it over again.

Source: *Everyday Circle Times.* Liz and Dick Wilmes. (Elgin, Illinois: Building Blocks Publications, 1983).

FIVE LITTLE BIRDS

Five little birds without any home.
   (hold up five fingers)
Five little trees in a row.
   (raise hands high over head)
Come build your nests in our branches tall.
   (cup hands)
We'll rock them to and fro.

TEN LITTLE FINGERS

I have ten little fingers and ten little toes.
(children point to portions of body as
they repeat words)
Two little arms and one little nose.
One little mouth and two little ears.
Two little eyes for smiles and tears.
One little head and two little feet.
One little chin, that makes _____
complete.

Science:

1. Height and Weight Chart

Design a height and weight chart for the
classroom. The children can help by
measuring each other. Record the
numbers. Later in the year measure the
children and record their progress. Note
the differences.

2. Using a Scale

Collect a variety of small objects and place
on the science table with a balancing
scale. The children can measure with the
scale noting the differences.

3. Temperature

Place an outdoor thermometer on the
playground. Encourage the children to
examine the thermometer. Record the
temperature. Mark the temperature on the
thermometer with masking tape. Bring the
thermometer into the classroom. Check the
thermometer again in half an hour. Show
the children the change in temperature.

Dramatic Play:

1. Grocery Store

In the dramatic play area, arrange a
grocery store. To do this, collect a variety
of empty boxes, paper bags, sales receipts,
etc. Removable stickers can be used to indicate the grocery prices. A cash register
and play money can also be added to
create interest.

2. Clock Shop

Collect a variety of clocks for the children
to explore. Using discarded clocks, with
the glass face removed, is an interesting
way to let the children explore numerals
and the internal mechanisms.

3. Telephoning

Prepare a classroom telephone book with
all the children's names and telephone
numbers. Contact your local telephone
company to borrow the training system.
The children can practice dialing their
own numbers as well as their classmates.

Arts and Crafts:

1. Marker Sets

Using rubber bands, bind two watercolor
markers together. Repeat this procedure
making several sets. Set the markers, including an unbound set, on the art table.
The children can use the bound marker
sets for creating designs on paper.

2. Clipping Coupons

Collect coupon flyers from the Sunday edition of the paper and magazines for this
activity. Place the flyers with scissors on a
table in the art area. If interested, the
children can cut coupons from the paper.

3. Coupon Collage

Clipped coupons, paste and paper can be
placed on a table in the art area.

4. Ruler Design

Collect a variety of rulers that are of different colors, sizes and types. Using paper
and a marking tool, the children can
create designs.

5. Numeral Cookie Cutter

Numeral cookie cutters should be provided with play dough.

Sensory:

Add to the sensory table colored water and a variety of measuring tools.

Math:

1. Number Chain

Cut enough strips of paper to make a number chain for the days of the month. During group time each day, add a link to represent the passage of time. Another option is to use the chain as a countdown by removing a link per day until a special day. This is an interesting approach to an upcoming holiday.

2. Silverware Set

Provide a silverware set. The children can sort the pieces according to sizes, shapes and/or use.

3. Constructing Numerals

Provide each interested child with a ball of playdough. Instruct children to form some numerals randomly. It would be important for teacher to monitor work and correct reversals. Then children can add the proper corresponding number of dots for that numeral just formed.

An extension of this activity would be to make cards with numerals. The children roll their playdough into long ropes that could be placed over the lines of the numerals.

Group Time (games, language):

1. Squirrels in the Park

Choose five children to be squirrels. The children should sit in a row while one child pretends to go for a walk in the park carrying a bag of peanuts. When the child who is walking approaches the squirrels, provide directions. These may include: feeding the first squirrel, the fifth, the third, etc.

2. Block Form Board

On a large piece of cardboard trace around one of each of the shapes of the blocks in the block area. Let children match blocks to the shape on the board.

3. Match Them

Show the child several sets of identical picture cards, squares, objects or flannel board pictures. Mix the items. Then have the children find matching pairs. One method of doing this is to hold up one item and have the children find the matching one.

4. Follow the Teacher

At group time, provide directions containing a number. For examples say 1 jump, 2 hops, 3 leaps, 4 tip-toe steps, etc. The numbers used should be developmentally appropriate for the children.

Cooking:

Peanut Butter Treats

1/4 cup margarine
1/4 cup peanut butter
1 cup raisins
40 regular-sized marshmallows
5 cups rice cereal

Melt the margarine over low heat. Add marshmallows and melt. Add the peanut butter and stir. Add the rice cereal and raisins. Stir until all ingredients are well mixed. Spread the mixture onto a buttered pan and press into a firm layer. Let cool and cut into squares.

MANIPULATIVES FOR MATH ACTIVITIES

buttons
beads
bobbins
craft pompoms
spools
shells
seeds (corn, soybeans)
shelled peanuts
toothpicks
pennies

checkers
crayons
golf tees
plastic caps from
    markers, milk con-
    tainers, plastic bottles
stickers
fishing bobbers
keys

small toy cars
plastic bread ties
marbles
cotton balls
bottle caps
poker chips
paper clips
clothespins
erasers

Records:

The following records can be found in preschool educational catalogs:

1. **Number Fun.** Melody House Records.

2. **We All Live Together Series—Volume 2.** "The Number Rock" Youngheart Records.

3. **We All Live Together Series—Volume 3.** "1, 2, Buckle My Shoe" Youngheart Records.

4. **Numbers.** Sesame Street Records.

Books and Stories:

The following books and stories can be used to complement the theme:

1. **Odds and Evens.** Thomas Clement O'Brian. (New York: Thomas Y. Crowell Company, 1971).

2. **Six Little Ducks.** Chris Conover. (New York: Thomas Y. Crowell Company, 1976).

3. **I Can Count.** Lynn N. Grundy. (Loughborough: Ladybird Books, 1970).

4. **Count and See.** Tana Hoban. (New York: Macmillan Publishing Company, 1963).

5. **3 x 3: Three by Three.** James Kruss. (New York: Macmillan Publishing Company, 1963).

6. **The Three Bears.** Paul Galdone. (New York: The Seabury Press, 1972).

7. **The Sesame Street Book of Numbers.** Children's Television Workshop. (New York: Little, Brown and Company, 1970).

8. **My Little Counting Book.** Margaret Yerian. (Racine, Wisconsin: Western Publishing Co., 1976).

9. **Two Little Bears.** YLLA. (New York: Harper and Row, 1954).

10. **Chicken Little Counts to Ten.** Margaret Friskey. (Chicago: Childrens Press, 1946).

11. **Over in the Meadow.** John Langstaff. (New York: Harcourt Brace Jovanovich, 1956).

12. **One, Two, Three for Fun.** Muriel Stanek. (Niles, IL: Albert Whitman and Co., 1967).

13. **One Dancing Drum.** Gail Kredenser. (New York: S.G. Phillips, 1971).

14. **Inch by Inch.** Leo Leonni. (New York: Astor-Honor, 1962).

15. **Number Men.** Louise True. (Chicago: Childrens Press, 1962).

16. **One Was Johnny.** Maurice Sendak. (New York: Harper & Row, 1962).

17. **The Doorbell Rang.** Pat Hutchins. (New York: Scholastic, 1986).

18. **Ten Items or Less.** Stephanie Calmenson. (New York: Golden Book, 1985).

19. **My One Book.** Jane Belk Moncure. (Chicago: Childrens Press, 1985).

20. **My Two Book.** Jane Belk Moncure. (Chicago: Childrens Press, 1985).

21. **My Three Book.** Jane Belk Moncure. (Chicago: Childrens Press, 1985).

22. **My Four Book.** Jane Belk Moncure. (Chicago: Childrens Press, 1985).

23. **My Five Book.** Jane Belk Moncure. (Chicago: Childrens Press, 1985).

24. **My Six Book.** Jane Belk Moncure. (Chicago: Childrens Press, 1986).

25. **My Seven Book.** Jane Belk Moncure. (Chicago: Childrens Press, 1986).

26. **My Eight Book.** Jane Belk Moncure. (Chicago: Childrens Press, 1986).

27. **My Nine Book.** Jane Belk Moncure. (Chicago: Childrens Press, 1986).

28. **My Ten Book.** Jane Belk Moncure. (Chicago: Childrens Press, 1986).

Puzzles:

The following puzzles can be found in preschool educational catalogs:

1. **"Number Inlays"** 10 pieces. Judy/Instructo.

2. **"Odd/Even Duck"** 20 pieces. Puzzle People.

3. **"Figure Fit"** 11 pieces. Childcraft.

4. **"Counting Bug"** 10 pieces. Childcraft.

5. **"Fingers and Toes Counting"** 6 pieces. Childcraft.

6. **"Birthday Sequence Puzzle"** 10 pieces. Childcraft.

38 NURSERY RHYMES

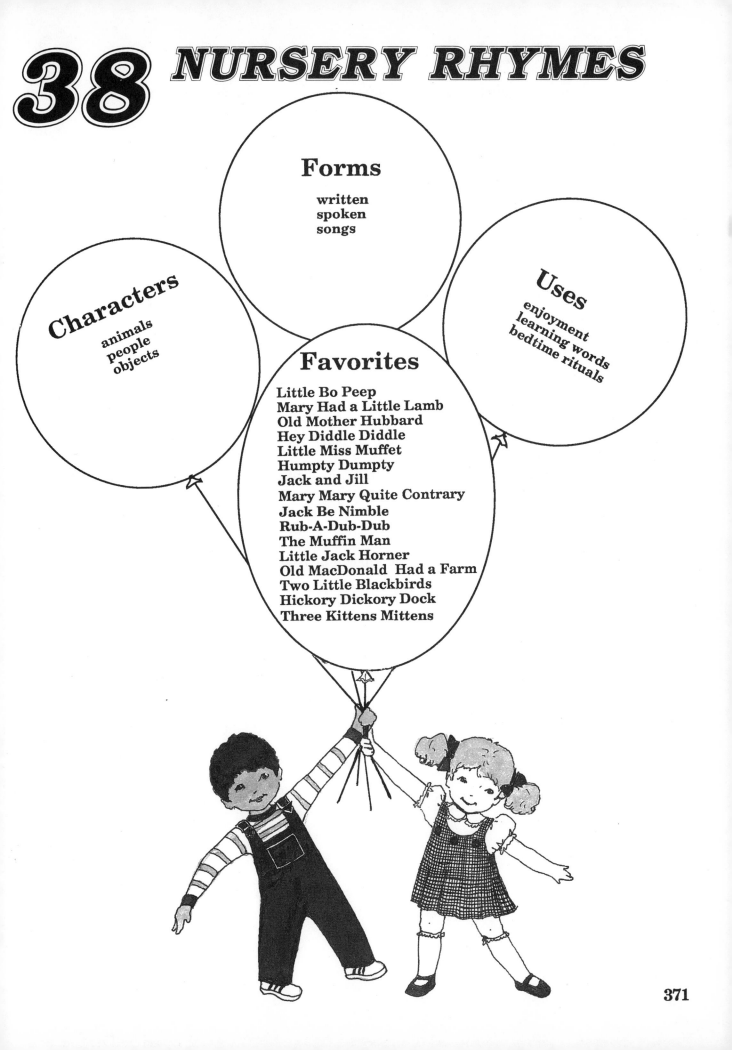

Forms

written
spoken
songs

Characters

animals
people
objects

Uses

enjoyment
learning words
bedtime rituals

Favorites

Little Bo Peep
Mary Had a Little Lamb
Old Mother Hubbard
Hey Diddle Diddle
Little Miss Muffet
Humpty Dumpty
Jack and Jill
Mary Mary Quite Contrary
Jack Be Nimble
Rub-A-Dub-Dub
The Muffin Man
Little Jack Horner
Old MacDonald Had a Farm
Two Little Blackbirds
Hickory Dickory Dock
Three Kittens Mittens

Theme Goals:

Through participating in the experiences provided by this theme, the children may learn:

1. Favorite nursery rhymes.

2. Uses of nursery rhymes.

3. Forms of nursery rhymes.

4. Characters portrayed in nursery rhymes.

Concepts for the Children to Learn:

1. Nursery rhymes are fun to listen to and say.

2. Nursery rhymes can contain real or pretend words.

3. Some nursery rhymes are about animals.

4. Some nursery rhymes help us learn numbers and counting.

5. Some nursery rhymes teach us about different people.

Vocabulary:

nursery rhyme—short, simple poem or rhyme.

Bulletin Board

The purpose of this bulletin board is to promote name recognition and call attention to the printed word. This is a check-in bulletin board. Each child is provided a bulletin board piece with their name printed on it. When they arrive each morning at school, they hang their name on the bulletin board. To create a "Find Your Mitten" bulletin board, cut a mitten out of tagboard for each child in the class. Three kittens can be constructed and attached to the bulletin board to represent the three little kittens who lost their mittens. Use a paper punch to cut a hole in the top of each mitten. Hang push pins on the bulletin board for the children to hang their mittens on during the course of the day.

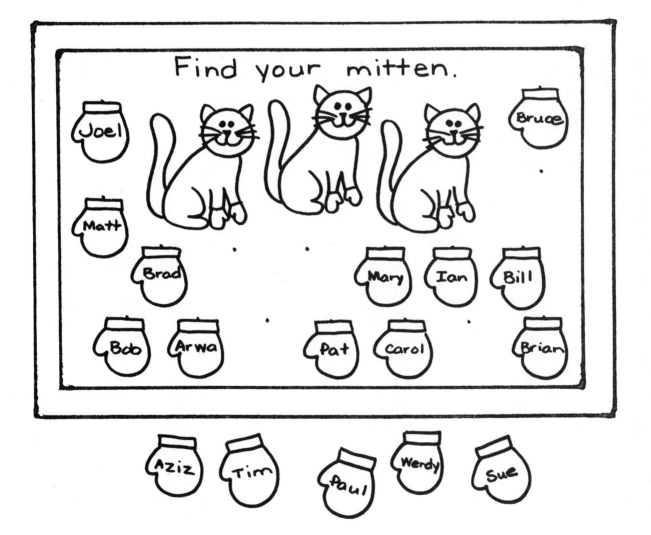

Parent Letter

Dear Parents,

In our classroom this week the curriculum will focus on nursery rhymes. These rhymes can serve as a bridge between the home and school. I'm sure many of you have shared favorite nursery rhymes with your child at home. Nursery rhymes are an easy introduction to poetry, as well as the concept of rhyming words.

At School This Week

We have a fun-filled week planned for our unit on nursery rhymes. A few highlights include:

* acting out various rhymes with puppets that represent different characters from familiar nursery rhymes.
* unraveling the riddle of the "Humpty Dumpty" nursery rhyme. (Why couldn't Humpty be put back together? Because Humpty was an egg!)
* creating "Little Miss Muffet" spiders in the art area.
* taking turns being nimble and quick as we jump over a candlestick to dramatize the rhyme of "Jack Be Nimble."

At Home

To foster concepts of the unit at home, try the following:

* Let your child help you crack eggs open to make scrambled eggs. Children like to feel that they have accomplished a grownup task when they crack the eggs.
* Sing or recite some of the many rhymes your child already knows such as "Jack and Jill" and "Mary Had a Little Lamb." These also develop an enjoyment of music and singing.

Have a good week!

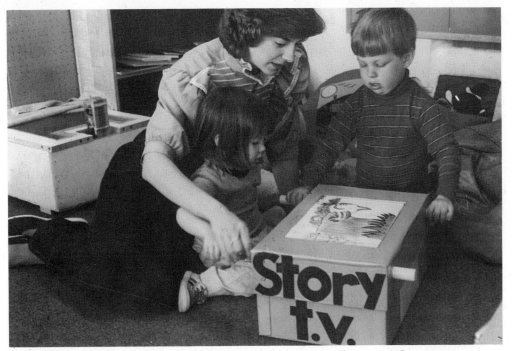

FIGURE 38 Nursery rhymes may be learned several ways.

Music:

1. **"Hickory Dickory Dock"** (traditional)

   Hickory dickory dock
   The mouse ran up the clock.
   The clock struck one, the mouse ran down,
   Hickory dickory dock.

2. **"The Muffin Man"** (traditional)

   Oh, do you know the muffin man,
   The muffin man, the muffin man?
   Oh, do you know the muffin man
   Who lives on Dreary Lane?

   Yes, I know the muffin man . . .

3. **"Two Little Blackbirds"** (traditional)

   Two little blackbirds sitting on a hill
   One named Jack. One named Jill.
   Fly away Jack. Fly away Jill.
   Come back Jack. Come back Jill.
   Two little blackbirds sitting on a hill.
   One named Jack. One named Jill.

4. **"Jack and Jill"** (traditional)

   Jack and Jill went up a hill
   To fetch a pail of water.

Jack fell down and broke his crown
And Jill fell tumbling after.

Fingerplays:

LITTLE JACK HORNER

Little Jack Horner
Sat in a corner
Eating a Christmas pie.
   (pretend you're eating)
He put in his thumb,
   (thumb down)
And pulled out a plum
   (thumb up)
And said, "What a good boy am I!"
   (say out loud)

PAT-A-CAKE

Pat-a-cake, Pat-a-cake, baker's man.
Bake me a cake as fast as you can!
   (clap hands together lightly)
Roll it
   (roll hands)
And pat it
   (touch hands together lightly)
And mark it with a "B"
   (write "b" in the air)
And put it in the oven for baby and me.
   (point to baby and to yourself)

WEE WILLIE WINKLE

Wee Willie Winkle runs through the town
  (pretend to run)
Upstairs, downstairs in his night gown,
  (point up, point down, then point to clothes)
Rapping at the window, crying through
the lock
  (knock in the air, peek through a hole)
"Are the children all in bed, for now it's
eight o'clock?"
  (shake finger)

OLD KING COLE

Old King Cole was a merry old soul
  (lift elbows up and down)
And a merry old soul was he.
  (nod head)
He called for his pipe.
  (clap two times)
He called for his bowl.
  (clap two times)
And he called for his fiddlers three.
  (clap two times then pretend to play violin)

HICKORY DICKORY DOCK

Hickory dickory dock
  (swing arms back and forth together,
  bent down low)
The mouse ran up the clock.
  (run fingers up your arm)
The clock struck one
  (clap, and then hold up one finger)
The mouse ran down.
  (run fingers down your arm)
Hickory dickory dock
  (swing arms back and forth together,
  bent down low)

Science:

1. Mary's Garden

A styrofoam cup with the child's name
printed on it and a scoop of soil should be
provided. Then let everyone choose a
flower seed. Be sure to save the seed
packages. The children can plant their
seed, water and care for it. When the
plant begins to grow, try to identify the
name of the plants by comparing them to
pictures on the seed packages.

2. Hickory Dickory Dock Clock

Draw and cut a large Hickory Dickory
Dock clock from cardboard. Move the
hands of the clock and see if the children
can identify the numeral.

3. Wool

Pieces of wool fabric mounted on cardboard can be matched with samples.

4. Pumpkin Tasters

Plan a Peter, Peter, Pumpkin Eater pumpkin tasting party.

Dramatic Play:

1. Baker

Baking props such as: hats, aprons, cookie
cutters, baking pans, rolling pins, mixers,
spoons and bowls can be placed in the
dramatic play area.

2. Puppets

A puppet theater can be placed in the
dramatic play area for the duration of the
unit. To add variety, each day a different
set of puppets can be added for the
children.

Arts and Crafts:

1. Spiders

Add black tempera paint to a playdough
mixture. In addition to the playdough, provide black pipe cleaners or yarn. Using
these materials, spiders or other objects
can be created.

2. Spider Webs

Cut circles of black paper to fit in the bottom
of a pie tin. Mix thin silver or white tempera
paint. Place a marble and two teaspoons of
paint on the paper. Gently tilt the pie tin,
allowing the marble to roll through the
paint, creating a spider web design.

3. Twinkle Twinkle Little Stars

The children can decorate stars with glitter. The stars can be hung from the ceiling and during group time sing "Twinkle, Twinkle, Little Star."

4. Little Boy Blue's Horn

Collect paper towel tubes. The tubes can be painted with tempera. When the tubes are dry, cover one end with tissue paper and secure with a rubber band. The children can use them as a horn.

Sensory:

Water and Pails

Add water, pails and scoopers to the sensory table.

Large Muscle:

1. Jack Be Nimble's Candlestick

Make a candlestick out of an old paper towel holder and tissue paper for the flame. Repeat the rhyme by substituting each child's name.

Jack be nimble. Jack be quick.
Jack jump over the candlestick.

2. Wall Building

Encourage the children to create a large wall out of blocks for Humpty Dumpty. Act out the rhyme.

Field Trips/Resource People:

1. Candlemaking

Invite a resource person to demonstrate candlemaking, or take a field trip to a craft center so that the children can view candles being made.

2. Greenhouse

Visit a florist or greenhouse to observe flowers and plants.

Math:

1. Puzzles

Draw or cut out several pictures of different nursery rhymes (Jack and Jill, Jack Be Nimble, etc.) and mount on tagboard. Laminate and cut each pictures into five to seven pieces. The children can match nursery rhyme puzzle pieces.

2. Rote Counting

Say or sing the following nursery rhyme to help the children with rote counting.

1, 2 buckle my shoe
3, 4 shut the door
5, 6 pick up sticks
7, 8 lay them straight
9, 10 a big fat hen.

3. Matching

Draw from one to ten simple figures from a nursery rhyme (mittens, candlesticks, pails, etc.) on the left side of a sheet of tagboard and the corresponding numeral on the right side. Laminate the pieces and cut each in half creating different shaped puzzle pieces. The children can match the number of figures to the corresponding numeral.

4. Mitten Match

Collect several matching pairs of mittens. Mix them up and have children match the pairs.

Social Studies:

Table Setting

On a sheet of tagboard, trace the outline of a plate, cup, knife, fork, spoon and napkin. Laminate. The children can match the silverware and dishes to the outline on the placemat in preparation for snack or meals. This activity can be extended by having the children turn the placemat over, and arrange the place setting without the aid of an outline.

Group Time (games, language):

Old Mother Hubbard's Doggie Bone Game

Save a bone or construct one from tagboard. Ask one child to volunteer to be the doggie. Seat the children in a circle with the doggie in the center and the bone in front of him. The doggie closes his eyes. A child from the circle quietly comes and steals the bone. When the child is reseated with the bone out of sight, the children will call

"Doggie, doggie, where's your bone? Someone took it from your home!"

The doggie gets three chances to guess who has the bone. If he guesses correctly, the child who took the bone becomes the doggie.

Cooking:

1. Bran Muffins

(Use with the "Muffin Man" rhyme)

3 cups whole wheat bran cereal
1 cup boiling water
1/2 cup shortening or oil
2 eggs
2 1/2 cups unbleached flour
1 1/2 cups sugar
2 1/2 teaspoons baking soda
2 cups buttermilk

Preheat the oven to 400 degrees. Line the muffin tins with paper baking cups. In a large bowl combine the cereal and boiling water. Stir in the shortening and eggs. Add the remaining ingredients. Blend well. Spoon the batter into cups about 3/4 full. Bake at 400 degrees for 18 to 22 minutes or until golden brown. Eat at snack and sing the "Muffin Man" song.

2. Humpty Dumpty Pear Salad

For each serving provide ½ pear, 1 lifesaver, 1 tablespoon mayonnaise, 2 cherries, 1 raisin and a lettuce leaf. The children can prepare their own salad. To do this each child puts a lettuce leaf on a plate and places a pear half on top of it, round side up. Then add the two cherries for eyes, a raisin for a nose and the piece of lifesaver candy for a mouth. Add mayonnaise to taste.

Source: *Let Loose on Mother Goose*. Terry Graham. (Incentive Publishing Company, 1982).

3. Cottage Cheese

1 gallon pasteurized skim milk (to make 1 to 1 1/2 pounds of cottage cheese)
salt
liquid rennet or a junket tablet

Heat the water to 80 degrees Fahrenheit in the bottom part of a double boiler. Use a thermometer to determine the water temperature. Do not guess.

Pour the skim milk into the top of the double boiler. Dilute 2 or 3 drops of liquid rennet in a tablespoon of cold water and stir it into the milk. If rennet is not available, add 1/8 of a junket tablet to a tablespoon of water and add it to the milk. Allow the milk to remain at 80 degrees, until it curdles in about 12 to 18 hours. During this period no special attention is necessary. If desired, the milk may be placed in a warm oven overnight. Place the curd in a cheese cloth over a container to drain the whey. Occasionally, pour out the whey that collects in the container so that the draining will continue. In 15 to 20 minutes, the curd will become mushy and will drain more slowly. When it is almost firm and the whey has nearly ceased to flow, the cheese is ready for salting and eating. Salt the cheese to taste. The cottage cheese can be spread on crackers for a snack.

4. Miss Muffet's Curds and Whey

2 cups whole milk
1 teaspoon vinegar

Warm milk and add vinegar. Stir as curds separate from the whey. Curds are the milk solids and the whey is the liquid that is poured off. You can let your children taste the whey but they probably will not be thrilled by it. Strain the curds from the whey, then dump the curds onto a paper towel and gently press the curds with more towels to get out the liquid. Sprinkle with salt and refrigerate. Eat as cottage cheese. You can also serve the curds at room temperature. Stir them until they are smooth. Add different flavorings (such as, cinnamon, orange flavoring, vanilla, etc). Use as a spread on crackers. Curds mixed with peanut butter is great. Serves 12 (2 crackers each).

Records:

The following records can be found in preschool educational catalogs:

1. **More Mother Goose with the Play-Along at Home Rhythm Band.** (A Disney Land Record, Walt Disney Production, 1962).

2. **Nursery Rhymes—Rhyming and Remembering.** Ella Jenkins.

Books and Stories:

The following books and stories can be used to complement the theme:

1. **The Best Mother Goose Ever.** Richard Scarry. (New York: Golden Press, 1982).

2. **Old MacDonald Had a Farm.** Abner Graboff. (New York: Scholastic Book Services, 1971).

3. **Mother Goose.** Wallace Tripp. (Boston: Little, Brown Company, 1976).

4. **The Tall Book of Mother Goose.** Feodor Rojankovsky. (New York, London: Harper and Brother, 1942).

5. **Old Mother Hubbard and Her Dog.** Evaline Ness. (New York: Holt, Reinhart, Winston, 1972).

6. **Mother Goose—A Treasury of Best Loved Rhymes.** Watty Peper. (New York: Platt and Munk, 1972).

7. **To Market, To Market.** Peter Spier. (New York: Doubleday and Company, Inc., 1967).

8. **A Mother Goose ABC in a Pumpkin Shell.** (New York: Harcourt, Brace and World, Inc., 1960).

9. **The Puffin Book of Nursery Rhymes.** Iona and Peter Opie. (New York: Penguin Books, 1963).

10. **Mother Goose Nursery Rhymes.** Arthur Rackham (ill.) (New York: Viking Press, 1975).

Puzzles:

The following puzzles can be found in preschool educational catalogs:

1. **"Woman in a Shoe"** 12 pieces. Judy/Instructo.

2. **"Little Miss Muffet"** 8 pieces. Judy/Instructo.

3. **"Little Bo Peep"** 9 pieces. Judy/Instructo.

4. **"Mary Had a Little Lamb"** 10 pieces. Judy/Instructo.

5. **"Jack and Jill"** 10 pieces. Judy/Instructo.

6. **"Hickory Dickory Dock"** 11 pieces. Judy/Instructo.

7. **"Hey Diddle Diddle"** 12 pieces. Judy/Instructo.

8. **"Little Boy Blue"** 12 pieces. Judy/Instructo.

9. **"Humpty Dumpty"** 17 pieces. Judy/Instructo.

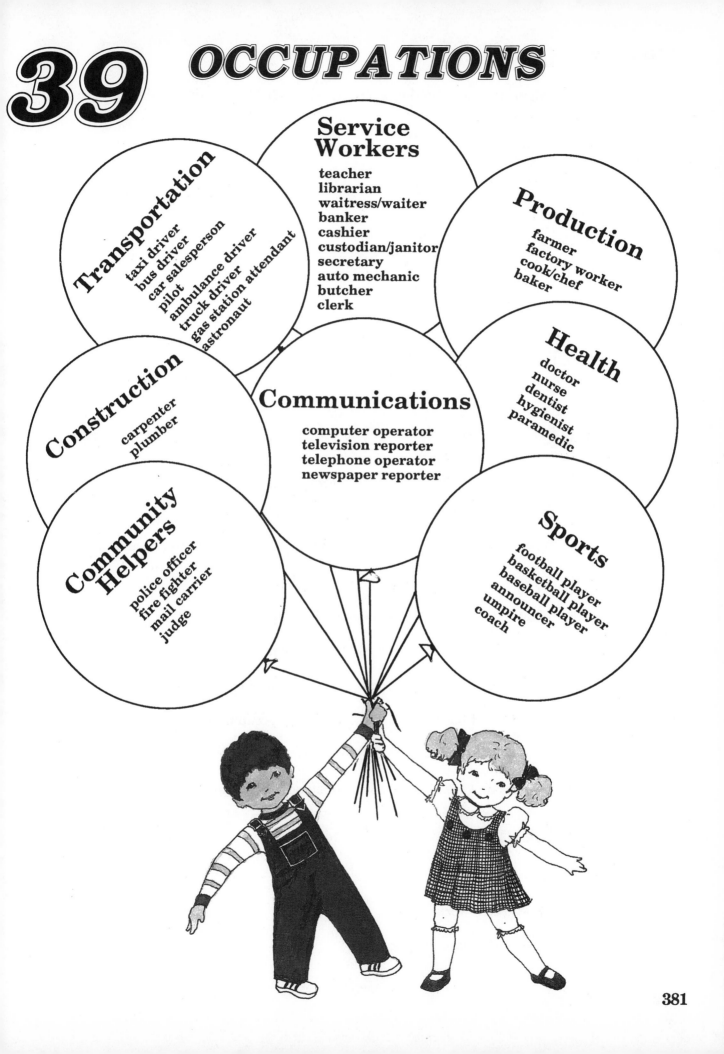

39 OCCUPATIONS

Service Workers

teacher
librarian
waitress/waiter
banker
cashier
custodian/janitor
secretary
auto mechanic
butcher
clerk

Transportation

taxi driver
bus driver
car salesperson
pilot
ambulance driver
truck driver
gas station attendant
astronaut

Production

farmer
factory worker
cook/chef
baker

Construction

carpenter
plumber

Communications

computer operator
television reporter
telephone operator
newspaper reporter

Health

doctor
nurse
dentist
hygienist
paramedic

Community Helpers

police officer
fire fighter
mail carrier
judge

Sports

football player
basketball player
baseball player
announcer
umpire
coach

381

Theme Goals:

Through participating in the experiences provided by this theme, the children may learn:

1. Occupations of community helpers.

2. Sports figure occupations.

3. Health occupations.

4. Transportation occupations.

5. Communications occupations.

6. Construction occupations.

7. Production occupations.

8. Service occupations.

Concepts for the Children to Learn:

1. An occupation is a job a person performs.

2. There are many different kinds of occupations.

3. Taxi drivers, pilots and ambulance drivers are transportation occupations.

4. Doctors, nurses and dentists are health occupations.

5. A community helper is someone who helps us.

6. Teachers, librarians and custodians are service occupations.

7. Cooks, factory workers and farmers are production occupations.

8. Football and baseball players are sports occupations.

9. Television and newspaper reporters are in communications occupations.

10. Builders and architects are in construction occupations.

Vocabulary:

1. **occupation**—the job a person performs to earn money.

2. **job**—type of work.

3. **service**—helping people.

Bulletin Board

The purpose of this bulletin board is to stress that men and women can be doctors, farmers, construction workers, teachers, judges, etc. To prepare the bulletin board, construct a boy and girl out of tagboard. Design several occupational outfits that may be worn by either sex. Color and laminate the pieces. Magnet pieces or push pins and holes could be used to affix clothing on children.

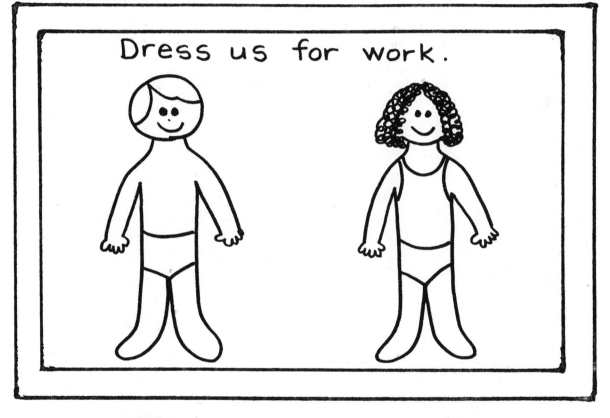

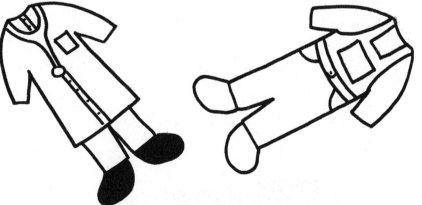

Parent Letter

Dear Parents,

Hello! This week at school we will be exploring a new unit on occupations. Through experiences provided by this theme the children will become aware of a great number of occupations and the way these workers help us today.

At School This Week

Some learning experiences this week include:

* listening to books and records about people in our neighborhoods.
* making occupation hats.
* visiting a police station on Wednesday at 2:00 p.m. Join us if you can!
* observing an ambulance and talking with a paramedic.
* designing a job chart for our classroom.

At Home

Page through magazines with your child. Discuss equipment and materials that are used in various occupations. Questions such as the following can be asked to stimulate thinking skills. Who might use a typewriter to perform a job? What occupations involve the use of a cash register? Your child might be interested in visiting your place of employment!

Have a good week!

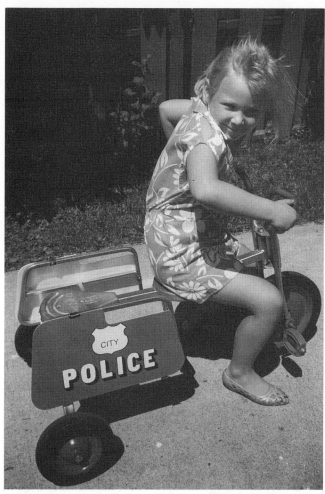

FIGURE 39 Being a police officer is just one of many occupations to choose from.

Fingerplays:

FARM CHORES

Five little farmers woke up with the sun.
It was early morning and the chores must
be done.
The first little farmer went out to milk the
cow.
The second little farmer thought he'd better
plow.
The third little farmer cultivated weeds.
The fourth little farmer planted more seeds.
The fifth little farmer drove his tractor round.
Five little farmers, the best that can be found.

TRAFFIC POLICEMAN

The traffic policeman holds up his hand.
  (hold up hand, palm forward)
He blows the whistle,
  (pretend to blow whistle)

He gives the command.
  (hold up hand again)
When the cars are stopped
  (hold up hand again)
He waves at me.
Then I may cross the street, you see.
  (wave hand as if indicating for someone
  to go)

THE CARPENTER

This is the way he saws the wood
  (right hand saws left palm)
Sawing, sawing, sawing.
This is the way he nails a nail
  (pound right fist on left palm)
Nailing, nailing, nailing.
This is the way he paints the house
  (right hand paints left palm)
Painting, painting, painting.

Dramatic Play:

1. **Hat Shop**

   Police officer hats, firefighter hats, construction worker hats, business person hats and other occupational related hats should be placed in the dramatic play area.

2. **Classroom Cafe**

   Cover the table in the dramatic play area with a tablecloth, provide menus, a tablet for the waitress to write on, a space for a cook, etc. A cash register and play money may also be added to encourage play.

3. **Hair Stylist**

   Collect empty shampoo bottles, curlers, combs, brushes, barrettes, ribbons, hair spray containers and magazines. Cut the cord off a discarded hair dryer and curling iron and place in the dramatic play area.

4. Our Library

Books on a shelf, a desk for the librarian, stamper and ink pad to check out books should be placed in the dramatic play area. A small table for children to sit and read their books would also add interest.

5. Workbench

A hammer, nails, saws, vices, a carpenter's apron, etc. should be added to the workbench. Eye goggles for the children's safety should also be included. Constant supervision is needed for this activity.

6. An Airplane

Create an airplane out of a large cardboard refrigerator box. If desired, the children can paint the airplane.

7. Post Office

A mailbox, letters, envelopes, stamps and mail carrier bags can be set up in the dramatic play or art area.

8. Fast-Food Restaurant

Collect bags, containers, and hats to set up a fast food restaurant.

9. A Construction Sight

Hard hats, nails, a hammer, large blocks and scrap wood can be provided for outdoor play. Cardboard boxes and masking tape should also be available.

10. Prop Boxes

The following prop boxes can be made by collecting the materials listed.

Police Officer

* badge
* hat
* uniforms
* whistle
* walkie-talkie

Mail Carrier

* letter bag
* letter/stamps
* uniforms
* mailbox
* envelopes
* paper
* pencil
* rubber stamp
* ink pad
* wrapped cardboard boxes

Firefighter

* boots
* helmet
* hose
* uniform
* gloves
* raincoat
* suspenders
* goggles

Doctor

* stethoscope
* medicine bottles
* adhesive tape
* cotton balls
* red cross armband
* chart holder

Arts and Crafts:

1. Mail Truck

Precut mail truck parts including: 1 rectangle, 1 square and 2 circles. The children can paste the pieces together and decorate. This activity is most appropriate for older children.

2. Occupation Vests

Cut a circle out of a large paper grocery bag. Then from the circle cut a slit down the center of the bag. Cut out arm holes. Provide felt-tip colored markers for the children to decorate the vests. They may elect to be a pilot, police officer, mail carrier, baker, flight attendant, doctor, firefighter etc.

3. Mail Pouch

Cut the top half off a large grocery bag. Use the cut away piece to make a shoulder strap. Staple it to the bag. The children can decorate the bag with crayons or markers.

Sensory:

The following materials can be added to the sensory table:

* sponge hair rollers with water
* wood shavings with scoops and scales
* sand with toy cars, trucks, airplanes
* pipes with water

Large Muscle:

Cut large cardboard boxes to make squad cars. Take the boxes and spray paint them either blue or white. Emblems can be constructed for the sides.

Field Trips/Resource People:

1. Take field trips to the following:

   * bank
   * library
   * grocery store
   * police station
   * doctor/dentist office
   * beauty salon/barber
   * courthouse
   * television/radio station
   * airport
   * farm
   * restaurant

2. Invite the following resource people to school:

   * police officer with squad car
   * firefighter with truck
   * ambulance driver with an ambulance
   * truck driver with truck
   * taxi driver with cab

Social Studies:

1. Occupation Pictures

Pin occupation pictures on classroom bulletin boards and walls.

2. A Job Chart

Make a chart containing classroom jobs. Include tasks such as feeding the class pet, watering plants, sweeping the floor, wiping tables, etc.

Group Time (games, language):

1. Brushes as Tools

Collect all types of brushes and place in a bag. The children can reach into the bag and feel one. Before removing it, the child describes the kind of brush. When using with younger children, limit the number of brushes. Also, before placing the brushes in the bag, show the children each brush and discuss its use.

2. Machines as Helpers Chart

Machines and tools help people work and play. Ask the children to think of all of the machines they or their parents use around the house. As they name a machine, list it on a chart and discuss how it is used.

3. Mail It

Play a variation of Duck, Duck, Goose. The children can sit in a circle. One child holds an envelope and walks around the circle saying "letter" as he taps each child on the head. When he gets to the one he wants to chase him, have the child drop the letter and say "Mail it!" Then both children run around the circle until they return to the letter. The chaser gets to "mail" the letter by walking around and repeating the game.

Cooking:

Cheese Hammers

cheese chunks
pretzel sticks

Cut cheese into small squares. Poke a pretzel into each cheese chunk. Just before you eat your "hammer,," say the fingerplay "Hammer and Saw" (see fingerplays).

Source: *Everyday Circle Times*. Liz and Dick Wilmes.

EXCURSIONS

Special excursions and events in an early childhood program give opportunities for widening the young child's horizons by providing children exciting direct experiences. The following places or people are some suggestions:

train station	tree farm	airport
dentist office	car wash	riding stable
post office	children's houses	barber shop
grocery store	garage mechanic	college dormitory
zoo	television studio	shoe repair shop
dairy	drug store	print shop
family garden	bakery	artist's studio
poultry house	hospital	bowling alley
construction site	meat market	department store windows
beauty shop	library	potter's studio
offices	apple orchard	teacher's house
animal hospital	farm	street repair site
fire station		

Records:

The following records can be found in preschool educational catalogs:

1. **These are the People in My Neighborhood.** Fred Rogers.

2. **We All Live Together.** Youngheart Records.

3. **My Street Begins at My House.** Ella Jenkins.

4. **Pretend.** Hap Palmer.

Books and Stories:

The following books and stories can be used to complement the theme:

1. **Simon Boom Gets a Letter.** V.R. Suhl. (Englewood Cliffs, NJ: Four Winds Press, 1976).

2. **What Can She Be? A Police Officer.** Gloria and Esther Goldreich. (New York: Lothrop, Lee and Shepard Company, 1975).

3. **A Letter to Amy.** Ezra Jack Keats. (New York: Harper and Row, 1968).

4. **The Little Fire Engine.** Graham Greene. (New York: Doubleday and Company, 1973).

5. **Red Light Says Stop.** Barbara Rinkoff. (New York: Lothrop, Lee and Shepard Company, 1974).

6. **Policeman Small.** Lois Lenski. (New York: Henry Z. Walck, 1962).

7. **Fire Girl.** Gibson Rich. (Old Westbury, CT: The Feminist Press, 1972).

8. **I Can Be An Animal Doctor.** Kathern Wentzel Lumley. (Chicago: Childrens Press, 1985).

9. **My Daddy Is a Nurse.** Mark Wandro. (Reading, MA: Addison-Wesley, 1981).

10. **My Mother the Mail Carrier.** Inez Maury. (Old Westbury, CT: Feminist Press, 1976).

11. **I Can Be a Secretary.** Dee Lillegard. (Chicago: Childrens Press, 1987).

12. **World At Work.** Robert Durham. (Chicago: Childrens Press, 1987).

Puzzles:

The following puzzles can be found in preschool educational catalogs:

1. **"Who Does What?"** Judy/Instructo.

2. **"Transportation Puzzles"**—set of ten puzzles including truck, bulldozer, tractor, etc. Judy/Instructo.

3. **Occupation puzzles**—multi-ethnic career puzzles. Judy/Instructo.

"firefighter"
"grocery cashier"
"telephone line person"
"mail carrier"
"farmer"
"nurse"
"dentist"
"doctor"
"police officer"
"mail carrier"
"carpenter"
"astronaut"
"school crossing guard"
"teacher"
"T.V. reporter"
"librarian"
"pilot"

"barber"
"lawyer and judge"
"car mechanic"
"construction worker"
"cashier"

4. **"Space Exploration"** Judy/Instructo.

5. **"Occupation Hats"** 6 pieces. Puzzle People.

6. **"Occupational Sandy, Occupational Jerry"** (available in white or black) Puzzle People.

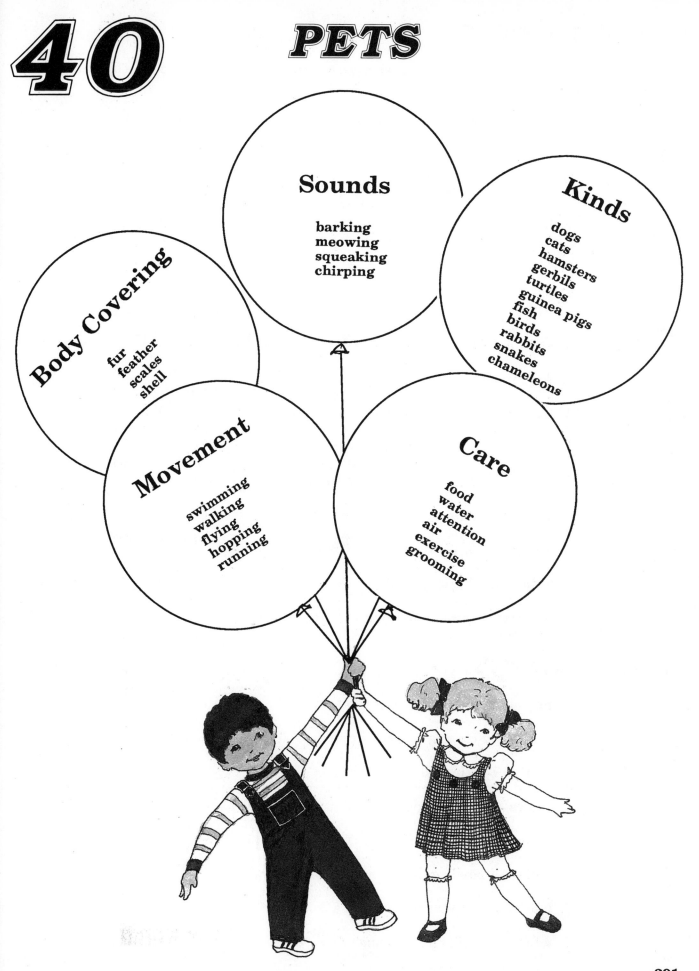

Sounds

barking
meowing
squeaking
chirping

Kinds

dogs
cats
hamsters
gerbils
turtles
guinea pigs
fish
birds
rabbits
snakes
chameleons

Body Covering

fur
feather
scales
shell

Movement

swimming
walking
flying
hopping
running

Care

food
water
attention
air
exercise
grooming

Theme Goals:

Through participating in the experiences provided by this theme, the children may learn:

1. Some animals are kept as pets.

2. Pet care.

3. Places pets live.

4. Body coverings of pets.

5. Sounds of pets.

6. Movements of pets.

Concepts for the Children to Learn:

1. An animal kept for enjoyment is called a pet.

2. Dogs, cats, fish, hamsters, gerbils and birds can all be pets.

3. Pets need food and water.

4. Barking, meowing, squeaking and chirping are pet sounds.

5. To move, pets may swim, walk, fly, hop or run.

6. The care of a pet depends on the type of animal.

7. Skin coverings on pets differ.

8. A veterinarian is a pet doctor.

Vocabulary:

1. **pet**—animal that is kept for pleasure.

2. **fur**—hairy coating of some animals.

3. **feathers**—skin covering of birds.

4. **scales**—skin covering of fish and other reptiles.

5. **veterinarian**—an animal doctor.

6. **collar**—a band worn around an animal's neck.

7. **leash**—a cord that attaches to a collar.

8. **whiskers**—stiff hair growing around the animal's nose, mouth and eyes.

Bulletin Board

The purpose of this bulletin board is to encourage the development of mathematical skills. The children can count the fish in each water piece and match it to the corresponding numbered fishbowl. To prepare the bulletin board, construct fishbowls out of white tagboard or construction paper. Write a numeral beginning with one on each fishbowl and the corresponding number of dots. Hang the fishbowls on the bulletin board. Next, construct pieces as illustrated that will fit on top of the fishbowl to represent water in the bowl. Draw fish to match the numerals in each bowl. The pieces can be attached to each other to hang on the bulletin board by using magnet pieces, or push pins and a paper punch.

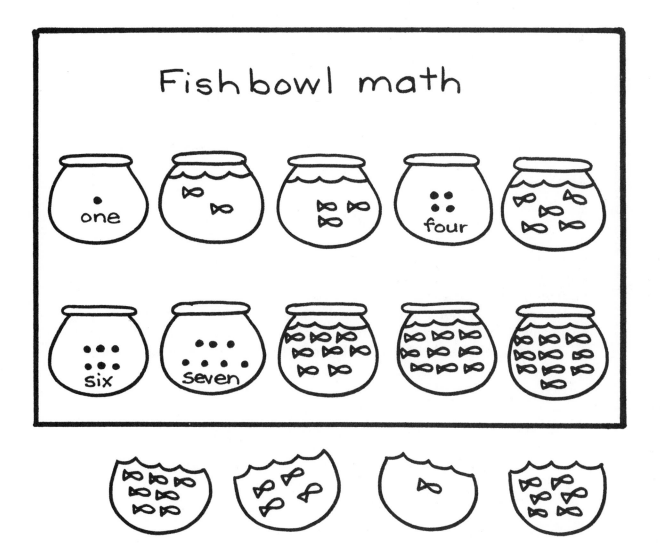

Parent Letter

Dear Parents,

Children are naturally curious about animals. Keeping that in mind, we will be starting a unit on pets this week and I'm sure that we'll be busy! The children will discover the kinds of animals most people keep as pets. They will also learn the care that is involved in having a pet.

At School This Week

The following are some of the learning experiences your child will participate in during our pet unit:

* making a special treat for Greta, our classroom gerbil.
* creating a large doghouse out of an appliance box for the dramatic play area.
* interacting with a variety of pets. Dani and Donny will bring their rabbit on Tuesday, and Cindy will bring her bird on Wednesday. If you are willing to bring your family pet to school to show the children, we welcome you. Contact me and we can arrange a time that would be convenient for you (and your pet).
* listening to the story *Clifford, The Big Red Dog* by Norman Bridwell.

At Home

Is your family considering adding a pet to your household? If so, there are many variables to be taken into consideration because not all households are meant to include pets. Allergies, fears and lifestyles are three things that need to be considered. Also, you will need to consider your child's readiness for a pet.

To develop fine motor skills, provide magazines and newspapers for your child to cut or tear out pictures of animals. These can be used to create an animal alphabet book or a collage to hang in your child's bedroom.

Have a good week!

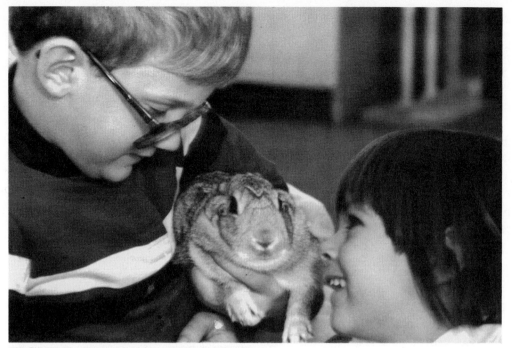

FIGURE 40 Rabbits make fun pets.

Music:

. "Rags"
(Sing this song to one of the children's favorite tunes)

I have a dog and his name is Rags.
   (point to self)
He eats so much that his tummy sags.
   (hold tummy)
His ears flip-flop and his tail wig-wags.
   (flip hands by ears and wag hands at back)
And when he walks he zigs and zags
   (put hands together and zig-zag them)

Flip-flop
Wiggle-waggle
Zig-zag   (Repeat the same actions)
Flip-flop
Wiggle-waggle
Zig-zag

. "Six Little Pets"
(Sing to the tune of "Six Little Ducks," a traditional early childhood song.)

Six little gerbils I once knew, fat ones, skinny ones, fair ones too. But the one little gerbil was so much fun. He would play until the day was done.

Six little dogs that I once knew, fat ones, skinny ones, fair ones too. But the one little dog with the brown curly fur, he led the others with a grr, grr, grr.

Six little fish that I once knew, fat ones, skinny ones, fair ones too. But the one little fish who was the leader of the crowd, he led the others around and around.

Six little birds that I once knew, fat ones, skinny ones, fair ones too. But the one little bird with the pretty little beak, he led the others with a tweet, tweet, tweet.

Six little cats that I once knew, fat ones, skinny ones, fair ones too. But the one little cat who was as fluffy as a ball, he was the prettiest one of all.

3. "Have You Ever Seen A Rabbit"
(Sing to the tune of "Have You Ever Seen A Lassie?")

Have you ever seen a rabbit, a rabbit, a rabbit?
Have you ever seen a rabbit go hopping around?
Go hopping, go hopping, go hopping, go hopping
Have you ever seen a rabbit go hopping around?

Fingerplays:

MY PUPPY

I like to pet my puppy.
  (pet puppy)
He has such nice soft fur.
  (pet puppy)
And if I don't pull his tail
  (pull tail)
He won't say "Grr!"
  (make face)

IF I WERE

If I were a dog
I'd have four legs to run and play.
  (down on all four hands and feet)
If I were a fish
I'd have fins to swim all day.
  (hands at side fluttering like wings)
If I were a bird
I could spread my wings out wide.
And fly all over the countryside.
  (arms out from sides fluttering like wings)
But I'm just me.
I have two legs, don't you see?
And I'm just as happy as can be.

THE BUNNY

Once there was a bunny
  (fist with two fingers tall)
And a green, green cabbage head.
  (fist of other hand)
"I think I'll have some breakfast," this
little bunny said.
So he nibbled and he cocked his ears to say,
"I think it's time that I be on my way."

SAMMY

Sammy is a super snake.
  (wave finger on opposite palm)
He sleeps on the shore of a silver lake.
  (curl finger to indicate sleep)
He squirms and squiggles to snatch a snack
  (wave finger and pounce)
And snoozes and snores till his hunger is
back.
  (curl finger on palm).

NOT SAY A SINGLE WORD

We'll hop, hop, hop like a bunny
  (make hopping motion with hand)
And run, run, run like a dog.
  (make running motion with fingers)
We'll walk, walk, walk like an elephant
  (make walking motion with arms)
And jump, jump, jump like a frog.
  (make jumping motions with arms)
We'll swim, swim, swim like a goldfish
  (make swimming motion with hand)
And fly, fly, fly like a bird.
  (make flying motion with arms)
We'll sit right down and fold our hands
  (fold hands in lap)
And not say a single word!

Science:

1. Pet Foods

Cut pictures of pets and pet foods and
place on the science table. Include different
foods such as meat, fish, carrots, lettuce,
nuts and acorns. The children can match
the food to a picture of the animal that
would eat each type of food.

2. Bird Feathers

Bird's feathers with a magnifying glass
can be placed on the science table for the
children to examine.

3. Hamster and Gerbil Pet Food

The children can assist in preparing the
pet food for hamsters or gerbles. The
recipe is as follows:

1/2 cup cracked corn
1/2 cup flour
1/4 cup water
1/2 teaspoon salt

Mix the water with flour in a bowl. Add
salt. Form into balls and roll into cracked
corn. Cool to harden. Serve once a day.

Source: *Critter's Kitchen*. Michelle
Reynolds. (New York: Athenum Publishing
Company, 1979).

Dramatic Play:

1. Pet Store

The children can all bring in their stuffed animals to set up a pet store. A counter, a cash register and several empty pet food containers should be provided to stimulate play.

2. Veterinarian Prop Box

Collect materials for a veterinarian prop box. Include a stethoscope, empty pill bottles, fabric cut as bandages, splints and stuffed animals.

Arts and Crafts:

1. Pet Sponge Painting

Cut sponges into a variety of pet shapes. Place on the art table with paper and a shallow pan of tempera paint.

2. Doghouse

Provide an old large cardboard box for the children to make a doghouse with adult supervision. They can cut holes, paint and decorate it. When dry, the doghouse can be moved into the dramatic play area or on the outdoor play yard.

3. Cookie Cutters and Playdough

Pet-shaped cookie cutters and playdough can be placed on the art table.

Sensory:

Minnows

Fill the sensory table with cold water. Place minnows purchased from a bait store into the water. The children will attempt to catch the minnows. Teachers should stress the importance of being gentle with the fish and follow through with limits set for the activity. After participating in this activity, the children should wash their hands.

Field Trips/Resource People:

1. Pet Show

Plan a pet show. Each child who wants to show a pet should sign up for a time and day. If children can all bring in a pet the same day have a big pet show. Award prizes for longest tail, longest ears, biggest, smallest, best groomed, loudest barker, most obedient, etc. Children who do not have a pet or cannot arrange to bring it to school can bring a stuffed toy.

2. Veterinarian

Invite a veterinarian to talk to the children about how a veterinarian helps pets and animals. Pet care can also be addressed.

3. Pet Store

Visit a pet store to observe types of pets, their toys and other accessories. Pictures can be taken on the trip and later placed on the bulletin board of the classroom.

4. Pet Groomer

Visit a pet groomer. Observe how the pet is bathed and groomed.

Social Studies:

1. Animal Sounds

Tape several animal sounds and play them back for the children to identify.

2. Feeding Chart

Design and prepare a feeding chart for the classroom pets.

3. Weekend Visitor

Let children take turns bringing class pets home on weekends. Prepare a card for each animal's cage outlining feeding and behavioral expectations.

Cooking:

Animal Cookies

1 1/2 cups powdered sugar
1 cup butter or margarine

1 egg
1 teaspoon vanilla extract
1/2 teaspoon almond extract
2 1/2 cups flour
1 teaspoon baking soda
1 teaspoon cream of tartar

Mix powdered sugar, margarine, egg and vanilla and almond extract. Mix in flour, baking soda and cream of tartar. Cover and refrigerate for 2 hours. Preheat oven to 375 degrees. Divide dough into halves. Roll out 1/2 inch thick on a lightly floured, cloth-covered board. Cut the dough into animal shapes with cookie cutters or let children cut. Place on lightly greased cookie sheet. Bake 7 to 10 minutes. Serve for snack.

Records:

The following records can be found in preschool educational catalogs:

1. **Walk Like The Animals.** Hap Palmer.

2. **Walter The Waltzing Worm.** Hap Palmer.

Books and Stories:

The following books and stories can be used to complement the theme:

1. **How Puppies Grow.** Millicent E. Selsam. (New York: Scholastic Book Service, 1971).

2. **One Kitten For Kim.** Adelaide Hoel. (Reading, MA: Addison-Wesley Publishing Company, 1969).

3. **Whose Mouse Are You?** Robert Kraus. (New York: Macmillan Publishing Company, 1970).

4. **The Playful Little Dog.** Jean Horton Bera. (New York: Wonder Book, 1951).

5. **Your Parakeet.** Larry and Polly Foster. (Chicago: Melmont Publishers, Inc., 1955).

6. **Bob Wanted a Pony.** Marguerite and Dorothy Bryan. (New York: Dodd, Mead and Company, 1948).

7. **My Puppy.** Polly and Larry Foster. (Chicago: Melmont Publishers, Inc., 1956).

8. **Friskey Try Again.** Charles Phillip Fox. (Chicago: Reilly and Lee Company, 1959).

9. **Pets Around The World.** Kathryn Jackson. (Chicago: Silver Burdett Company, 1957).

10. **Pets.** Alme Ratzesberger. (Chicago: Rand McNally and Company, 1954).

11. **Corduroy.** Don Freedman. (New York: The Viking Press, 1968).

12. **Clifford, The Big Red Dog.** Norman Bridwell. (New York: Scholastic Book Services, 1972).

13. **Theodore.** Edward Ormondroyd. (New York: Parnassus Press, 1966).

14. **Joey's Cat.** Robert Burch. (New York: The Viking Press, 1969).

Puzzles:

The following puzzles can be found in preschool educational catalogs:

1. Animal Parent and Baby Puzzles Judy/Instructo.

   "Monkey and Baby" 6 pieces.
   "Pig and Piglets" 7 pieces.
   "Horse and Foal" 7 pieces.
   "Penguin Families" 8 pieces.

2. **"Kitten"** 5 pieces. Judy/Instructo.

3. **"Fish"** 6 pieces. Judy/Instructo.

4. **"Dog"** 9 pieces. Judy/Instructo.

5. **"Rabbit"** 11 pieces. Judy/Instructo.

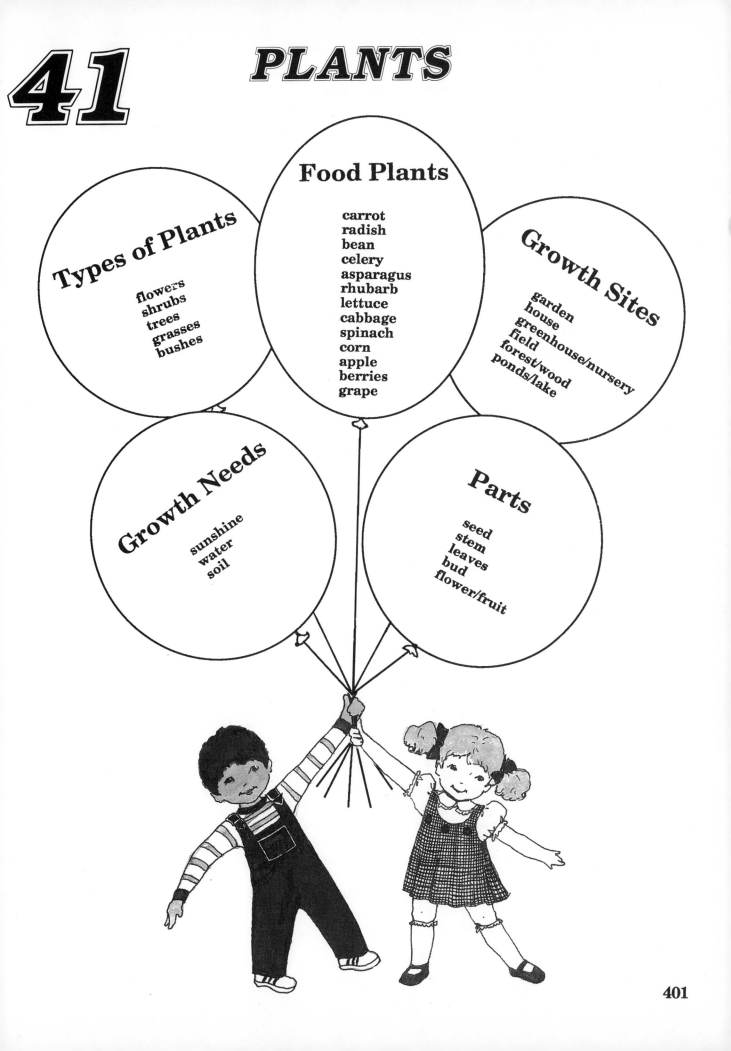

41 PLANTS

Food Plants

carrot
radish
bean
celery
asparagus
rhubarb
lettuce
cabbage
spinach
corn
apple
berries
grape

Types of Plants

flowers
shrubs
trees
grasses
bushes

Growth Sites

garden
house
greenhouse/nursery
field
forest/wood
ponds/lake

Growth Needs

sunshine
water
soil

Parts

seed
stem
leaves
bud
flower/fruit

Theme Goals:

Through participating in the experiences provided by this theme, the children may learn:

1. Types of plants.

2. Growth of plants.

3. The parts of a plant.

4. Plant growth sites.

5. Plants that provide food.

Concepts for the Children to Learn:

1. Plants are living things that grow.

2. There are many kinds of plants.

3. Plants grow from seeds.

4. Plants need water, sunlight and soil to grow.

5. People and animals eat some types of plants.

6. The parts of a plant are the stem, roots, leaves, flower/fruit and seeds.

7. There are different sizes, colors and shapes of seeds.

Vocabulary:

1. **plant**—living thing, usually green, that grows and changes.

2. **stem**—part of the plant that supports the leaves and grows upward.

3. **leaf**—part of the plant that grows on the stem.

4. **root**—part of the plant that grows into the soil.

5. **seed**—part of plant that can grow into another plant.

6. **vegetable**—a plant grown for food.

7. **fruit**—edible plant product that has seeds.

8. **flower**—a colored plant part that contains seeds.

9. **garden**—ground for growing plants.

10. **sprout**—first sign of growth.

Bulletin Board

The purpose of this bulletin board is to foster numeral recognition. To prepare the bulletin board, construct flower pots out of construction paper. Color each pot and draw dots on it as illustrated. Hang the pots on the bulletin board. Next, construct the same number of flowers as pots with stems. In the center of each flower, write a numeral. The children can place each flower in the flower pot with the corresponding number of dots.

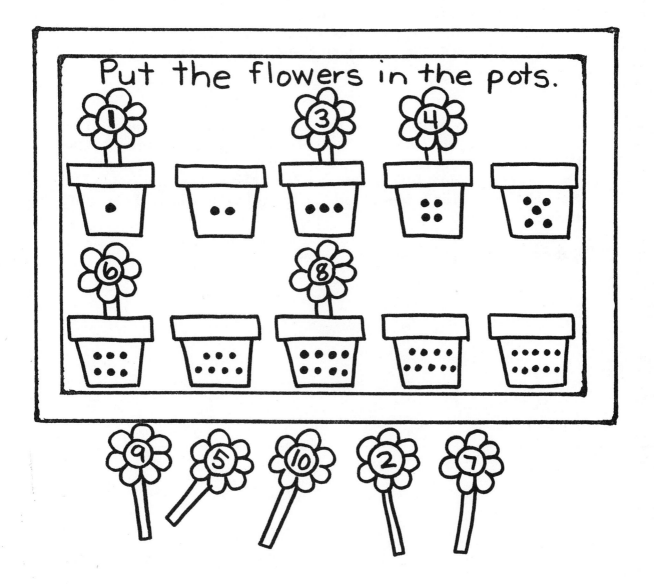

Parent Letter

Dear Parents,

This week at school we will be focusing on plants. Through the unit the children will become aware of the parts of a plant as well as discover where plants can be grown and what plants can be eaten.

At School This Week

Some of the learning experiences planned for our week on plants include:

* listening to the story *The Plant Sitter* by Gene Zion
* sprouting alfalfa seeds to add to a salad.
* walking around our play yard to collect plants.
* playing hopscotch in the shape of a flower.

At Home

There are many ways to foster the concepts of this unit at home. If you have plants, let your child help water them. If you are planning to start a garden, section off a small portion for your child to grow plants.

At mealtimes, identify various parts of plants that are eaten. For example, we eat the leaves of lettuce, the stems of celery, the root of a carrot, and so on.

Have a good week!

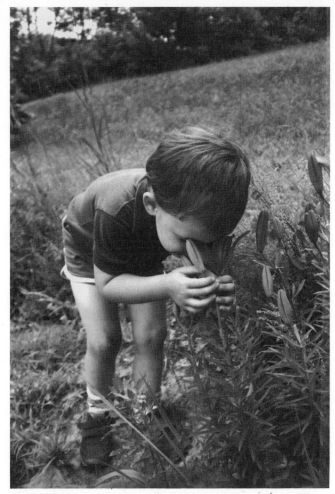

FIGURE 41 Some plants smell so good!

Music:

1. **"The Seed Cycle"**
(Sing to the tune of "The Farmer in the Dell")

The farmer sows his seeds.
The farmer sows his seeds.
Hi-ho the dairy-o
The farmer sows his seeds.

Other verses:
The wind begins to blow...
The rain begins to fall...
The sun begins to shine...
The seeds begin to grow...
The plants grow big and tall...
The farmer cuts his corn...
He puts it in his barns...
And now the harvest is in...

Children can dramatize the parts for each verse.

2. **"This is the Way We Rake the Garden"**
(Sing to the tune of: "Here We Go Round the Mulberry Bush")

This is the way we rake the garden,
Rake the garden, rake the garden.
This is the way we rake the garden,
So early in the morning.

Other verses:
This is the way we plant the seeds...
This is the way the rain comes down...
This is the way we hoe the weeds...
This is the way the garden grows...
This is the way we pick the vegetables...
This is the way we eat the vegetables...

3. **"The Farmer in the Dell"** (traditional)

Fingerplays:

MY GARDEN

This is my garden.
   (extend one hand forward, palm up)
I'll rake it with care
   (make raking motion on palm with other hand)
And then some flower seeds
   (make planting motion with thumb and index fingers)
I'll plant in there.

The sun will shine
   (make circle above head)
And the rain will fall
   (let fingers flutter down to lap)
And my garden will blossom
   (cup hands together, extend upward slowly until fingers stand straight)
And grow straight and tall.

PLANTS

Plants need care to help them grow
Just like boys and girls you know.
Good soil, water, sunshine bright.
Then watch them pop overnight.

Science:

1. **Watch Seeds Grow**

Two identical plastic transparent plates and blotting paper are needed for this

405

activity. Moisten the blotting paper. Then lay the wet paper on one of the plates. On the top of the paper plate place various seeds—corn, peas, squash, bean, etc. Place the other plate over the seeds to serve as a cover. Tie the plates together tightly. Stand the plate on the edge in a pan containing 1/2 inch water. Watch the seeds sprout and grow.

2. Colored Celery

In clear containers place several celery stalks with leaves. In each container add 3 inches of water and drop a different color of food coloring. The leaves of the celery should turn colors in a few hours. Try splitting a celery stalk in half, but do not split the stalk all the way up to the top. Put one half of the stalk in red water, and the other half in blue water. Watch what happens to the leaves.

3. Sunlight Experiment

Place seeds in two jars. Place one jar in a dark place such as a closet or cupboard and avoid watering it. Keep the other jar in a sunny area and water it frequently. Which one grew? Why?

4. Growing Bean Plants

Each child can grow a bean plant.

5. Tasting Plants

Various fruits and vegetables grown from plants should be provided for the children to taste and smell.

6. Feely Box

In the feely box, place different parts of a plant such as root, stem, leaves, flowers, fruit and buds. The children can feel and verbally identify the part of the plant before looking at it.

7. Root a Vegetable

Place a potato or carrot in a jar, root end down so that one-third is covered by water. A potato can be held upright by inserting toothpicks or nails in at three points. This can be rested on the rim of the jar. The children can water as needed. Roots should grow out from the bottom and shoots from the top. Then plant the root in soil for an attractive plant.

8. Beans

Soak dry navy beans in a jar of water overnight. The next day compare soaked beans with dry beans. Note the difference in texture and color. Open some bean seeds that were soaked. A tiny plant should be inside the seed. These can be placed under a microscope for closer observation.

9. Budding Branches

Place a branch that has buds ready to bloom in a jar of water on the science table. Let the children observe the buds bloom. Notice that after all the stored food of the plant is used the plant will die.

Dramatic Play:

1. Greenhouse

Provide materials for a greenhouse. Include window space, pots, soil, water, watering cans, seeds, plants, posters, work aprons, garden gloves, a terrarium and seed packages to mount on sticks.

2. Jack and the Beanstalk

Act out the story *Jack and the Beanstalk*. The children can dramatize a beanstalk growing.

3. Vegetable-Fruit Stand

Display plastic fruits and vegetables. Set up a shopping area with carts, cash registers and play money. Provide a balance scale for children to weigh the produce.

406

4. Garden Planting

Plant a small garden outdoors. Provide seeds, watering cans, garden tools, gloves and garden hats.

Arts and Crafts:

1. Grass Hair

Save 1/2-pint milk cartons. The children can decorate the outside of the carton like a face. Place soil in the cartons and add grass seeds. After approximately 7 days the grass will start to grow, and it will look like hair. If the grass becomes too long, have the child give it a haircut.

2. Flower Collage

Collect flowers and weeds. Press the flowers and weeds between paper and books. Dry them for 7 to 10 days. The children can use the pressed foliage to create their own collages on paper plates or construction paper.

3. Seed Pictures

Supply the children with paper, paste or glue, and various kinds of seeds. Included may be grass, beans and popcorn seeds. The children can express their own creativity through self-created designs.

4. Nature Tree

Cut a branch off a tree and place in a pail of plaster of paris. The children can decorate the tree with a ribbon and different forms of plant life that they have collected or made. Included may be flowers, plants, fruits, vegetables and seeds.

5. Leaf Rubbings

Place a thin piece of paper over a leaf. Rub gently with the long side of a crayon.

6. Easel Ideas

Cut easel paper into different shapes such as:

* leaves
* flower
* flower pots
* fruits and vegetables

7. Egg Carton Flowers

Use egg cartons and pipe cleaners to make flowers. To make the flower stand up, place a pipe cleaner into the egg carton as well as a styrofoam block.

8. Muffin Liner Flowers

Use paper muffin tin liners to make flowers.

9. Hand and Foot Flowers

Create a flower by using the child's hands and feet. Trace and cut two left and right hands and one set of left and right feet. Put one set of hands together to form the top of the flower and the other set (facing down) to form the bottom side. Add a circle to the middle. Cut a stem from green paper and add the green feet, as leaves. This makes a cute Mother's Day idea. Mount on white paper.

Math:

1. Charting Growth

The children can observe the growth of a small plant by keeping a chart of its growth. Record the date of the observation and the height. For convenience, place the chart near the plant table.

2. Flower Pot Match Game

Construct flower pots. The number constructed will depend upon the developmental appropriateness. Write a numeral on each, beginning with the numeral one. Then make the same number of flowers, varying from one petal to the total number of flower pots constructed. The children match the flower pot to the flower with the same number of petals.

3. Counting and Classifying Seeds

Place a variety of seeds on a table. Encourage the children to count and classify them into groups. To assist in counting and classifying, an egg carton with each section given a number from 1 to 12 may be helpful. Encourage the children to observe the numeral and place a corresponding number of seeds in each section.

4. Plant Growth Seriation

Construct pictures of plants through stages of growth. Begin with a seed, followed by the seed sprouting. The third picture should be the stem erupting from the soil surface. Next a stem with leaves can be constructed. Finally flowers can be added to the last picture. This could also be made into a bulletin board.

5. Seed Match

Collect a variety of seeds such as corn, pumpkin, orange, apple, lima bean, watermelon, pea and peach. Cut several rectangles out of white tagboard. On the top half of each rectangle draw one of the seed types you have collected. Encourage the children to sort the seeds matching them to those seeds glued on the individual cards.

Social Studies:

1. Plant Walk

Walk around the neighborhood and try to identify as many plants as you can.

2. Play Yard Plants

Make a map of the play yard. The children can collect a part of each plant located in the playground. The plant samples can be mounted on the map.

3. Planting Trees

Plant a tree on your playground. Discuss the care needed for trees.

4. Family Tree

Make a Family Tree by mounting a bunch of branches in a pail of dirt. Each child

can bring in a family picture to be placed on a leaf shape and hung on the tree branches.

Large Muscle:

1. Leaf Jumping

Cut out eight large leaves from tagboard. Arrange the leaves on a pattern on the floor. Encourage the children to jump from one leaf to another. This game could also be played outdoors by drawing the leaves on the sidewalk with chalk.

2. Flower Hopscotch

Design a hopscotch in the form of a flower. Use chalk on a sidewalk outdoors or masking tape can be used indoors to make the form.

3. Vegetable, Vegetable, Plant

Play Vegetable, Vegetable, Plant as a variation of Duck, Duck, Goose.

4. Raking and Hoeing

Provide the children with hoes and rakes to tend to the play yard.

Field Trips/Resource People:

1. Greenhouse

Visit a greenhouse or a tree nursery to observe the different plants and trees and inquire about their care.

2. Farm

Plan a visit to a farm. While there, observe the various forms of plant life.

3. Florist

Visit a florist. Observe the different colors, types and sizes of flowering plants.

Group Time (games, language):

Feltboard Fun

Construct felt pieces representing the stages of a flower's growth. Include a bulb, seed, cuttings, root, stem, leaves and a flower. During group time, review the name and purpose of each part with the children. The children can take turns coming up to the flannel board and adding the pieces. After group time, the felt pieces should be left out so that the child can reconstruct the growth during self-selected activity period.

Cooking:

1. Vegetable Tasting Party

Prepare raw vegetables for a tasting party. Discuss the color, texture and flavor of each vegetable.

2. Sprouts

Provide each interested child with a small jar. Fill the bottom with alfalfa seeds. Fill the jar with warm water and cover with cheesecloth and a rubberband. Each day rinse and fill the jar with fresh warm water. In three or four days the seeds will sprout. The sprouts may be used on sandwiches or salads at lunch time.

3. Latkes (Potato Pancakes)

2 potatoes, peeled and grated
1 egg, slightly beaten
1/4 cup flour
1 teaspoon salt
cooking oil

Mix the ingredients in a bowl. Drop the mixture by tablespoons into hot oil in an electric skillet. Brown on both sides. Drain on paper towels.

4. Ground Nut Soup (Nigeria)

1 large tomato
1 large potato
1 onion
2 cups water
1 beef boullion cube
1 cup shelled, unsalted roasted peanuts
1/2 cup milk
2 tablespoons rice

Peel potato and onion. Dice potato, tomato and onion. Place in saucepan with the water and boullion cube. Boil, covered, for 30 minutes. Chop and add the peanuts, milk and rice to the boiling mixture. Stir. Lower heat and simmer 30 minutes. Serves 6 to 8.

Records:

The following records can be found in preschool educational catalogs:

1. **Let's Sing Along with Mother Goose.** Side 2. "Oats, Peas, Beans and Barley Grow." (Record Guild of America; Farmingdale, New York).

2. **Great Bedtime Stories: Jack and the Beanstalk.** (New York: A.A. Records Inc.).

3. **Walt Disney Presents a Child's Garden of Verses.** "The Little Nut Tree," (Walt Disney Productions, U.B.A.).

Books and Stories:

The following books and stories can be used to complement the theme:

1. **Mushroom in the Rain.** Mirra Ginaburg. (New York: Macmillan Publishing Company, 1974).

2. **Dandelion.** Svatas Ladislav. (New York: Doubleday and Company Inc., 1976).

3. **Now You Know: Many Plants.** Anne R. Neighoff. (Chicago: Encyclopedia Britannica, 1973).

4. **Our Terrariums.** Herbert Wong and Matthew Vessel. (Reading, MA: Addison-Wesley Publishing Company, 1969).

5. **Seeds and More Seeds.** Millicent Selsam. (New York: Harper and Row Publishers, 1959).

6. **Seeds by the Wind and Water.** Jordan Helene. (New York: Thomas Y. Crowell Company, 1962).

7. **Busy Seeds.** Irma Black. (New York: Holiday House, Inc., 1970).

8. **A Tree is a Plant.** Clyde Robert Bulla. (New York: Thomas Y. Crowell Company, 1960).

9. **Who Goes There in My Garden?** Ethel Collier. (New York: Young Scott Books, 1963).

10. **The Turnip.** Janina Domanska. (New York: Macmillan Publishing Company, 1969).

11. **Where Does Your Garden Grow?** August Goldin. (New York: Thomas Y. Crowell, 1967).

12. **The Flower.** Mary Louise Downer. (New York: William R. Scott, Inc., 1955).

13. **The Giving Tree.** Shel Silverstein. (New York: Harper and Row Publishing Company, 1964).

14. **The Plant Sitter.** Gene Zion. (New York: Harper and Row Publishing Company, 1959).

15. **The Tiny Seed.** Eric Carle. (Natick, MA: Picture Book Studio, 1987).

16. **A First Look at the World of Plants.** Millicent E. Selsam and Joyce Hunt. (New York: Walker & Co., 1978).

17. **Little Green Pumpkins.** Christa Chevalier. (Niles, IL: Albert Whitman and Company, 1981).

Puzzles:

The following puzzles can be found in preschool educational catalogs.

1. **"Fruits"** Judy/Instructo.

2. **"Vegetables"** Judy/Instructo.

3. **"Sunflower Sequence Puzzle"** Kaplan.

4. **"Tree"** Judy/Instructo.

42 PUPPETS

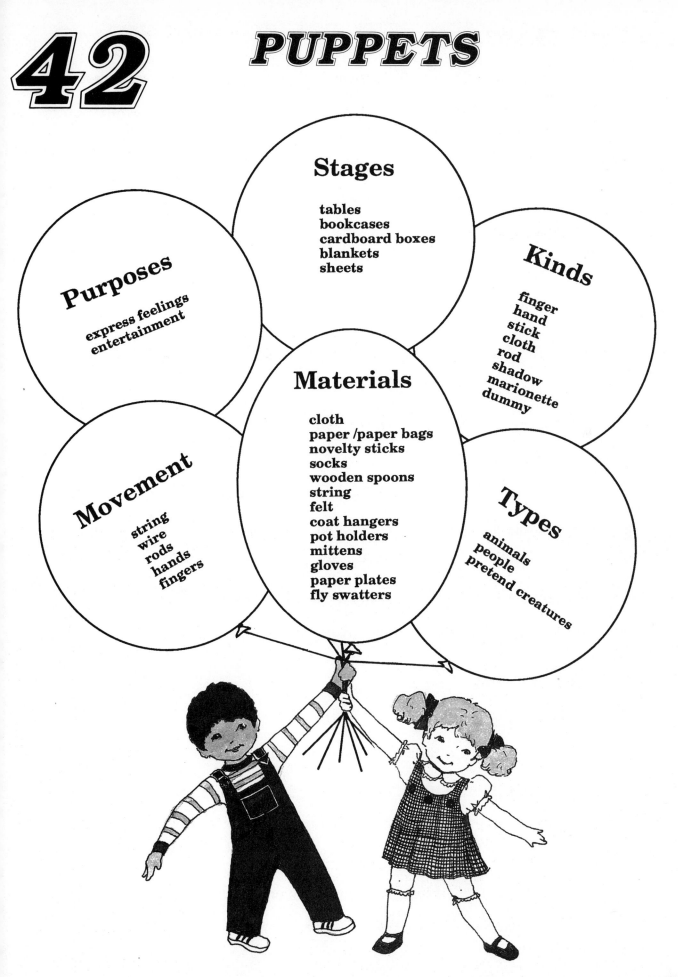

Stages

tables
bookcases
cardboard boxes
blankets
sheets

Purposes

express feelings
entertainment

Kinds

finger
hand
stick
cloth
rod
shadow
marionette
dummy

Materials

cloth
paper /paper bags
novelty sticks
socks
wooden spoons
string
felt
coat hangers
pot holders
mittens
gloves
paper plates
fly swatters

Movement

string
wire
rods
hands
fingers

Types

animals
people
pretend creatures

411

Theme Goals:

Through participating in the experiences provided by this theme, the children may learn:

1. The purpose of using puppets.

2. Kinds of puppets.

3. Types of puppets.

4. Materials used to make puppets.

5. Ways of moving puppets.

6. Types of puppet stages.

Concepts for the Children to Learn:

1. Puppets can be fun.

2. We can use puppets to express feelings.

3. People talk for puppets.

4. Puppets can be made from paper, cloth or even wood.

5. Puppets can be made to look like animals, people or pretend creatures.

6. Puppets can be moved with hands or fingers.

7. Mittens, gloves and paper plates can all be made into puppets.

8. Large boxes can be used for puppet stages.

Vocabulary:

1. **puppet**—a toy that is moved by the hand or finger.

2. **marionette**—a puppet with strings for movement.

3. **puppet show**—a story told with puppets.

4. **puppeteer**—a person who makes a puppet move and speak.

5. **puppet stage**—a place for puppets to act.

6. **entertainment**—things we enjoy seeing and listening to.

7. **imaginary**—something that is not real.

Bulletin Board

The purpose of this bulletin board is to show a variety of puppets. The children's expressive language skills will be stimulated by interacting with the puppets. Design the bulletin board by constructing about five or six simple puppets for the children to take off the bulletin board to play with. Include a fly swatter puppet, a paper bag puppet, hand puppet, sock puppet and a wooden spoon puppet. Hooks or push pins can be used to attach the puppets to the bulletin board.

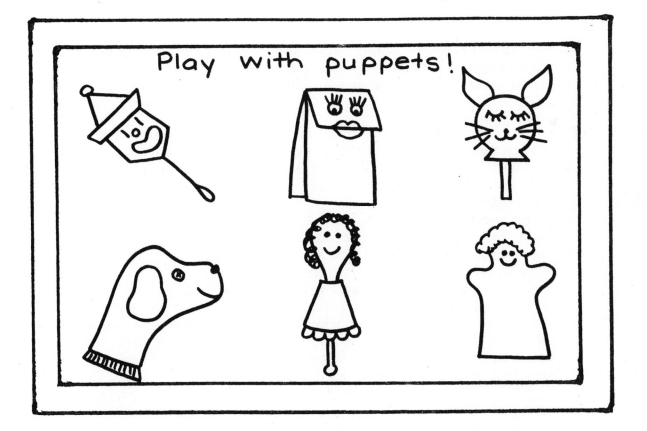

Parent Letter

Dear Parents,

We will be enjoying a unit on puppets this week. Puppets are magical and motivating to young children. Sometimes a child will respond or talk to a puppet in a situation when he might not talk to an adult or other child. Through learning experiences involving puppets, the children will become aware of the different types of puppets and materials that can be used to make puppets. They will express themselves creatively and imaginatively.

At School This Week

Some of this week's plans include:

* creating our own puppets with a variety of materials.
* using the puppet stage throughout the week, putting on puppet shows for one and all.
* exploring various types of puppets, including finger, hand, stick, shadow and marionette puppets.

At Home

The children enjoy retelling familiar stories and making up original stories for puppet characters. To stimulate this type of play, you and your child can make simple puppets at home with objects found around the house.

Paper Bag Puppets—Using small paper lunch bags, children can use crayons or markers to create a puppet. The fold in the bag can be used as the mouth. After the child's hand is in the bag, the puppet can talk. Yarn scraps can easily be glued on for hair and construction paper scraps can add a decorative touch.
Sock Puppets—I'm sure you have a couple of socks around the house that seem to have lost their mate. (Does your dryer eat socks, too?) Depending on your child's skills and how much supervision you can provide— eyes, a nose and hair of a variety of materials (yarn, buttons, fabric) can either be sewn or glued on. Insert your hand and your puppet is ready!
Stick Puppets—Make story characters' faces or bodies on heavy paper or on cardboard with crayons, markers or paint. Cut the figures out and attach them with strong glue or tape to a ruler, popsicle stick, tongue depressor or any stick that can be used to hold the puppet and move it. A large box or table can serve as the puppet stage.

Enjoy your week!

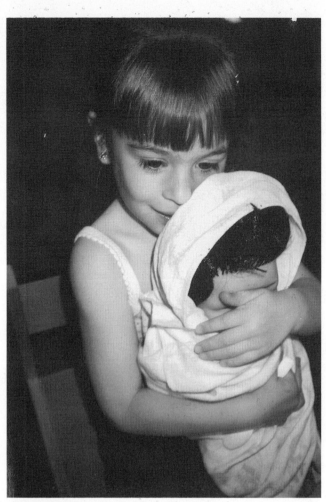

FIGURE 42 Puppets are fun to make and play with.

Music:

"Eensy Weensy Spider" (traditional)

Fingerplays:

CATERPILLAR CRAWLING

One little caterpillar crawled on my shoe.
Another came along and then there were two.
Two little caterpillars crawled on my knee.
Another came along and then there were three.
Three little caterpillars crawled on the floor.
Another came along and then there were four.
Four little caterpillars watch them crawl away.
They'll all turn into butterflies some fine day.

This fingerplay can be told using puppets made from felt or tagboard.

Source: *The Everything Book.* Valerie Indenbaum and Marcia Shapior. (Chicago: Partner Press, 1983).

SPECKLED FROGS

Five green speckled frogs
Sitting on a speckled log
Eating the most delicious bugs,
Yum, Yum!
  (rub tummy)

One jumped into the pool
Where it was nice and cool
Now there are four green speckled frogs.

Repeat until there are no green speckled frogs.

This finger play can be told using puppets made from felt or tagboard.

CHICKADEES

Five little chickadees sitting in a door
  (hold up hand)
One flew away and then there were four
  (put down one finger at a time)
Four little chickadees sitting in a tree
One flew away and then there were three.
Three little chickadees looking at you.
One flew away and then there were two.
Two little chickadees sitting in the sun.
One flew away and then there was one.
One little chickadee sitting all alone.
He flew away and then there were none.

This fingerplay can be told using puppets made from felt or tagboard.

Science:

1. **Classify Puppets**

During group time let the children classify the various puppets into special categories such as animals, people, insects, imaginary things, etc.

2. Button Box

A large box of buttons should be provided. The children can sort the buttons according to color, size or shape into a muffin tin pan or egg carton.

Dramatic Play:

1. Puppet Show

A puppet stage should be available throughout the entire unit in the dramatic play area. Change or add the puppets on a regular basis using as many different kinds of puppets as possible.

2. Puppet Shop

A variety of materials should be provided for the children to construct puppets. Include items such as buttons, bows, felt, paper bags, cloth pieces, socks, tongue depressors, etc.

Arts and Crafts:

1. Making Puppets

Puppets can be made from almost any material. Some suggestions are listed here:

* cotton covered with cloth attached to a tongue depressor.
* paper sacks stuffed with newspaper.
* a cork for a head with a hole in it for a finger.
* socks.
* cardboard colored with crayon attached to a tongue depressor.
* fly swatter.
* oatmeal box attached to a dowel.
* nylon pantyhose stretched over a hanger bent into an oval shape.
* empty toilet paper and paper towel rolls.

2. Puppet Stages

Puppet stages can be made from the following materials:

* boxes, including tempera paint and markers for decorating.
* large paper bags.
* half gallon milk carton.
* towel draped over an arm.
* towel draped over the back of a chair.
* blanket covering a card table.

Sensory:

Sensory Table

During this unit add to the sensory table all of the various materials that puppets are made of:

* string
* buttons
* felt
* toilet paper rolls
* cardboard
* paper
* sticks
* wood shavings

Large Muscle:

1. Creative Movement

Demonstrate how to manipulate a marionette. Then have the children pretend that they are marionettes and that they have strings attached to their arms and legs. Say, "Someone is pulling up the string that is attached to your arm, what would happen to your arm?" Allow the children to make that movement. Continue with other movements.

2. Large Puppets

Large puppets such as stick or rod puppets can provide the children with a lot of large muscle movement.

3. Pin the Nose on the Puppet

This game is a variation of the traditional Pin the Tail on the Donkey.

Field Trips/Resource People:

1. Puppet Show

Place puppets by the puppet stage to encourage the children to put on puppet shows.

2. Puppeteer

Invite a puppeteer to visit the classroom and show the children the many uses of puppets.

Math:

1. Examine a Puppet

With the children, examine a puppet and count all the various parts of it. Count its eyes, legs, arms, stripes on its shirt, etc. Discuss how it was constructed.

2. Puppet Dot to Dot

Draw a large puppet on a sheet of tagboard. Laminate or cover the tagboard sheet with clear adhesive paper. A grease pencil or felt-tip watercolor marker should be provided for the children to draw. Also felt scraps should be available to remove grease markers. Otherwise, a damp cloth or paper towel should be available.

Social Studies:

Occupation Puppets

Introduce various types of occupation puppets. Ask the children to describe each.

Group Time (games, language):

Puppet Show

Using your favorite classroom stories, put on a puppet show. The children can volunteer to be the various characters. Pre-tape the story so that the children can listen to it while they practice. This might be a good activity to invite parents to attend.

Cooking:

1. Puppet Faces

Make open-faced sandwiches using peanut butter or cream cheese spread onto a slice of bread or a bun. Carrot curls can be used to represent hair. Raisins and green or purple grape halves can be used for the eyes, nose and mouth.

2. Dog Puppet Salad

Place a pear half onto the plate. Two apple slices can be added to resemble a dog's ears hanging down. Then raisins or grape halves can be used to represent the eyes and nose of a dog.

Record:

The following record can be found in preschool educational catalogs:

Puppet Parade. Melody House Records. "The Little Red Hen Operetta"

Books and Stories:

The following books and stories can be used to complement the theme:

1. **Pinocchio and His Puppet Show Adventure.** Walt Disney Productions. (New York: Random House, 1973).

2. **The Adventures of Pinocchio.** Carlo Collodi. (New York: Macmillan Publishing, 1963).

3. **Marionettes on Stage.** Leonard Suib. (New York: Harper and Row, 1975).

4. **You Can Put on a Show.** Lewy Olfson. (New York: Sterling Publishing Company, 1975).

Puzzles:

The following puzzles can be found in preschool educational catalogs:

1. **"Pinocchio"** Judy/Instructo.

2. **"Puppet"** Judy/Instructo.

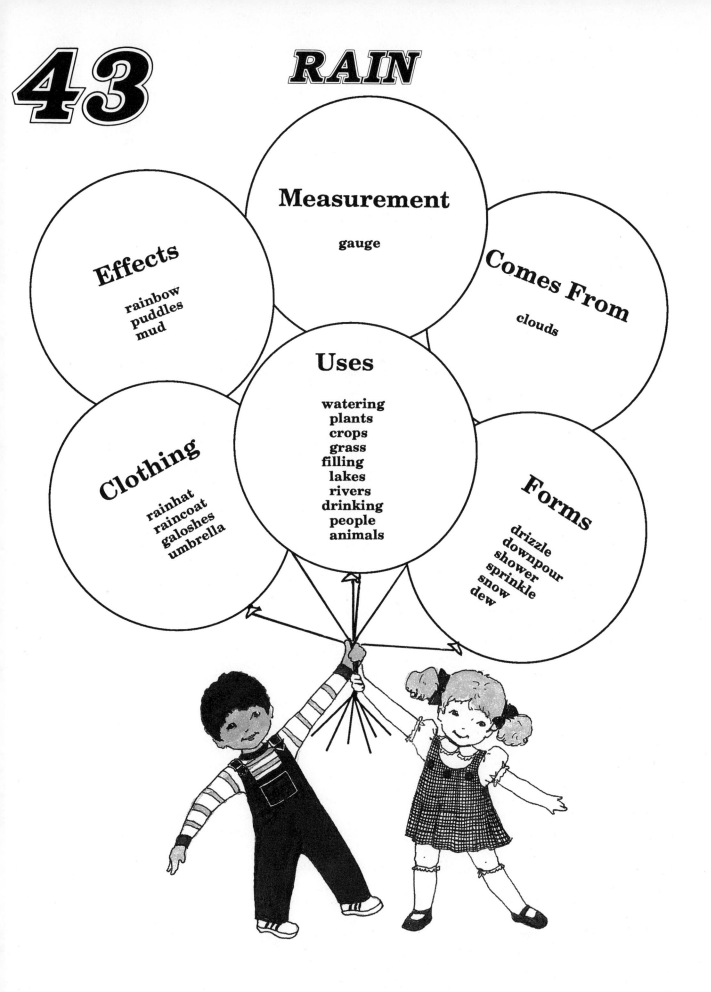

43 RAIN

Measurement
gauge

Effects
rainbow
puddles
mud

Comes From
clouds

Uses
watering
plants
crops
grass
filling
lakes
rivers
drinking
people
animals

Clothing
rainhat
raincoat
galoshes
umbrella

Forms
drizzle
downpour
shower
sprinkle
snow
dew

Theme Goals:

Through participating in the experiences provided by this theme, the children may learn:

1. Uses of rain.

2. Effects of rain.

3. Clothing worn for protection from the rain.

4. Forms of rain.

5. Origin of rain.

6. The tool used for the measurement of rain.

Concepts for the Children to Learn:

1. Rain falls as a liquid from the clouds.

2. Rain can fall in the form of drizzle, snow or a shower.

3. Rain can be used for watering lawns and filling lakes.

4. A rainbow sometimes appears when it rains while the sun is shining.

5. A rainbow is colorful.

6. An umbrella is used in the rain to keep us dry.

7. Raincoats, hats and galoshes are rain clothing.

8. Puddles can form during a rainfall.

9. The amount of rain can be measured in a water gauge.

10. Farmers need rain to water the crops.

Vocabulary:

1. **rain**—water that falls from the clouds.

2. **rainbow**—a colorful sight formed when the sun shines while it is raining.

3. **puddle**—rain collection on the ground.

4. **umbrella**—a shade for protection against rain.

5. **snow**—frozen rain.

6. **gauge**—a tool for measuring rain.

Bulletin Board

The purpose of this bulletin board is to develop an awareness of sets, as well as to identify written numerals. Construct clouds out of gray tagboard. Write a numeral on each cloud. Cut out and laminate. Next, trace and cut cloud shadows from construction paper. Attach the shadows to the bulletin board. A set of raindrops, from one to ten, should be attached underneath each cloud shadow. Magnet pieces or push pins and holes in the cloud piece can be used for the children to match each cloud to it corresponding shadow, using the raindrops as a clue.

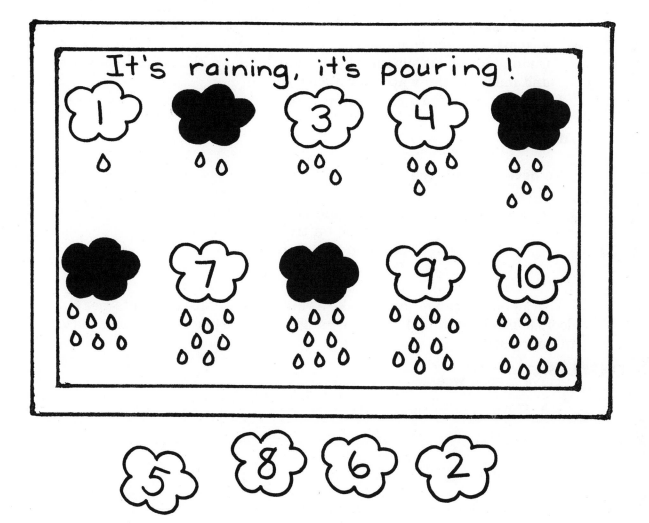

Parent Letter

Dear Parents,

"Rain, rain, go away. Come again some other day." is a familiar nursery rhyme. It is one that we may often hear this week as a unit on rain begins. Throughout the week the children will become aware of the uses and forms of rain as well as how rainbows are created.

At School This Week

The following activities are just a few that have been planned for the rain unit:

* a visit by TV 8's weatherman. Tom Hector will be coming at 2:00 pm on Tuesday to show us a video made for preschoolers that depicts various weather conditions.
* finding out about evaporation by setting out a shallow pan of water and marking the water level each day.
* creating a rainbow on a sunny day outdoors with a garden hose.

At Home

To develop language skills practice this rain poem with your child:

> Rain on the green grass
> And rain on trees.
> Rain on the rooftops,
> But not on me!!

Use an empty can or jar to make a rain gauge. Place the container outdoors to measure rainfall. Several gauges could be placed in various places in your yard.

Have a good week!

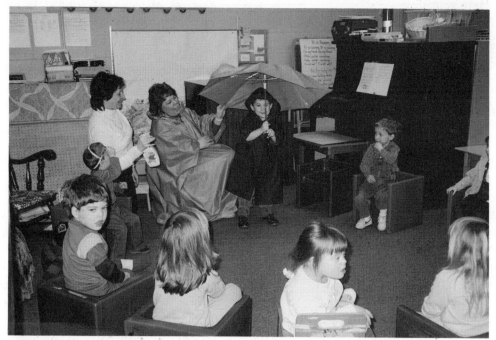

FIGURE 43 Getting ready for the rain indoors!

Music:

"Rainy"
(Sing to the tune of "Bingo")

There was a day when we got wet
and rainy was the weather
R-A-I-N-Y R-A-I-N-Y R-A-I-N-Y
and rainy was the weather.

Repeat each verse eliminating a letter and
substituting it with a clap until the last
chorus is all claps to the same beat.

Fingerplays:

LITTLE RAINDROP

This is the sun, high up in the sky.
  (hold hands in circle above head)
A dark cloud suddenly comes sailing by.
  (slide hands to side)
These are the raindrops.
  (make raining motion with fingers)
Pitter patter down.
Watering the flowers,
  (pouring motion)
Growing on the ground.
  (hands pat the ground)

RAINY DAY FUN

Slip on your rain coat.
  (pretend to put coat on)
Pull up your galoshes.
  (pull up galoshes)
Wade in puddles,
Make splishes and sploshes.
  (make stomping motions)

THUNDERSTORM

Boom, bang, boom, bang!
  (clap hands)
Rumpety, lumpety, bump!
  (stomp feet)
Zoom, zam, zoom, zam!
  (swish hands together)
Rustles and bustles
  (pat thighs)
And swishes and zings!
  (pat thighs)
What wonderful noises
A thunderstorm brings.

RAIN

From big black clouds
  (hold up arms)
The raindrop fell.
  (pull finger down in air)

Drip, drip, drip one day,
  (hit one finger on palm of hand)
Until the bright sunlight changed them
Into a rainbow gay!
  (make a rainbow with hands)

Source of first four fingerplays: *Everyday Circle Times*. Dick and Liz Wilmes.

THE RAIN

I sit before the window now
  (seat yourself, if possible)
And I look out at the rain.
  (shade your eyes and look around)
It means no play outside today
  (shake head, shrug)
So inside I remain.
  (rest chin on fist, look sorrowful)
I watch the water dribble down
  (follow up-to-down movements with eyes)
And turn the brown grass green.
  (sit up, take notice)
And after a while I start to smile
At Nature's washing machine.
  (smile, lean back, relax)

Source: *Finger Frolics—Finger Plays for Young Children*. Cromwell Hibner Faitel.

Science:

1. Tasting Water

Collect tap water, soda water, mineral water and distilled water. Pour the different types of water in into paper cups and let children taste them. Discuss the differences.

2. Evaporation

The children can pour water into a jar. Mark a line at the water level. Place the jar on a window ledge and check it everyday. The disappearance is called evaporation.

3. Catching Water

If it rains one day during your unit, place a bucket outside to catch the rain. Return the bucket to your science table. Place a bucket of tap water next to the rain water and compare.

4. Color Mixing

Using water and food coloring or tempera, mix the primary colors. Discuss the colors of the rainbow.

Dramatic Play:

1. Rainy Day Clothing

Umbrellas, rain coats, hats, galoshes and a tape containing rain sounds should be added to the dramatic play area. Use caution when selecting umbrellas for this activity. Some open quickly and can be dangerous.

2. Weather Station

A map, pointer, adult clothing and pretend microphone should be placed in the dramatic play area. The children can play weather person. Pictures depicting different weather conditions can be included.

Arts and Crafts:

1. Eyedropper Painting

Paint with eyedroppers as an application tool and water colored with food coloring.

2. Waxed Paper Rainbows

Cut wax paper in the shape of large rainbows. Then prepare red, yellow, green and blue crayon shavings. After this, the children can sprinkle the crayon shavings on one sheet of waxed paper. Place another sheet of waxed paper on the top of the sheet with sprinkled crayon. Finally, the teacher should place a linen towel over the top of the waxed paper sheets. A warm iron should be applied to meet the two pieces together. Cool and attach a string. Hang from the window.

3. Rainbow Yarn Collage

Using rainbow-shaped paper and rainbow-colored yarn, the children can make rainbow yarn collages.

4. Thunder Painting

Tape record a rain or thunderstorm. Leave this tape with a tape recorder and earphones at the easel. Grey, black and white paint can be provided. Let the children listen to the rainstorm and paint to it. Ask the children how the music makes them feel.

5. Rainbow Mobiles

Pre-cut rainbow arcs. On these, the children can paste styrofoam packing pieces. After this, they can paint the pieces. Display the mobiles in the room.

Sensory:

Add to the sensory table:

* water with scoops, cups and spoons.
* sand and water (make puddles in the sand).
* rainbow-colored sand, rice and pasta.
* rainwater

Large Muscle:

Worm Wiggle

The purpose of this game is to imitate worm motions. Show the children how to lie on their stomachs, holding their arms in at at their sides. The children should try to move forward without using their hands or elbows like a worm would wiggle.

Field Trips/Resource People:

1. Reflection

Take a walk after it rains. Enjoy the puddles, overflowing gutters and swirls of water caught by sewers. Look in the puddles. Does anyone see a reflection? Look up in the sky. Do you see any clouds, the sun or a rainbow? What colors are in a rainbow?

2. The Weather Person

Take a field trip to a television station and see what equipment a weather person uses.

Math:

Rainbow Match

Fabrics of all the colors of the rainbow can be cut into pieces. The children can sort these and group them into different colors, textures and sizes.

Group Time (games, language):

1. Creative Thinking

Read this poem to your children and then ask them, "Why didn't I get wet?" You may have to read the poem again or you may have to encourage the children to use their imagination since the answer is not in the poem.

RAIN

Rain on green grass
and rain on the tree.
Rain on the rooftop,
But not on me!

Source: *Everyday Circle Times.* Liz and Dick Wilmes. (Building Block Publications).

2. Jump In Puddles

This game is played like Musical Chairs. The puddles are made from circles on the floor with one child in each and one less circle than children so one child is out of the circles. On the signal, "Jump in the puddles," the children have to switch puddles. The child who was out has a chance to get in a puddle. The child who does not get into a puddle waits until the next round. This can be played indoors or outdoors. Hula hoops could also be used in small groups of four children using three hoops.

Miscellaneous:

1. **Cut and Tell Story: "The Rainbow's End"**

   Source: *Cut and Tell Scissor Stories for Spring*. Jean Warren. (Totline Press, Warren Publishing House. P.O. Box 2255, Everett, WA 98203).

2. **Flannelboard Stories**

   Source: *Flannel Graphs—Flannel Board fun for Little Ones*. Jean Stangl. (A division of David S. Lake Publishers, Belmont, CA).

Cooking:

Rainbow Fruits

Serve a different colored snack each day. An example would be to correspond with the colors of the rainbow.

* strawberries
* oranges
* lemon finger gelatin (see a gelatin box for recipe)
* blueberries added to yogurt
* grape juice
* grapes or blackberries
* lettuce salad

Records:

The following records can be found in preschool educational catalogs:

1. **Color Me a Rainbow.** Melody House Records.

2. **Follow the Clouds.** Melody House Records.

3. **Raindrops.** Melody House Records.

4. **Adventures in Sound.** Melody House Records.

Books and Stories:

The following books and stories can be used to complement the theme:

1. **How to Make a Cloud.** Jeanne Bendick. (New York: Parent's Magazine Press, 1971).

2. **It's Raining Said John Twining.** N.M. Bodecker. (New York: Atheneum, 1973).

3. **Storms.** Ray Broekel. (Chicago: Childrens Press, 1982).

4. **Thunderstorm.** Mary Szilagyi. (New York: Bradbury, 1985).

5. **Run to the Rainbow.** Margaret Hillert. (Chicago: Follett Publishing Company, 1981).

6. **Clouds.** Roy Wandelmaier. (Mahwah, NJ: Troll Associates, 1985).

7. **The Cloud Book.** Tomie dePaola. (New York: Holiday House, 1975).

8. **Weather.** Robert and Imelda Updegraff. (New York: Penguin Books, 1982).

9. From Ice to Rain. Marlene Reidel. (Minneapolis, MN: Carolrhoda, 1981).

Puzzles:

The following puzzles can be found in preschool educational catalogs:

1. "Rainbow" Lauri.

2. "Rain" 4 pieces. Judy/Instructo.

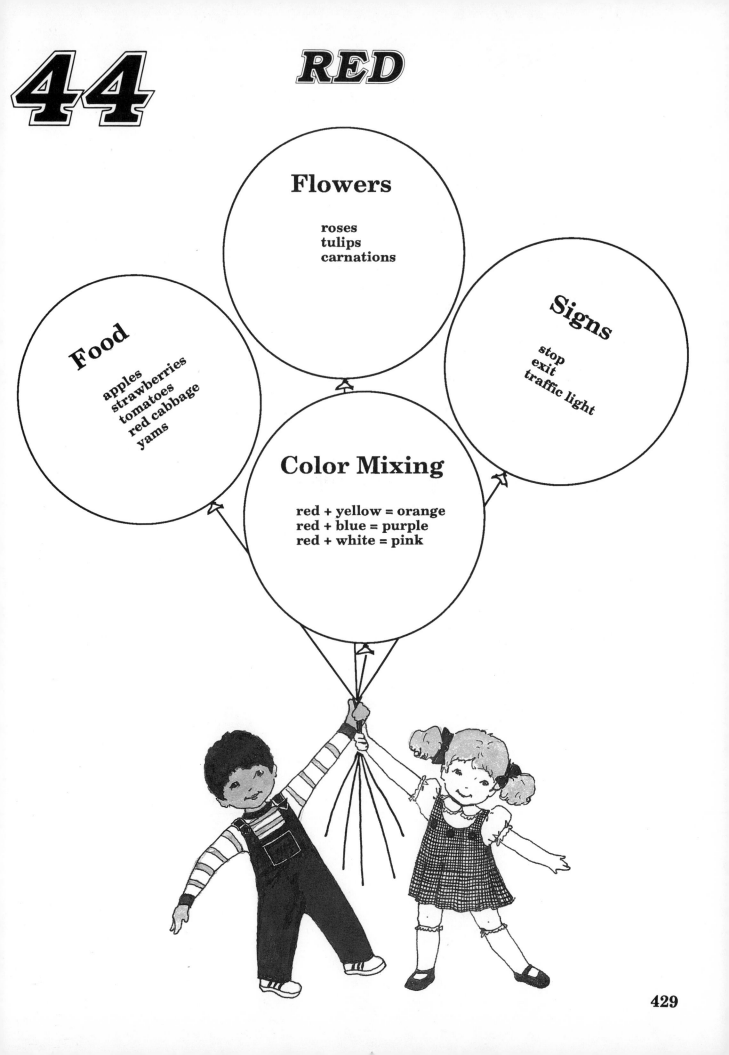

Flowers

roses
tulips
carnations

Signs

stop
exit
traffic light

Food

apples
strawberries
tomatoes
red cabbage
yams

Color Mixing

red + yellow = orange
red + blue = purple
red + white = pink

Theme Goals:

Through participating in the experiences provided by this theme, the children may learn:

1. Red is a color.

2. Some foods are red.

3. Many objects are red.

4. Red can be mixed with other colors to make different colors.

Concepts for the Children to Learn:

1. Red is a primary color.

2. Some foods, such as tomatoes and strawberries, are 'red.

3. Red and yellow mixed together make orange.

4. Red and blue mixed together make purple.

5. Red and white mixed together make pink.

6. Some fire trucks and fire hydrants are red.

7. A stop sign is colored red.

8. Some roses, tulips and carnations are red.

Vocabulary:

1. **red**—a primary color.

2. **primary colors**—red, yellow and blue.

Bulletin Board

The purpose of this bulletin board is to reinforce the mathematical skills of matching sets of objects to a written numeral. Green produce baskets or other small baskets can be hung on the bulletin board for a strawberry counting bulletin board. Attach baskets to the bulletin boards using staples or push pins. Collect small plastic strawberries, or make strawberries out of tagboard. On each basket mark a numeral. The children can place the appropriate number of strawberries into each basket.

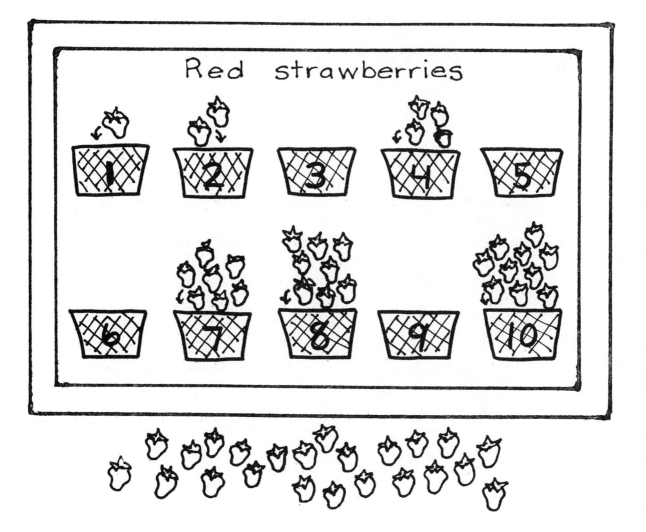

Parent Letter

Dear Parents,

Colors are everywhere and they make our world beautiful. That's why this week we'll be focusing on a specific color—red! It's a popular color with young children and many objects in our world are red. The experiences provided this week will also help the children become aware of colors that are formed when mixed with red.

At School This Week

A few of this week's experiences include:

* mixing the color red with yellow and blue to make orange and purple.
* setting up an art store in the dramatic play area where the children can act out the buying and selling of art supplies.
* exploring red colored crayons, markers, pencils, chalk, paint, and paper.
* filling the sensory table with red goop.

At Home

To reinforce the concepts in this unit, try the following activities at home with your child:

* To develop observation skills look around your house with your child for red items. How many red objects can you find in each room?
* Prepare red foods for meals such as apples, strawberries, tomatoes and jam.
* Prepare red ice cubes to cool your drinks. To do this, just add a few drops of red food coloring to the water before freezing it.

Have a colorful week!

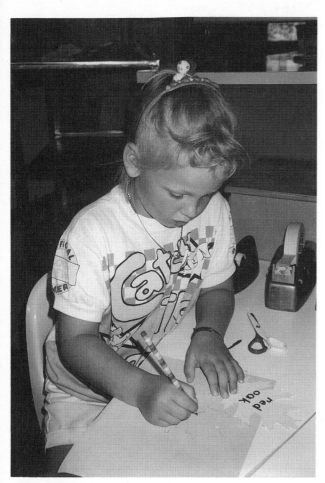

FIGURE 44 Red is a color that can be found on oak leaves.

Fingerplays:

TULIPS

Five little tulips–red and gay
  (hold up hand)
Let us water them every day.
  (make sprinkle motion with other hand)
Watch them open in the bright sunlight.
  (cup hand, then open)
Watch them close when it is night.
  (close hand again).

MY APPLE

Look at my apple, it's red and round.
  (make ball shape with hands)
It fell from a tree down to the ground
  (make downward motion)
Come let me share my apple, please do!
  (beckoning motion)
My mother can cut it right in two—

(make slicing motion)
One half for me and one half for you
  (hold out 2 hands, sharing halves)

FIVE RED APPLES

Five red apples in a grocery store.
  (hold up five fingers)
Bobby bought one, and then there were four
  (bend down one finger)
Four red apples on an apple tree.
Susie ate one, and then there were three.
  (bend down one finger)
Three red apples. What did Alice do?
Why, she ate one, and then there were two.
  (bend down one finger)
Two red apples ripening in the sun;
Timmy ate one, and then there was one
  (bend down one finger)
One red apple and now we are done;
I ate the last one, and now there are none.
  (bend down last finger)

Science:

Mixing Colors

Place 2 or 3 ice cube trays and cups filled with red, yellow and blue colored water on the science table. Using an eyedropper, the children can experiment mixing colors in the ice cube trays. Smocks should be provided to prevent stained clothing.

Dramatic Play:

1. **Art Store**

Set up an art supplies store. Include paints, crayons, markers, paper, chalk, brushes, money and cash register.

2. **Fire Station**

Firefighter's hats can be added to the dramatic play area.

3. **Colored Hats**

After reading *Caps for Sale* by Esphyr Slobodykina, set out colored hats for children to retell the story.

Arts and Crafts:

1. Red Paint

Red and white paint can be provided at the easels. By mixing these colors, children can discover shades of red.

2. Red Crayons, Markers, etc.

Red markers, crayons and chalk can be placed on a table in the art area. The children can observe the similarities and differences of these various items.

3. Red Paper

Watercolors and red paper can be placed on a table in the art area.

4. Red Crayon Rubbings

Red crayons, red paper or both can be used to do this activity. Place an object such as a penny, button or leaf under paper. Use the flat edge of a crayon to color over the item. An image of the object will appear on the paper.

5. Paint Blots

Fold a piece of paper in half. Open up and place a spoon of red paint on the inside of the paper. Refold paper and press flat. Reopen and observe the design. Add two colors such as blue and yellow and repeat process to show color mixing.

6. Paint Over Design

Paint over a crayon picture with watery red paint. Observe how the paint will not cover it.

7. Glitter Pictures

The children make a design using glue on a piece of paper. Then shake red glitter onto glue. Shake the excess glitter into a pan.

8. Red Fingerpaint

Red fingerpaint and foil should be placed on an art table. Yellow and blue paint can be added to explore color mixing.

Sensory:

1. Red Water

Fill the sensory table with water and red food coloring. The children can add coloring and observe the changes.

2. Red Shaving Cream

Shaving cream with red food coloring added can be placed in the sensory table. During self-selected play the children can explore the shaving cream.

3. Red Goop

Mix together red food coloring, 1 cup cornstarch and 1 cup water in sensory table.

4. Red Silly Putty

Mix together red food coloring, 1 cup liquid starch, and 2 cups white glue. This mixture usually needs to be continuously stirred for an extended period of time before it jells.

Large Muscle:

1. Ribbon Dance

Attach strips of red crepe paper to short wooden dowels or unsharpened pencils to make ribbons. The children can use the ribbons to move to their favorite songs.

2. Red Bird, Red Bird

The children should form a circle by holding hands. Then choose a child to be a bud and start the game. Children chant:

Red bird, red bird through my window
Red bird, red bird through my window
Red bird, red bird through my window
Oh!

The bird goes in and out, under the children's arms. The bird stops on the word "Oh" and bows to the child facing him. This child becomes the new bird. The color of the bird can be determined by the color of the clothing of each child picked to be the bird.

Field Trips/Resource People:

1. Art Store

Visit an art store. Observe all the red items for sale.

2. Take a Walk

Take a walk around the neighborhood and look for red objects.

3. Floral Shop

Visit a floral shop and specifically observe red flowers.

4. Fire Station

Visit a fire station. Note the color of the engine, hats, sirens, etc.

5. Resource People

Invite the following resource people to the classroom:

* artist
* gardener
* firefighter

Math:

1. Color Cards

Construct color cards that start with white and gradually become cherry red. The children can sequence the cards from white to red or red to white. Discontinued sample color cards could be obtained from a paint store.

2. Bead Stringing

Yarn and a variety of colored beads should be available to the children. After initial exploration, the children can make patterns with beads. Example: red, yellow, red, yellow, red.

3. Colored Bags

Place three bags labeled red, yellow, blue and a variety of blocks on a table. The children can sort the blocks by placing them in the matching colored bag.

Social Studies:

1. Discussion about Colors

During group time discuss colors and how they make us feel. Hold up a color card and ask a child how it makes him feel.

2. Color Chart

Construct a "My Favorite Color Is..." chart. Encourage each child to name their favorite color. After each child's name, print his favorite color with a colored marker. Display the chart in the classroom.

3. Colored Balloons

Each child should be provided with a balloon. The balloons should be the colors of the rainbow: red, orange, yellow, green, blue and purple. Arrange the children in the formation of a rainbow. Children with red balloons should stand together, etc. Take a picture of the class. Place the picture on the bulletin board.

Group Time (games, language):

1. Colored Jars

Collect five large jars. Fill 3 with red water, 1 with yellow water and 1 with blue water. Show children the 3 red jars. Discuss the color red. Discuss that it can make other colors too. Show them the yellow jar. Add yellow to red. What happens? Add blue water to other red jar. What happens? Discuss color mixing.

2. Play Red Light, Green Light

Pick one child to be your traffic light. Place the "traffic light" about 30 feet away from the other children facing away from chldren who have formed a long line. With back to children, the traffic light says "green light." Children try to creep towards the traffic light. Traffic light may then say "red light" and turn towards the children. Children must freeze. The traffic light tries to see if any children are still at the starting line. The game continues with "green light." The first child to reach the traffic light becomes the new light.

Cooking:

1. Raspberry Shrub

Thaw and cook 4 packages of 10-ounce frozen raspberries for 10 minutes. Rub the cooked raspberries through strainer with wooden spoon. Cool. Add 1 can (6 ounces) of frozen lemonade concentrate, thawed. Just before serving, stir in 2 quarts of ginger ale, chilled. Makes 24 servings, about 1/2 cup each.

2. Red Pepper Paste—West Africa

1/4 cup dry red wine
1 teaspoon ground red pepper
3/4 teaspoon salt
1/4 teaspoon ground ginger
1/8 teaspoon ground cardamon
1/8 teaspoon ground coriander
1/8 teaspoon ground nutmeg
1/8 teaspoon cloves
1/8 teaspoon ground cinnamon
1/8 teaspoon black pepper
1/8 of a medium onion
1 small clove garlic
1/4 cup paprika

Place all ingredients except paprika in blender container. Cover and blend on high speed until smooth, scraping the sides of the blender frequently. Heat paprika in 1 quart saucepan for 1 minute. Add spice mixture gradually, stirring until smooth. Heat, stirring occasionally, until hot, about 3 minutes. Cool.

3. Pink Dip

Mix 2/3 cup mayonnaise or salad dressing, 2 tablespoons Red Pepper Paste and 1 tablespoon lemon juice. Serve with celery sticks.

Source: *Betty Crocker's International Cookbook*. (New York: Random House, 1980).

Records:

The following records can be found in preschool educational catalogs:

1. **Learning Basic Skills Through Music. Volume 1.** Hap Palmer.

2. **Learning Basic Skills Through Music. Volume 2.** Hap Palmer.

3. **I Know the Colors in the Rainbow.** Ella Jenkins.

Books and Stories:

The following books and stories can be used to complement the theme:

1. **My Red Umbrella.** Robert Bright. (New York: William Morrow, 1959).

2. **Red is for Apple.** Beth G. Hoffman. (New York: Random House, 1966).

3. **Caps for Sale.** Esphyr Slobodo. (Reading, MA: Addison-Wesley, 1947).

4. **Is It Red? Is It Yellow? Is It Blue?** Tana Hoban. (New York: William Morrow and Company, Inc., 1978).

5. **My Slippers are Red.** Charlotte Steiner. (New York: Alfred A. Knopf, 1957).

6. **The Red Woolen Blanket.** Bob Graham. (Boston: Little, Brown & Co., 1987).

7. **Hiram's Red Shirt.** Mable Watts. (New York: Golden Press, 1981).

8. **The Red Jacket Mix-Up.** Ari Hill. (New York: Golden Press, 1986).

9. **I Dance in My Red Pajamas.** Edith Thacher Hurd. (New York: Harper and Row, 1982).

Puzzles:

The following puzzles can be found in preschool educational catalogs.

1. **"Lobster"** 9 pieces. Childcraft.

2. **"Great Big Fire Engine"** 18 pieces. Judy/Instructo.

3. **"Two Apples"** 2 pieces. Childcraft.

4. **"Apple Tree"** 3 pieces. Childcraft.

5. **"Traffic Safety Puzzles"** 5 pieces. Judy/Instructo.

6. **"Ladybug"** 5 pieces. Judy/Instructo.

SAFETY

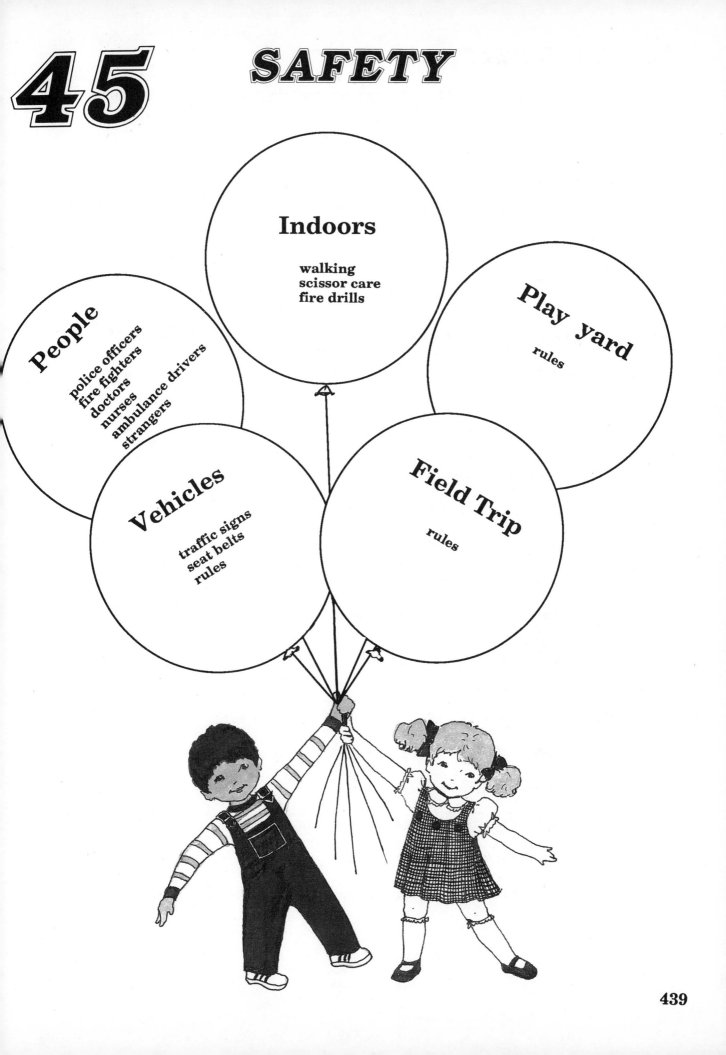

Indoors

walking
scissor care
fire drills

Play yard

rules

People

police officers
fire fighters
doctors
nurses
ambulance drivers
strangers

Vehicles

traffic signs
seat belts
rules

Field Trip

rules

Theme Goals:

Through participating in the experiences provided by this theme, the children may learn:

1. Indoor safety precautions.

2. Play yard safety.

3. People who keep us safe.

4. Field trip safety.

5. Vehicle safety.

Concepts for the Children to Learn:

1. We walk indoors.

2. Play yard rules help keep us safe.

3. We have special rules for field trips.

4. Fire drills prepare us for emergencies.

5. Scissors need to be handled carefully.

6. Wearing a seat belt is practicing car safety.

7. Traffic signs help prevent accidents.

8. Police officers, firefighters, doctors, nurses, and ambulance drivers help keep us safe.

9. Only talk to people you know.

Vocabulary:

1. **safety**—freedom from danger.

2. **sign**—a lettered board.

3. **seatbelt**—strap that holds a person in a vehicle.

4. **rule**—the way we are to act.

5. **fire drill**—practicing leaving the building in case of a fire.

Bulletin Board

The purpose of this bulletin board is to call attention to safety signs. The children are to match the safety sign with its outline on the board. To prepare this bulletin board, construct six safety signs out of tagboard, each a different shape. Color appropriately and laminate. Trace the outline of these signs onto black construction paper to create shadow signs as illustrated. Staple the shadow signs to the bulletin board. Punch holes in the safety signs using a hole punch. The children can match the shape of the safety signs to the shadow signs by hanging them on the appropriate push pins.

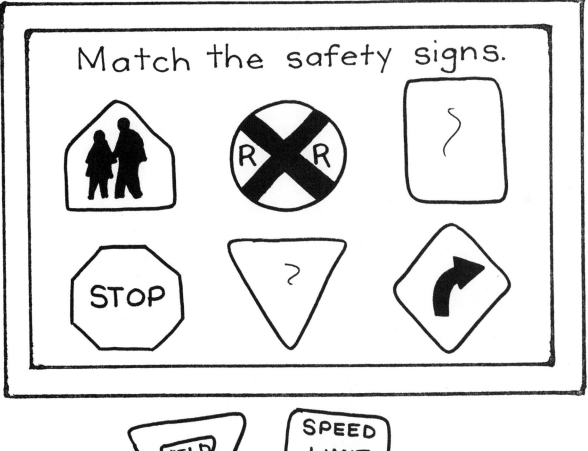

Parent Letter

Dear Parents,

This week at school we will be starting a unit on safety. We will be learning about safety at school, at home and outdoors. Through this unit the children will also become more aware of traffic signs and their importance.

At School This Week

A few of the activities planned for the week include:

* taking a safety walk to practice crossing streets.
* counting the number of traffic signs that are in our school neighborhood.
* visiting the fire station on Tuesday morning. We will be leaving at 9:30 and should return to school by 11:00.

At Home

One of the songs we will be learning follows. It will help your child become aware of the purpose and colors of a traffic light. You may enjoy singing the song at home with your child. The song is sung to the tune of "Twinkle, Twinkle, Little Star." The words are as follows:

> Twinkle, twinkle, traffic light,
> Standing on the corner bright.
> When it's green it's time to go.
> When it's red it's stop, you know.
> Twinkle, twinkle, traffic light,
> Standing on the corner bright.

Have a safe week!

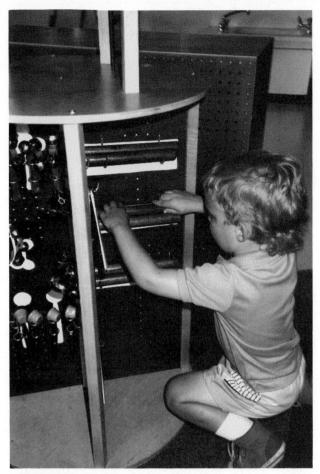

FIGURE 45 It's important to keep safety in mind while putting toys away.

Music:

1. **"Twinkle, Twinkle, Traffic Light"**
(Sing to the tune of "Twinkle, Twinkle, Little Star")

Twinkle, twinkle, traffic light,
Standing on the corner bright.
When it's green it's time to go.
When its red it's stop, you know.
Twinkle, twinkle, traffic light,
Standing on the corner bright.

2. **"Do You Know the Police Officer"**
(Sing to the tune of "The Muffin Man")

Oh, do you know the police officer,
The police officer, the police officer?
Oh, do you know the police officer
Who helps me cross the street?

This song can be extended. For example,
the song can be continued substituting

"who helps me when I'm lost" or "who
helps one cross the street."

3. **"We Are Safe"**
(Sing to the tune of "Mulberry Bush")

This is the way that we are safe
We are safe, we are safe.
This is the way that we are safe
Every day of the year.

This is the way we cross the street—
Look left, then right, left then right.
This is the way we cross the street—
Look left, then right for safety.

This is the way we ride in the car—
Sit up straight, buckle your belt.
This is the way we ride in the car—
Buckle your belt for safety.

Resource: *Everyday Circle Time.* Liz and
Dick Wilmes. (Illinois: Building Blocks
Publication, 1983).

Fingerplays:

SILLY TEDDY BEAR

Silly little teddy bear
Stood up in a rocking chair.
  (make rocking movement)
Now he has to stay in bed
  (lay head on hands)
With a bandage round his head.
  (circular movement of hand around head)

CROSSING STREETS

At the curb before I cross
I stop my running feet
  (point to feet)
And look both ways to left and right
  (look left & right)
Before I cross the street.
Lest autos running quietly
Might come as a surprise.
I just don't listen with my ears
  (point to ears)
But look with both my eyes.
  (point to eyes)

443

RED LIGHT

Red light, red light what do you say?
I say, "Stop and stop right away!"
  (hold palm of hand up)
Yellow light, yellow light what do you say?
I say, "Wait till the light turns green."
Green light, green light what do you say?
I say "Go, but look each way."
Thank you, thank you, red, yellow, green
Now I know what the traffic light means.

FIVE POLICE OFFICERS

Five strong police officers standing by a store.
One became a traffic cop, then there were four.
Four strong police officers watching over me.
One took a lost boy home, then there were three.
Three strong police officers all dressed in blue.
One stopped a speeding car and then there were two.
Two strong police officers, how fast they can run.
One caught a bad man and then there was one.
One strong police officer saw some smoke one day.
He called the firefighter who put it out right away.

THE CROSSING GUARD

The crossing guard keeps us safe
As he works from day to day.
He holds the stop sign high in the air,
For the traffic to obey.
And when the cars have completely stopped
And its as safe as can be,
He signals us to walk across
The street very carefully.

Science:

1. Sorting for Safety

Collect empty household product containers. Include safe and dangerous items such as cleaning supplies, orange juice containers, etc. Place all the items in one large box. The children can separate the containers into "safe" and "dangerous" categories. Younger children may be able to separate the containers into edible and non-edible categories.

2. All About Me

On a table place identification items. Prepare a separate card for each child. Record the following information on the cards:

* height
* weight
* color hair
* color eyes
* fingerprint
* signature (if child can or a teacher can help)

Dramatic Play:

1. Fire Engine

A large cardboard box can be decorated by the children as a fire engine with yellow or red tempera paint. When the fire engine is dry, place it in the dramatic play area with short hoses and firefighter hats. This prop could also be placed outdoors, weather permitting.

2. Prop Boxes

Develop prop boxes such as:

Firefighter
bell
jacket/uniform
boots
whistle
hose
oxygen mask
hats

Police Officer
hat
badges
handcuffs
stop sign (for holding)

3. Firefighter Jackets

Construct firefighter jackets out of large paper bags. Begin by cutting three holes. One half is used for the child's head at the top of the bag. Then cut two large holes for arms. These props may encourage the children to dramatize the roles of the firefighters.

4. Seat Belts

Collect child-sized car seats. Place them around like chairs, letting the children adjust them for themselves or their dolls.

Arts and Crafts:

1. Firefighter Hats

Cut firefighter hats out of large sheets of red construction paper for the children to wear.

2. Easel Painting

On the easel, place cut out shapes of fire hats or boots.

3. Traffic Lights

Construct stop and go lights out of shoeboxes. Tape the lid to the bottom of the box. Cover with black construction paper and have children place green, yellow and red circles in correct order on the box. The red circle should be placed on the top, yellow in the middle and green on the bottom.

4. Officer Hats and Badges

Police officer hats and badges can be constructed out of paper and colored with crayons or felt-tip watercolor markers.

Sensory:

1. Pumps and Hoses

Water pumps, hoses and water can be placed in the sensory table.

2. Trucks

Small toy fire trucks and police cars can be placed in the sensory table with sand.

Large Muscle:

1. Safety Walk

Take a safety walk. Practice observing traffic lights when crossing the street. Point out special hazards to the children.

2. Stop, Drop and Roll

Practice Stop, Drop, and Roll with the children. This will be valuable to them if they are ever involved in a fire and their clothes happen to catch on fire. Usually a firefighter will teach them this technique while visiting the fire station.

Field Trips/Resource People:

1. Firefighter

Invite a firefighter to the classroom. Ask him to bring firefighter clothing and equipment and to discuss each item.

2. Police Car

Invite a police officer to visit the classroom. Ask him to bring a police car to show the children.

Math:

1. Sequencing Hats

Draw pictures of three police hats. Make each picture identical except design three different sizes. The children can sequence the objects from largest to smallest or smallest to largest. Discuss the sizes and ask which is largest? smallest? middle?

2. Safety Items

Walk around the school and observe the number of safety items. Included may be exit signs, fire drill posters, fire extinguishers, sprinkler systems, fire alarm/drill bells, etc.

Social Studies:

1. Safety Pictures and Signs

Post safety pictures and signs around the room.

2. Stop and Go Light

Draw a large stop and go light on a piece of tagboard. Color with felt-tip markers. Print the following across from the corresponding colors:

Green means go we all know
Yellow means wait even if you're late,
Red means stop!

3. Safety Signs

Take a walk and watch for safety signs. Discuss the colors and letters on each sign.

Group Time (games, language):

Toy Safety

Collect a variety of unsafe toys that may have sharp edged block, broken wagon, etc. During group time discuss the dangers of each toy.

Cooking:

1. Banana Rounds

4 medium bananas
1/2 tablespoon honey
1/8 teaspoon nutmeg
1/8 teaspoon cinnamon
1/4 cup wheat germ

The children can peel the bananas and then slice them with a plastic knife. Measure the spices, wheat germ and honey. Finally, mix them with the bananas. Chill. Serves 8.

2. Stop Signs

eight-sided crackers
peanut butter
jelly

Spread a thin layer of peanut butter and jelly on each cracker.

3. Yield Signs

triangle crackers
yellow cheese

Cut yellow cheese into triangles. Put the cheese on the crackers.

Records:

The following records are available through preschool educational catalogs:

1. **Learning Basic Skills Through Music, Health and Safety.** (Freeport, New York: Activity Records Inc).

2. **Look At My World Record.** "Fire Station." Kathy Lencinski Poelker.

Books and Stories:

The following books and stories can be used to complement the theme:

1. **Watch Out.** Harold Longman. (New York: Parents Press Magazine, 1968).

2. **Let's Find Out About Safety.** Martha and Charles Shapp. (New York: Franklin Watts, Inc., 1975).

3. **Try It Again Sam.** Judith Viorst. (New York: Lothrop, Lee and Shepard Company, 1970).

4. **I Read Signs.** Tana Hokan. (New York: Greenwillow Books, 1983).

5. **The Fire Cat.** Esther Averill. (New York: Harper & Row Publishers, 1966).

6. **You Can Say "No!"** Rick Chacon. (Huntington Beach, CA: Teacher Created Materials, Inc., 1985).

7. **Safety Can Be Fun.** Munro Leaf. (Philadelphia: J. B. Lippencott, 1961).

8. **Curious George Goes To The Hospital.** Margaret and H. A. Rey. (Boston: Houghton Mifflin Company 1976).

9. **Mr. Clumbsy.** Roger Hargreaves. (Los Angeles: Publishers Company, 1978).

10. **The Fireman.** Rich Gibson. (New York: Feminist Press, 1972).

11. **About Our Friendly Helpers.** Hefflefinger and Hoffman. (Chicago: Melmont Publishers).

12. **The Yellow Balloon.** Edward Fenton. (New York: Doubleday and Company, 1967).

13. **Strangers.** Dorothy Chlad. (Chicago: Childrens Press, 1982).

14. **When There is a Fire ... Go Outside.** Dorothy Chlad. (Chicago: Childrens Press, 1982).

15. **When I Cross the Street.** Dorothy Chlad. (Chicago: Childrens Press, 1982).

16. **When I Ride in a Car.** Dorothy Chlad. (Chicago: Childrens Press, 1983).

17. **Playing on the Playground.** Dorothy Chlad. (Chicago: Childrens Press, 1987).

Puzzles:

The following puzzles can be found in preschool educational catalogs:

1. **"Safety Puzzle"** 5 pieces. Judy/Instructo.

2. **"Police Officer Puzzle"** 16 pieces. Judy/Instructo.

3. **"Firefighter Puzzle"** 11 pieces. Judy/Instructo.

4. **"Traffic Light"** 6 pieces. Puzzle People.

46 SCISSORS

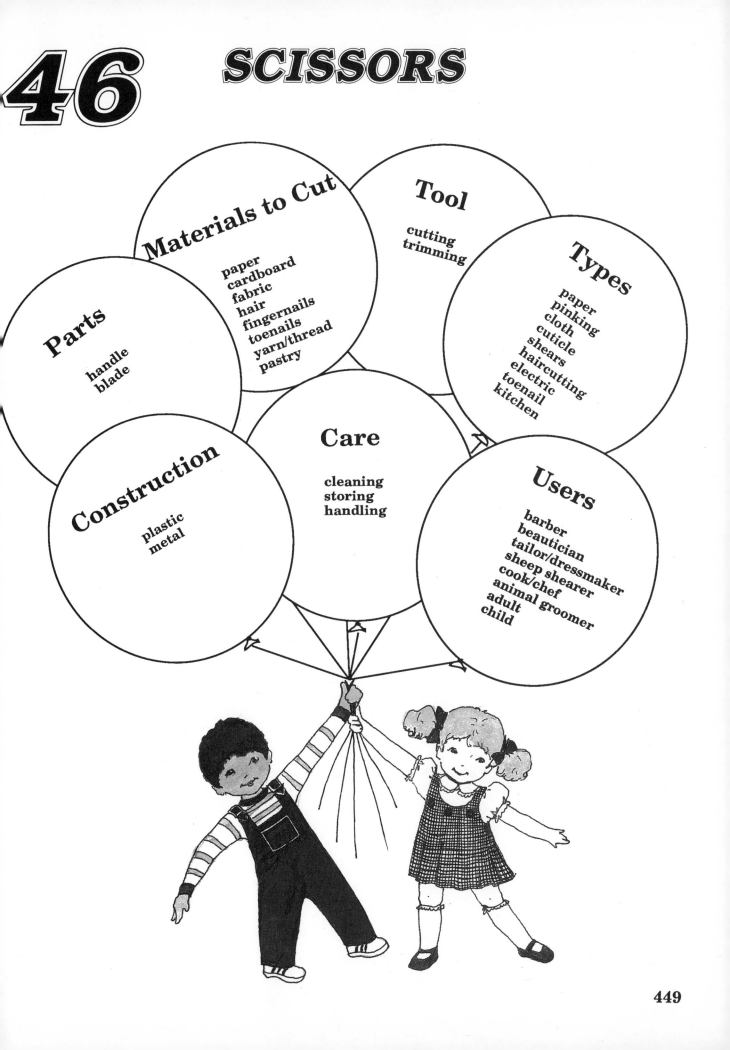

Materials to Cut

paper
cardboard
fabric
hair
fingernails
toenails
yarn/thread
pastry

Tool

cutting
trimming

Types

paper
pinking
cloth
cuticle
shears
haircutting
electric
toenail
kitchen

Parts

handle
blade

Construction

plastic
metal

Care

cleaning
storing
handling

Users

barber
beautician
tailor/dressmaker
sheep shearer
cook/chef
animal groomer
adult
child

Theme Goals:

Through participating in the experiences provided by this theme, the children may learn:

1. Parts of scissors.

2. Uses of scissors.

3. Materials that can be cut with scissors.

4. Care of scissors.

5. People who use scissors.

6. Sizes and shapes of scissors.

Concepts for the Children to Learn:

1. Scissors are tools.

2. Scissors help us do our work.

3. Scissors cut paper, fingernails, hair and material.

4. There are many types of scissors.

5. Some people need scissors for their job.

6. Hand motions make scissors cut.

7. Scissors need to be handled carefully.

Vocabulary:

1. **blade**—cutting edge of scissors.

2. **pinking shears**—sewing scissors.

3. **shears**—large scissors.

Bulletin Board

The purpose of this bulletin board is to have the children match the colored scissors to the corresponding colored skein. To prepare the bulletin board, construct six scissors out of tagboard. With felt-tip markers, color each one a different color, and laminate. Fasten the scissors to the top of the bulletin board. Next, construct six skeins of yarn out of tagboard. Color each skein a different color to correspond with the scissors. Attach the skeins to the bottom part of the bulletin board. Fasten a string to each of the scissors and a push pin to each of the skeins of yarn.

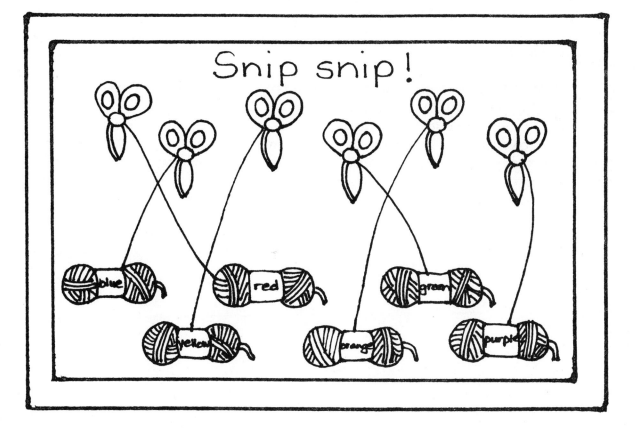

Parent Letter

Dear Parents,

Snip, snip, snip! This sound will be frequently heard in the classroom during the week as we start a unit on scissors. Through the experiences provided the children will be introduced to various kinds and uses of scissors. They will also learn the proper care and safety precautions to consider when handling and using scissors.

At School This Week

Some activities related to scissors this week include:

* discussing safety and proper uses of scissors.
* experimenting cutting with different kinds of scissors.
* cutting a variety of materials such as yarn, fabric, paper, wallpaper and aluminum foil.
* visiting Tom's Barber Shop on Wednesday morning. We will be leaving at 10:00 am and expect to watch a haircut demonstration. Also, we will observe the tools and equipment used by a barber.

At Home

Children need many experiences working with scissors before they are able to master cutting skills. Each child will learn this skill at his own rate. To assist your child, save scraps of paper and allow your child to practice cutting with them using child-sized scissors. Once the cutting skills have been mastered, your child may enjoy cutting coupons out of newspaper sections or magazines.

Have a good week!

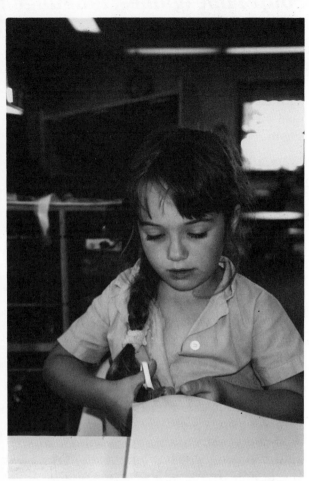

FIGURE 46 Scissors have many different uses, such as cutting paper.

Fingerplay:

OPEN SHUT THEM

Open shut them, open shut them.
   (use index and middle finger to make
   scissors motion)
Give a little snip, snip, snip.
   (three quick snips with fingers)
Open shut them, open shut them.
   (repeat scissors motion)
Make another clip.
   (make another scissor motion)

Science:

1. Scissor Show

Place a variety of scissors on an overhead projector. Encourage the children to describe each by naming and explaining its use.

2. Shadow Profiles

Tape a piece of paper on a wall or bulletin board. Stand a child in front of the paper. Shine a light source to create a shadow of the head. Trace each child's shadow. Provide scissors for the children to cut out their own shadows.

3. Weighing Scissors

On the science table, place a variety of scissors and a scale. The children should be encouraged to note the differences in weight.

Dramatic Play:

1. Beauty Shop

Set up a beauty shop in the dramatic play area. Include items such as curling irons, hairdryers, combs, brushes and wigs. Also include a chair, plastic covering, and Beauty Shop sign. A cash register and money can be added to encourage play.

2. Tailor/Dressmaking Shop

Materials that are easy to cut should be provided. Likewise, a variety of scissors should be placed next to the material. Older children may want to make doll clothes.

3. Bake Shop

Playdough, scissors, and other cooking tools can be placed on a table. If desired, make paper baker hats and a sign.

4. Dog Groomer

A dog grooming area can be set up in the dramatic play corner with stuffed animals, brushes and combs. If available, cut off the cord of an electric dog shaver and provide for the children.

Arts and Crafts:

1. Scissor Snip

Strips of paper with scissors can be provided for snipping.

2. Cutting

For experimentation, a wide variety of materials and types of scissors can be added to the art area for the children.

Sensory:

Playdough

Scissors can be placed next to the playdough in the sensory area.

Field Trips/Resource People:

1. Hair Stylist

Visit a hair stylist. While there, observe a person's hair being cut. Notice the different scissors that are used and how they are used.

2. Pet Groomer

Invite a pet groomer to class. If possible, arrange for a dog to be groomed.

Math:

Shape Sort

Cut out different colored shapes. Place the shapes on a table for the children to sort by color, shape and size.

Group Time (games, language):

Scissor Safety

Discuss safety while using scissors. The children can help make a list of "How we use our scissors safely." Display chart in room.

Cooking:

Pretzels

1 1/2 cups warm water
1 envelope yeast
4 cups flour
1 teaspoon salt
1 tablespoon sugar
coarse salt
egg

Mix the warm water, yeast and sugar together. Set this mixture aside for 5 minutes. Pour salt and flour into a bowl. Add the yeast mixture to make dough. Roll the dough into a long snake form. Cut the dough into smaller sections using scissors. The children can then form individual shapes with dough. Brush egg on the shapes with pastry brush and sprinkle with salt. Preheat the oven and bake pretzels at 425 degrees for 12 minutes.

PASTES

Bookmaker's Paste

1 teaspoon flour
2 teaspoons cornstarch
1/4 teaspoon powdered
    alum
3 ounces water

Mix dry ingredients. Add water slowly, stirring out all lumps. Cook over slow fire (preferably in a double boiler), stirring constantly. Remove when paste begins to thicken. It will thicken more as it cools. Keep in covered jars. Thin with water if necessary.

Cooked Flour Paste

1 cup boiling water
1 tablespoon powdered
    alum
1 pint cold water
1 pint flour
1 heaping teaspoon oil of
    cloves
oil of wintergreen
    (optional)

To 1 cup boiling water add powdered alum. Mix flour and fold in

---

water until smooth; pour mixture gradually into boiling alum water. Cook until it has a bluish cast, stirring all the time. Remove from fire, add oil of cloves and stir well. Keep in air-tight jars. Thin when necessary by adding water. A drop or two of oil of wintergreen may be added to give the paste a pleasing aroma.

Colored Salt Paste

Mix 2 parts salt to 1 part flour. Add powdered paint and enough water to make a smooth heavy paste. Keep in air-tight container.

Crepe Paper Paste

Cut or tear 2 tablespoons crepe paper of a single color. The finer the paper is cut, the smoother the paste will be. Add 1/2 tablespoon flour, 1/2 tablespoon salt and enough water to make a paste. Stir and squash the mixture until it is as smooth as possible. Store in air-tight container.

Books and Stories:

The following books and stories can be used to complement the theme:

1. **The Emperor's New Clothes.** Hans Christian Anderson. (New York: Golden Press, 1966).

2. **The Shoemaker and the Elves.** The Brothers Grimm. (New York: Scribner, 1960).

3. **Jeremy's First Haircut.** Linda Walvoord Girard. (Niles, IL: Albert Whitman and Co., 1986).

4. **I Can Be A Beautician.** Dee Lillegard. (Chicago: Childrens Press, 1987).

Puzzle:

The following puzzle can be found in preschool educational catalogs:

"Barber" Judy/Instructo.

47

SHAPES

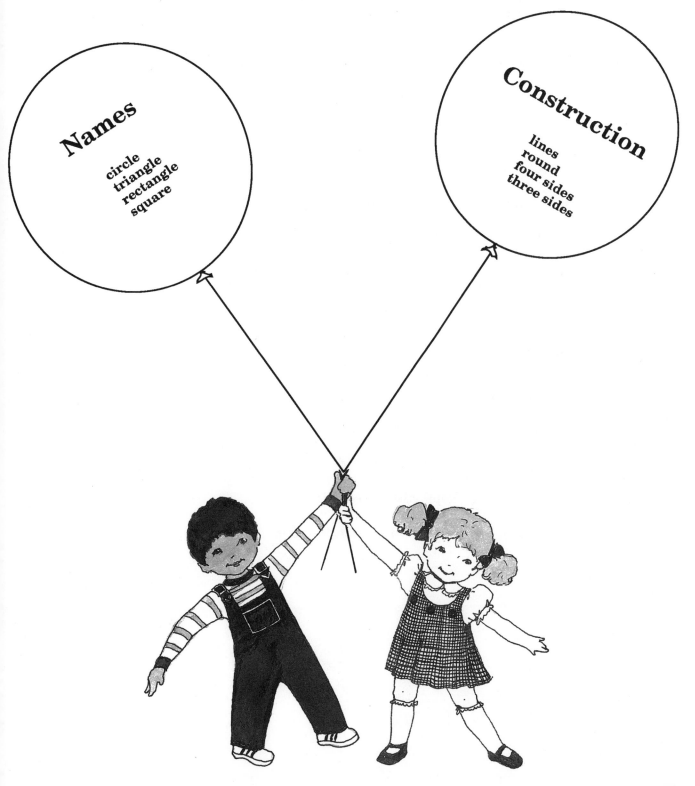

Names

circle
triangle
rectangle
square

Construction

lines
round
four sides
three sides

Theme Goals:

Through participating in the experiences provided by this theme, the children may learn:

1. The names of basic shapes.

2. Identification of basic shapes.

3. Objects have shapes.

Concepts for the Children to Learn:

1. There are many shapes of different sizes and colors in our world.

2. Some shapes have names.

3. A circle is round.

4. Triangles have three sides.

5. Rectangles and squares have four sides.

6. All objects contain one or more shapes.

7. We can draw lines to make shapes.

Vocabulary:

1. **circle**—a shape that is round.

2. **rectangle**—a shape with four sides.

3. **square**—a shape with four sides of equal length.

4. **triangle**—a shape with three sides.

5. **line**—a mark made with a pencil, crayon, etc. to make a shape.

Bulletin Board

The purpose of this bulletin board is to have the child make a shape train. To prepare the bulletin board use the model shown to construct a train using basic shapes. Color the shapes and laminate. Trace laminated shapes onto black construction paper to construct shadow shapes. Staple shadow shapes onto board in train pattern. By using magnets the children can affix the colored shape pieces to the shadows.

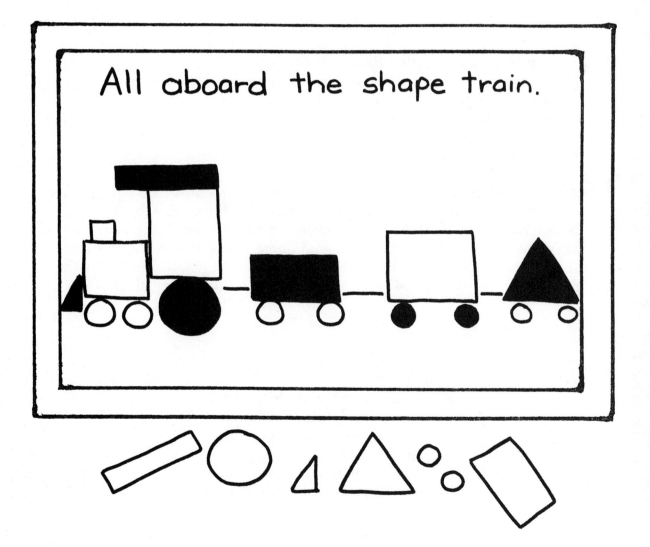

Parent Letter

Dear Parents,

Hello again! This week a unit will be introduced on shapes. Our world consists of shapes. The children will become aware of this on an introductory walk around the block. They will become familiar with the names of shapes and will also classify objects according to shape. Consequently, the children will be more aware of all the shapes in our world. In addition, the children that are developmentally ready will practice drawing some of the basic shapes.

At School This Week

Some of the fun-filled learning activities scheduled for this week include:

* playing a game called Shape Basket Upset.
* listening to the story *Shapes and Things* by Tana Hoban.
* feeling and identifying objects by shape in a feely box.
* making and baking cookies of various shapes.

At Home

You can reinforce the activities included in this unit into your home by observing shaped objects in your house. Each day at school we will have a special shape theme. Your child can bring in an object from home to fit the shape of the day. I will send home the shape the night before so you and your child will have time to look for an object. The following fingerplay can be recited to foster language and memory skills.

Circle and Square

Close my eyes, shut them tight.
  (close eyes)
Make a circle with my one hand.
  (make a circle with one hand)
Keep them shut; make it fair.
  (keep eyes shut)
With my other hand, make a square.
  (make a square with other hand)

Have a fun week!

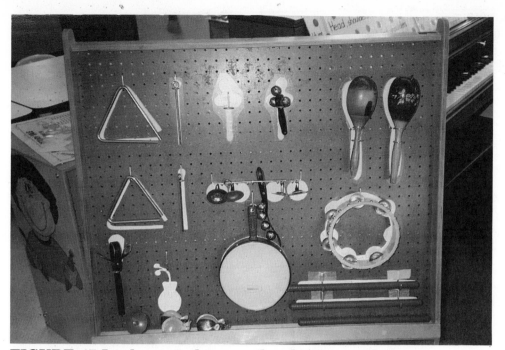

FIGURE 47 Look around to see the shapes around you.

Music:

The following songs can be found in *Music for Today's Young Children*. Butler, Talmadge, Kirland, Terry, Leach. (Broadman Press, 1975).

1. "Colors, Shapes, and Numbers"

2. "Different Shapes"

Fingerplays:

RIGHT CIRCLE, LEFT SQUARE

Close my eyes, shut them tight.
  (close eyes)
Make a circle with my one hand.
  (make circle with one hand)
Keep them shut; make it fair.
  (keep eyes shut)
With my other hand, make a square.
  (make square with other hand)

LINES

One straight finger makes a line.
  (hold up one index finger)
Two straight lines make one "t" sign.
  (cross index fingers)

Three lines made a triangle there
  (form triangle with index fingers
  touching and thumbs touching)
And one more line will make a square.
  (form square with hands)

DRAW A SQUARE

Draw a square, draw a square
Shaped like a tile floor.
Draw a square, draw a square
All with corners four.

DRAW A TRIANGLE

Draw a triangle, draw a triangle
With corners three.
Draw a traingle, draw a triangle
Draw it just for me.

DRAW A CIRCLE

Draw a circle, draw a circle
Made very round.
Draw a circle, draw a circle
No corners can be found.

WHAT AM I MAKING?

This is a circle.
  (draw circle in the air)

This is a square.
  (draw square in the air)
Who can tell me
What I'm making there?
  (draw another shape in the air)

Science:

1. Feely Box

Cut many shapes out of different materials such as felt, cardboard, wallpaper, carpet, etc. Place the shapes into a feely box. The children can be encouraged to reach in and identify the shape by feeling it before removing it from the box.

2. Evaporation

Pour equal amounts of water into a large round and a small square cake pan. Mark the water level with a grease pencil. Allow the water to stand for a week. Observe the amount of evaporation.

3. Classifying Objects

Collect four small boxes. Mark a different shape on each box. Include a circle, triangle, square and rectangle. Then cut shapes out of magazines. The children can sort the objects by placing them in the corresponding boxes.

4. What Shape Is It?

Place objects with distinct shapes in the feely box such as marbles, dice, pyramid, deck of cards, book, ball, button, etc. Encourage the children to reach in and identify the shape of the object they are feeling before they pull it out.

Dramatic Play:

1. Baker

Provide playdough, cake pans and cookie cutters.

2. Puppets

A puppet prop box should be placed in the dramatic play area. If available a puppet stage should be added. Otherwise a puppet stage can be made from cardboard.

Arts and Crafts:

1. Sponge Painting

Cut sponges into the four basic shapes. The children can hold the sponges with a clothespin. The sponge can be dipped in paint and printed on the paper. Make several designs and shapes.

2. Shape Mobiles

Trace shapes of various sizes on colored construction paper. If appropriate, encourage the children to cut the shapes from the paper and punch a hole at the top of each shape. Then, put a piece of string through the hole and tie onto a hanger. The mobiles can be hung in the classroom for decoration.

3. Easel Ideas

Feature a different shape of easel paper each day at the easel.

4. Shape Collage

Provide different colored paper shapes and glue for the children to create collages from shapes.

5. Stencils

Prepare individual stencils of the basic shapes. The children can use the stencils for tracing.

6. My Shape Book

Stickers, catalogs and magazines should be placed on the art table. Also prepare booklets cut into the basic shapes. Encourage the children to find, cut and glue the round objects in each shape book.

Sensory:

Add the following items to the sensory table:

1. marbles and water
2. different shaped sponges and water
3. colored water
4. scented water
5. soapy water

Large Muscle:

1. Walk and Balance

Using masking tape, outline the four basic shapes on the floor. The children can walk and balance on the shapes. Older children may walk forwards, backwards, and sideways.

2. Hopscotch

Draw a hopscotch with chalk on the sidewalk outdoors. Masking tape can be used to form the grid on the floor indoors.

Field Trips/Resource People:

Shape Walk

Walk around the school neighborhood. During the walk, observe the shapes of the traffic signs and houses. After returning to the school or center, record the shapes observed on a chart.

Math:

1. Wallpaper Shape Match

From scraps of old wallpaper, cut out two sets of basic shapes. Then mix all the pieces. The children can match the sets by pattern and shape.

2. Shape Completion

On several pieces of white tagboad draw a shape, leaving one side, or part of a circle, unfinished or dotted. Laminate the

tagboard. The children can complete the shape by drawing with watercolor markers or grease pencils. Erase with a damp cloth.

Group Time (games, language):

1. Shape Hunt

Throughout the classroom hide colorful shapes. The children can each find a shape.

2. Twister

On a large old bed sheet, secure many shapes of different colors, or draw the shapes on with magic markers. Make a spinner. Have children place parts of their bodies on the different shapes.

3. Shape Day

Each day highlight a different shape. Collect related items that resemble the shape of the day and display throughout the classroom. During group time, have each child find an object in the classroom that is the same shape as the shape of the day.

Cooking:

1. Shaped Bread and Peanut Butter

The children can cut bread with different shaped cookie cutters. Spread peanut butter or other toppings on the bread.

2. Fruit Cut-outs

1/2 cup sugar
4 envelopes unflavored gelatin
2 1/2 cups pineapple juice, apple juice, orange juice, grape juice or fruit drink

In a mixing bowl, stir the sugar and gelatin with rubber scraper until well mixed. Pour fruit juice into a 1-quart saucepan. Put the pan on the burner. Turn the burner to high heat. Cook until the juice boils. Turn burner off. Pour boiling fruit juice over sugar mixture. Stir with a rubber scraper until all the gelatin is dissolved. Pour into a 13 inch x 9 inch x 2 inch pan. Place in the refrigerator and chill until firm. Cookie cutters can be used to make shapes. Enjoy! This activity requires close supervision.

3. Shape Snacks

Spread cheese or peanut butter onto various shaped crackers and serve.
Serve cheese cut into circles, triangles, squares and rectangles.
Serve vegetable circles—cucumbers, carrots, zucchini.
Cut fruit snacks into circles—bananas, grapefruit wedges, apple slices, grapes and serve.

4. Nachos

4 flour tortillas
3/4 cup grated cheese
1/3 cup chopped green pepper (optional)

With clean kitchen scissors, cut each tortilla into 4 or 6 triangle wedges. Place on a cookie sheet and sprinkle the tortilla wedges with the cheese. Garnish with green pepper if desired. Bake in a 350 degree oven for 4 to 6 minutes or until the cheese melts. Makes 16 to 20 nachos.

5. Swedish Pancakes

3 eggs
1 cup milk
1 1/2 cups flour
1 tablespoon sugar
1/2 teaspoon salt
4 tablespoons butter
1 cup heavy cream
2 tablespoons confectioner's sugar or a
   12-ounce jar of fruit jelly

Using a fork or whisk, beat the eggs lightly in a large mixing bowl. Add half the milk. Fold in the flour, sugar and salt. Melt the butter and add it, the cream and the remaining milk to the mixture. Stir well. Lightly grease a frying pan or griddle, and place it over medium-high heat on a hot plate or stove. Carefully pour small amounts of the mixture onto the frying pan or griddle. Cook until the pancakes are golden around the edges and bubbly on top. Turn the pancakes over with a spatula and cook until the other sides are golden around the edges. Remove to a covered plate. Repeat until all the mixture is used. Sprinkle pancakes lightly with confectioner's sugar, or spread fruit jelly over them. Makes 3 dozen pancakes.

TO TEACH MATH CONCEPTS

Before a child can learn the more abstract concepts of arithmetic, he must be visually, physically and kinesthetically aware of basic quantitative concepts. Included could be:

Form Discrimination	large	high
	larger	low
circle	heavy	thick
square	light	thin
triangle	in	front
rectangle	out	back
	over	behind
Vocabulary	under	all
	top	none
big	bottom	some
little	long	first
small	short	last
smaller	tall	middle

near	more	slow
far	less	up
above	through	down
below	around	most
many	fast	least
few		

Records:

The following records can be found in preschool educational catalogs:

1. **We All Live Together Series—Volume 3.** "Shapes" Youngheart Records.

2. **We All Live Together Series—Volume 1.** "Round in a Circle" Youngheart Records.

3. **My World Is Round.** Melody House Records.

Books and Stories:

The following books and stories can be used to complement the theme:

1. **The Circle Sarah Drew.** Peter and Sarah Barrett. (New York: Scroll Press, 1970).

2. **The Line Sophie Drew.** Peter and Sarah Barrett. (New York: Scroll Press, 1972).

3. **The Square Ben Drew.** Peter and Sarah Barrett. (New York: Scroll Press, 1970).

4. **Circles, Triangles, Squares.** Tana Hoban. (New York: Macmillan Publishing Company, 1979).

5. **Round and Round and Round.** Tana Hoban. (New York: Macmillan Publishing Company, 1974).

6. **Listen to a Shape.** Marcia Brown. (New York: F. Watts, 1979).

7. **Shape and Form.** Albert W. Porter. (Worcester, MA: Davis Publications, 1974).

8. **Lines and Shapes.** Solveig Paulson Russell. (New York: Henry Z. Walck, Inc., 1965).

9. **It Looked Like Spilt Milk.** Charles Green Shaw. (New York: Harper and Row, 1947).

10. **The Sesame Street Book of Shapes.** (New York: New American Library, 1971).

11. **The Little Circle.** Ann Atwood. (New York: Scribner Press, 1967).

12. **Shapes and Things.** Tana Hoban. (New York: Macmillan Publishing Company, 1970).

13. **Shapes.** John Feiss. (New York: Bradbury Press, Inc., 1974).

14. **Round and Round and Square.** Fredun Shapur. (New York: Abelard-Schuman Company, 1963).

15. **A Wing on a Flea: A Book About Shapes.** Ed Emberley. (Boston, MA: Little, Brown, 1961).

16. **Shapes, Shapes, Shapes.** Tana Hoban. (New York: Greenwillow Books, 1986).

17. **I Know About Shapes.** Dick Bruna. (Los Angeles: Price, Stern and Sloan, 1984).

18. **The Shape of Me and Other Stuff.** Dr. Seuss. (New York: Beginner Books, 1973).

19. **Round in a Circle.** Yvonne Hooker. (New York: Grosset and Dunlap, 1982).

20. **Roly Goes Exploring.** Philip Newth. (New York: Philomel Books, 1981).

21. **Boxes! Boxes!** L.E. Fisher. (New York: The Viking Press, 1984).

22. **A, B, See!** Tara Hoban. (New York: Greenwillow Books, 1982).

Puzzles:

The following puzzles can be found in preschool educational catalogs:

1. **"Fit-a-Shapes"** Lauri.

2. **"Sorting Box"** (shapes) Childcraft.

3. **"Shape Discs"** Lauri.

4. **"Shapes"** 4 pieces. Puzzle People.

5. **"Traffic Light"** 6 pieces. Puzzle People.

48

SPORTS

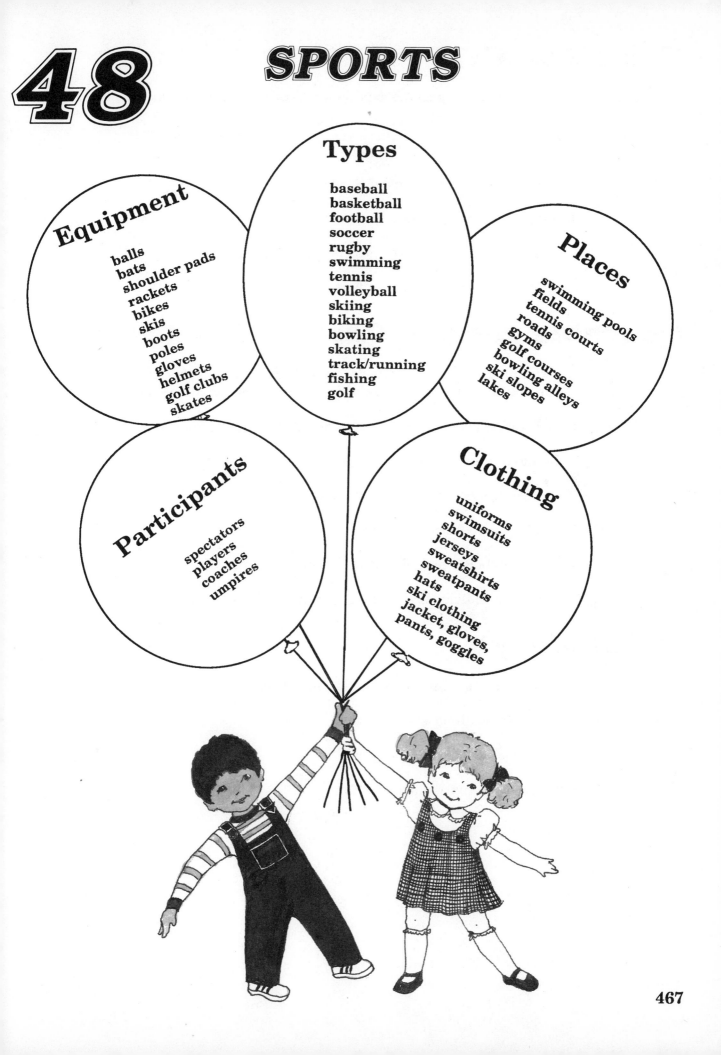

Types

baseball
basketball
football
soccer
rugby
swimming
tennis
volleyball
skiing
biking
bowling
skating
track/running
fishing
golf

Equipment

balls
bats
shoulder pads
rackets
bikes
skis
boots
poles
gloves
helmets
golf clubs
skates

Places

swimming pools
fields
tennis courts
roads
gyms
golf courses
bowling alleys
ski slopes
lakes

Participants

spectators
players
coaches
umpires

Clothing

uniforms
swimsuits
shorts
jerseys
sweatshirts
sweatpants
hats
ski clothing
jacket, gloves,
pants, goggles

Theme Goals:

Through participating in the experiences provided by this theme, the child may learn:

1. Places used for sports participation.

2. Types of sports people play.

3. Types of equipment used for sports.

4. Kinds of clothing worn for sports participation.

5. There are many people who participate in sports.

Concepts for the Children to Learn:

1. Swimming pools, playing fields, tennis courts, roads, gyms, golf courses, bowling lanes, lakes and ski slopes are all places that are used for sports.

2. Spectators, players and coaches are all sports participants.

3. Baseball, biking, football and golf are all types of sports.

4. Balls, bikes and golf clubs are sports equipment.

5. Uniforms are worn when playing some sports.

6. Some sports are played indoors, others outdoors.

7. There are individual and team sports.

Vocabulary:

1. **team**—a group of people who play together.

2. **uniform**—clothing worn for some sports.

3. **ball**—equipment used for sports.

4. **sport**—an activity played for fun.

Bulletin Board

The purpose of this bulletin board is to have the children hang the numeral ball on the glove that has the corresponding number of dots. To prepare the bulletin board construct baseball mitts out of brown tagboard. Attach dots starting with one on each of the gloves. The number of gloves prepared and dots will depend upon the developmental maturity of the children. Hang the gloves on the bulletin board. Next construct white baseballs. Write a numeral, starting with one, on each of the balls.

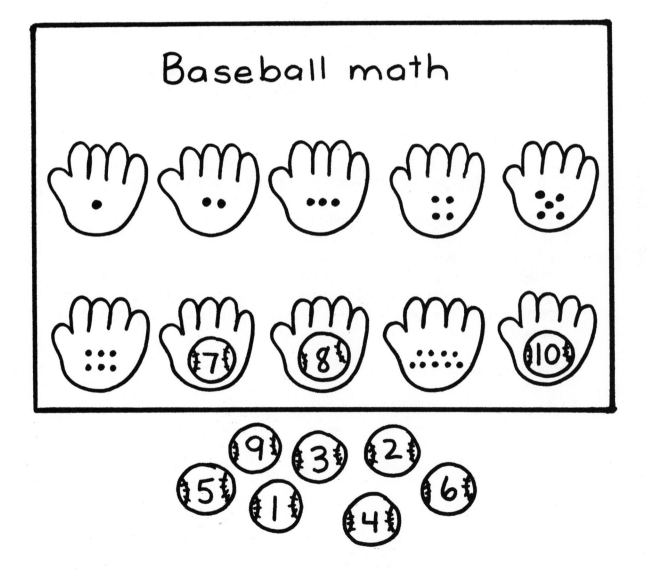

Parent Letter

Dear Parents,

Sports will be the focus of this week's unit. Through the experiences provided, the children will become familiar with sports equipment and clothing. They will also recognize sports as a form of exercise.

At School This Week

Activities planned for the week to foster sports concepts include:

* exploring balls used in different sports and classifying them into groups by size, color and ability to bounce and roll.
* trying on a variety of clothing used in different sports including a swim cap, goggles, shoulder and leg/knee pads, helmets, gloves and uniforms.
* skating in the room by wrapping squares of waxed paper around our feet and attaching it with a rubber band around our ankles. Our feet will then easily glide over the carpet!

At Home

You can incorporate sports concepts at home this week by

* looking through sports magazines with your child and pointing out the equipment that is used or the clothing that is worn. This will develop your child's observation skills.
* observing a sporting event with your child, such as basketball, baseball or football. Likewise, let your child watch you participate in a sport!
* participating in a sport together. Your child will enjoy spending special time with you!

Have a great week!

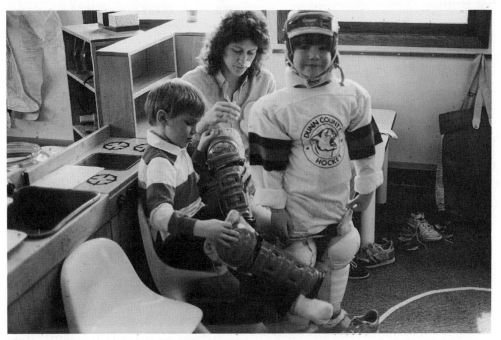

FIGURE 48 Getting ready for the big game

Fingerplays:

HERE IS A BALL

Here's a ball
  (make a circle with your thumb and
  pointer finger)
And here's a ball
  (make a bigger circle with two thumbs
  and pointers)
And a great big ball I see.
  (make a large circle with arms)
Now let's count the balls we've made,
One, two, three.
  (repeat)

FOOTBALL PLAYERS

Five big football players standing in the
locker room door.
One had a sore knee
And then there were four.

Four big football players down on their knees.
One made a touchdown
And then there were three.

Three big football players looking up at you.
One made a tackle
And then there were two.

Two big football players running in the sun.
One was off sides
And then there was one.

One big football player standing all alone.
He decided to go home
And then there was none.

Science:

1. **Feely Box**

Place a softball, hardball, golf ball and
tennis ball in a feeley box. The children
can reach into the box, feel and try to
guess the type of ball.

2. **Ball Bounces**

Observe the way different balls move.
Check to see if footballs, basketballs and
soccer balls can be bounced. Observe to see
if some go higher than others. Also repeat
using smaller balls such as tennis balls,
baseballs and golf balls.

3. **Wheels**

Observe the wheels on a bicycle. If possible bring a bike to the classroom and
demonstrate how peddling makes the
wheels move.

471

4. Examining Balls

Observe the composition of different balls. Ask the children to identify each. Then place the balls in water. Observe to see which ones float and which ones sink.

5. Types of Grass

Place real grass and artifical turf on the science table. The children can feel both types of grass and describe differences in texture.

Dramatic Play:

1. Baseball

Baseball caps, plastic balls, uniforms, catcher's mask and gloves can be placed in the dramatic play area.

2. Football

Balls, shoulder pads, uniforms and helmets can be provided for the children to use outdoors.

3. Tennis

Tennis rackets, balls, visors, sunglasses and shorts for the children can be placed outdoors. A variation would be to use balloons for balls and rackets made from hangers with a nylon pantyhose pulled around the hanger.

4. Skiing

Ski boots and skis can be provided for the children to try on.

5. Skating

Waxed paper squares for children to wrap around their feet and ankles can be provided. The children can attach the waxed paper with rubberbands around their ankles. Encourage the children to slide across the carpeting.

Arts and Crafts:

1. Easel Ideas

Cut easel paper in various sports shapes:

* baseball glove
* baseball diamond
* tennis racket
* bike
* tennis shoe
* football
* baseball cap
* football helmet
* all different sizes of balls

2. Baseball Glove Lacing

Prepare pre-cut baseball gloves out of brown construction paper. The older children might be able to cut them out themselves. Punch holes with a paper punch around the outer edge of the paper. Using yarn, let the children lace in and out of the holes of the gloves. Tie a knot at the end to secure the yarn.

3. Collages

Using sports related magazines, encourage the children to cut out various pictures. These pictures can be pasted onto another piece of paper.

4. Ball Collages

Balls used in various sports come in all different sizes. Using construction paper or wallpaper, cut the paper in various round shapes, as well as football shapes. Encourage the children to paste them on a large piece of construction paper and decorate.

5. Golf Ball Painting

Place a piece of paper in a shallow tray or pie tin. Spoon two or three teaspoons of thin paint onto the paper. Then, put a golf ball or ping-pong ball in the tray and tilt the pan in a number of directions, allowing the ball to make designs in the paint.

Sensory:

1. Swimming

Add water to the sensory table with dolls or small people figures.

2. Weighing Balls

Fill the sensory table with small balls, such as golf balls, styrofoam balls, wiffle balls or tennis balls. Add a balance scale so that the children can weigh the balls.

3. Measuring Mud and Sand

Add a mud and sand mixture to the sensory table with scoops and spoons.

4. Feeling Turf

Line the bottom of the sensory table with artificial turf.

Large Muscle:

1. Going Fishing

Use a large wooden rocking boat, or a large box that two to three children can sit in. Make fish out of construction paper or tagboard, and attach paper clips to the top. Tie a magnet to a string and pole. The magnet will attract the fish.

2. Kickball

Many sports involve kicking a ball. Discuss these sports with the children. Then provide the children with a variety of balls to kick. Let the children discover which balls go the farthest and which are the easiest to kick.

3. Sports Charades

Dramatize various sports including swimming, golfing, tennis and bike riding.

4. Golfing

Using a child-sized putter and regular golf balls, the children hit golf balls. This is an outdoor activity that requires a lot of teacher supervision.

5. Beach Volleyball

Use a large beach ball and a rope or net in a central spot outdoors. Let the children volley the beach ball to one another.

Field Trips/Resource People:

Suggested trips include:

1. a football field
2. a baseball field
3. tennis court
4. health (fitness) club
5. stadium
6. a swimming pool
7. the sports facilities of a local high school or college

Math:

1. Ball Sort

Sort various balls by size, texture and color.

2. Hat Sorting

Sort hats such as baseball cap, football helmet, biking helmet, visor, etc. by color, size, texture and shape.

Group Time (games, language):

"What's Missing"

Provide the children in a large group with a tray of sports equipment such as a ball, baseball glove, golf ball, sunglasses, goggles, etc. Let the children examine the tray of items. Then have the children close their eyes and place their heads in their laps. Remove one item from the tray and see if the children can guess what is missing. This activity will be more successful if the numbers are related to the age of the child. For example, with two-year-old children, use only two items. Three-year-olds may be successful with an additional item. If not, remove one.

473

Cooking:

Cheese Balls

    8 ounces cream cheese, softened
1 stick of butter, softened

2 cups grated cheddar cheese
1/2 package of onion soup mix

Blend all of the ingredients together. Shape the mixture into small balls. Roll the balls in chopped nuts if desired.

Records:

The following records can be found in preschool educational catalogs:

1. **And the Beat Goes on for Physical Education.**

2. **Coordination Skills.**

3. **Exercise is Kids' Stuff.**

4. **Fitness Fun for Everyone.**

5. **Have a Ball!**

6. **Jumpnastics**

Books and Stories:

The following books and stories can be used to complement the theme:

1. **Circles, Triangles and Squares.** Tana Hoban. (New York: Macmillan, 1974).

2. **Curious George Rides a Bike.** H.A. Rey. (Boston: Houghton Mifflin Company, 1952).

3. **Curious George Gets a Medal.** H.A. Rey. (Boston: Houghton Mifflin Company, 1957).

4. **Fast-Slow, High-Low.** Peter Spier. (New York: Doubleday, 1972).

Puzzles:

The following puzzles can be found in preschool educational catalogs:

1. **"Bicycle"** Judy/Instructo.

2. **"Boat"** Judy/Instructo.

3. **"Things with Wheels"** Judy/Instructo.

4. **"Roller Skate Champ"** Judy/Instructo.

5. **"Gym"** Judy/Instructo.

6. **"Park"** Judy/Instructo.

7. **"Sports"** Judy/Instructo.

8. **"Riding Bikes"** Judy/Instructo.

9. **"Playing Ball"** Judy/Instructo.

10. **"Pony Riding"** Judy/Instructo.

11. **"Fishing Hole"** Judy/Instructo.

49

SPRING

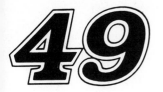

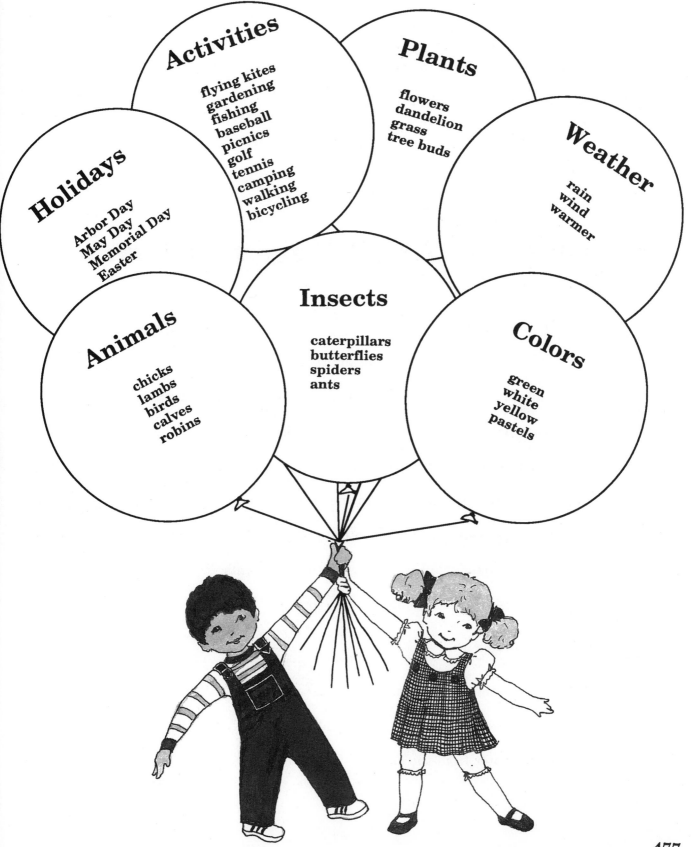

Activities

flying kites
gardening
fishing
baseball
picnics
golf
tennis
camping
walking
bicycling

Plants

flowers
dandelion
grass
tree buds

Holidays

Arbor Day
May Day
Memorial Day
Easter

Weather

rain
wind
warmer

Animals

chicks
lambs
birds
calves
robins

Insects

caterpillars
butterflies
spiders
ants

Colors

green
white
yellow
pastels

Theme Goals:

Through participating in the experiences provided by this theme, the children may learn:

1. Spring colors.

2. Spring weather.

3. Plants that grow in the spring.

4. Insects seen during the spring.

5. Springtime holidays.

6. Spring animals.

7. Spring activities.

Concepts for the Children to Learn:

1. Spring is a season.

2. It rains in the spring.

3. Light colors are seen during the spring.

4. Caterpillars and butterflies are insects seen in the spring.

5. Some holidays are celebrated in the spring.

6. Chicks, lambs and birds are springtime animals.

7. Some people go on picnics in the spring.

8. Many gardens are planted in the spring.

9. Flowers, dandelions and grass are spring plants.

10. Gardens are often planted in the spring.

Vocabulary:

1. **spring**—the season that comes after winter and before summer.

2. **garden**—a place where plants and flowers are grown.

3. **rain**—water from the clouds.

Bulletin Board

The purpose of this bulletin board is to have the children place the proper number of ribbons on each kite tail. To do this, they need to look at the number of dots on the kite. Construct kites and print the numerals beginning with one and the corresponding number of dots on each. Construct ribbons for the tails of the kites as illustrated. Color the kites and tails and laminate. Staple kites to bulletin board. Affix magnetic strips to each kite as the string. Affix a magnetic piece in the middle of each ribbon.

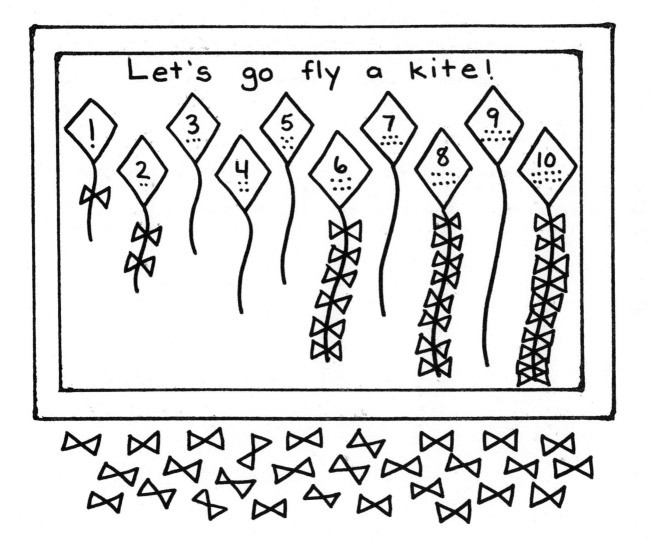

Parent Letter

Dear Parents,

The temperature is slowly rising, and there are patches of green grass on the playground. In other words, spring is here! And spring is the subject we will be exploring this week at school. Throughout the week, the children will become more aware of the many changes that take place during this season, as well as common spring activities.

At School This Week

Some of this week's learning experiences include:

* finding a suitable place on the playground to plant flowers.
* taking a walk around the neighborhood to observe signs of spring.
* planting grass seed in empty egg shells at the science table.
* creating pictures and designs with pastel water color markers in the art area.

At Home

To foster concepts of spring at home, save seeds from fruits such as oranges and apples. Assist your child in planting the seeds. Your child can also sort the seeds by color, size or type to develop classification skills. The seeds could also be used for counting. Happy seed collecting!

Until next week!

Music:

1. "Catch One If You Can"
(Sing to the tune of "Skip To My Lou")

Butterflies are flying. Won't you try and catch one?
Butterflies are flying. Won't you try and catch one?
Butterflies are flying. Won't you try and catch one?
Catch one if you can.

Raindrops are falling. Won't you try and catch one?
Raindrops are falling. Won't you try and catch one?
Raindrops are falling. Won't you try and catch one?
Catch one if you can.

2. "Signs of Spring"
(Sing to the tune of "Muffin Man")

Do you see a sign of spring,
A sign of spring, a sign of spring?
Do you see a sign of spring?
Tell us what you see.

3. Let's Be Windmills
(Sing to the tune of "If I Were a Lassie")

Oh I wish I were a windmill, a windmill, a windmill.
Oh I wish I were a windmill. I know what I'd do.
I'd swing this way and that way, and this way and that way.
Oh I wish I were a windmill, when the wind blew.

Fingerplays:

SEE, SEE, SEE

See, see, see
  (shade eyes with hands)
Three birds are in a tree.
  (hold up three fingers)
One can chirp
  (point to thumb)
And one can sing.
  (point to index finger)
One is just a tiny thing.
  (point to middle finger, then rock baby bird in arms)
See, see, see
Three birds are in a tree
  (hold up three fingers)

Look, look, look
  (shade eyes)
Three ducks are in a brook.
  (hold up three fingers)
One is white, and one is brown.
One is swimming upside down.
  (point to a finger each time)
Look, look, look
Three ducks are in a brook.
  (hold up three fingers)

THIS LITTLE CALF

(extend fingers, push each down in succession)

This little calf eats grass.
This little calf eats hay.
This little calf drinks water.
This little calf runs away.
This little calf does nothing
But just lies down all day.
  (rest last finger in palm of hand)

RAINDROPS

Rain is falling down.
Rain is falling down.
  (raise arm, flutter fingers to ground, tapping the floor)
Pitter-patter
Pitter-patter
Rain is falling down.

CREEPY CRAWLY CATERPILLAR

A creepy crawly caterpiller that I see
  (shade eyes)
Makes a chrysalis in the big oak tree.
  (make body into a ball)
He stays there and I know why
  (slowly stand up)
Because soon he will be a butterfly.
  (flap arms)

MY GARDEN

This is my garden.
  (extend one hand forward, palm up)
I'll rake it with care
  (make raking motion on palm with three other fingers)
And then some flower seeds
I'll plant there.
  (planting motion)
The sun will shine
  (make circle with hands)
And the rain will fall.
  (let fingers flutter down to lap)
And my garden will blossom
And grow straight and tall.
  (cup hands together, extend upwards slowly)

CATERPILLAR

The caterpillar crawled from a plant, you see.
  (left hand crawls up and down right arm)
"I think I'll take a nap," said he.
So over the ground he began to creep
  (right hand crawls over left arm)
To spin a chyrsallis, and he fell asleep.
  (cover right fist with left hand)
All winter he slept in his bed
Till spring came along and he said.
"Wake up, it's time to get out of bed!"
  (shake fist and pointer finger)
So he opened his eyes that sunny spring day.
  (spread fingers and look into hand)
"Look I'm a butterfly!" ... and he flew away.
  (interlock thumbs and fly hands away)

Science:

1. Alfalfa Sprouts

Each child who wishes to participate should be provided with a small paper cup, soil and a few alfalfa seeds. The seeds and soil can be placed in the cup and watered. Place the cups in the sun and watch the sprouts grow. The sprouts can be eaten for snack. A variation is to plant the sprouts in eggshells as an Easter activity.

2. Weather Chart

A weather chart can be constructed that depicts weather conditions such as sunny, rainy, warm, cold, windy, etc. Attach at least two arrows to the center of the chart so that the children can point the arrow at the appropriate weather conditions.

3. Thermometers

On the science table place a variety of outdoor thermometers. Also post a thermometer outside of a window, at a low position, so the children can read it.

4. Sprouting Carrots

Cut the large end off a fresh carrot and place it in a small cup of water. In a few days, a green top will begin to sprout.

5. Nesting Materials

Place string, cotton, yarn and other small items outside on the ground. Birds will collect these items to use in their nest building.

6. Grass Growing

Grass seeds can be sprinkled on a wet sponge. Within a few days the seeds will begin to sprout.

7. Ant Farm

An ant farm can by made by using a large jar with a cover. Fill the jar 2/3 full with sand and soil, and add ants. Punch a few air holes in the cover of the jar, and secure the cover to the top of the jar. The children can watch the ants build tunnels.

Dramatic Play:

1. Fishing

Using short dowels prepare fishing poles with a string taped to one end. Attach a magnet piece to the loose end of the string. Then construct fish from tagboard. Attach a paper clip to each fish. The magnet will attract the paper clip, allowing the children to catch the fish. Add a tackle box, canteen, hats and life jackets for interest.

2. Garden

A small plastic hoe, rake and garden shovels can be placed outdoors to encourage gardening. A watering can, flower pots, seed packages and sun hats will also stimulate interest.

3. Flower Shop

Collect plastic flowers, vases, wrapping paper, seed packages and catalogs and place in the dramatic play area. A cash register and play money can be added.

4. Spring Cleaning

Small mops, brooms, feather dusters and empty pails can be placed in the dramatic play area. A spray bottle filled with blue water which can be used to wash designated windows can also be provided.

Arts and Crafts:

1. Butterfly Wings

Fold a sheet of light colored paper in half. Show the children how to paint on only one side of the paper. The paper can be folded again and pressed. The result will be a symmetrical painting. Antennas can be added using crayons and markers to make butterflies.

2. Pussy Willow Fingerprints

Trace around a tongue depressor with a colored marker. Then using ink pads or fingerpaint, the children can press their finger on the ink pad and transfer their fingerprint to the paper. This will produce pussy willow buds.

3. Caterpillars

Cut egg cartons in half. Place them on the art table with short pieces of pipe cleaners, markers and crayons. From these materials, the children can make caterpillars.

4. Kites

Provide diamond-shaped construction paper, string, paper punch, crepe paper, glue, glitter and markers. For older children, provide the paper with a diamond already traced. This provides them an opportunity for practicing finger motor skills. The children can create kites, and use them outdoors.

Sensory:

The following items can be added to the sensory table:

* string, hay, sticks and yarn to make birds' nests
* tadpoles and water
* dirt with worms
* seeds
* water and boats
* ice cubes to watch them melt

Large Muscle:

1. Windmills

The children can stand up, swing their arms from side to side and pretend to be windmills. A fan can be added to the classroom for added interest. Sing the song "Let's Be Windmills" which is listed under music.

2. Puddles

Construct puddles out of tagboard and cover with aluminum foil. Place the puddles on the floor. The children can jump from puddle to puddle. A variation would be to do this activity outside, using chalk to mark puddles on the ground.

3. Caterpillar Crawl

During a transition time, the children can imitate caterpillar movements.

Field Trips/Resource People:

1. Nature Walk

Walk around your neighborhood, looking for signs of spring. Robins and other birds are often first signs of spring and can usually be observed in most areas of the country.

2. Farm

Arrange a field trip to a farm. It is an interesting place to visit during the spring. Ask the farmer to show you the farm equipment, buildings, crops and animals.

Math:

1. Seed Counting

On an index card, mark a numeral. The number of cards prepared will depend upon the developmental appropriateness for the children. The children are to glue the appropriate number of seeds onto the card.

2. Insect Seriation

Construct flannelboard pieces representing a ladybug, an ant, a caterpillar, a butterfly, etc. The children can arrange them on the flannelboard from smallest to largest.

Social Studies:

1. Animal Babies

Collect pictures of animals and their young. Place the adult animal pictures in one basket and the pictures of the baby animals in another basket. The children can match adult animals to their offspring.

2. Spring Cleanup

Each child should be provided with a paper bag to collect litter on a walk to a park, in your neighborhood or even on your playground. The litter should be discarded when you return to the center. Also the children should be instructed to wash their hands.

3. Dressing for Spring

Flannelboard figures with clothing items should be provided. The children can dress

the figures for different kinds of spring weather.

4. Spring Clothing

Collect several pieces of spring clothing such as a jacket, umbrella, hat, galoshes, and short-sleeved shirts. Add these to the dramatic play area.

Group Time (games, language):

1. What's Inside?

Inside a large box, place many spring items. Include a kite, an umbrella, a hat, a fishing pole, etc. Select an item without showing the children. Describe the object and give clues of how the item can be used. The children should try to identify the item.

2. Insect Movement

During transition time, ask the children to move like the following insects: worm, grasshopper, spider, caterpillar, butterfly, bumblebee, etc.

Cooking:

1. Lemonade

1 lemon
2 to 3 tablespoons sugar
1 1/4 cups water
2 ice cubes

Squeeze lemon juice out of lemon. Add the sugar and water. Stir to dissolve the sugar. This makes one serving. Adjust the recipe to accommodate your class size.

2. Watermelon Popsicles

Remove the seeds and rind from a watermelon. Puree the melon in a blender or food processor. Pour into small paper cups. Insert popsicle sticks and freeze. These fruit popsicles can be served at snack time.

SCIENCE ACTIVITIES

Twenty-five other interesting science activities include:

1. Observe **food forms** such as potatoes in the raw, shredded or sliced form. Fruits can be juiced, sliced or sectioned.

2. **Prepare tomatoes** in several ways, such as sliced, juiced, stewed, baked and pureed.

3. **Show corn** in all forms including on the cob, popcorn, fresh cooked and canned.

4. **Sort** picture cards into piles, living and non-living.

5. **Tape record voices.** Encourage the children to recognize each others' voices.

6. **Tape record familiar sounds** from their environment. Include a teaching clock, telephone ringing, doorbell, toilet flushing, horn beeping, etc.

7. Take the children on a **sensory walk**. Prepare by filling dishpan-sized containers with different items. Foam, sand, leaves, pebbles, mud, cold and warm water and grains can be used. Have the children remove their shoes and socks to walk through.

8. **Enjoy a nature walk.** Provide each child with a grocery bag and instructions to collect leaves, rocks, soil, insects, etc.

9. Provide the children with **bubbles**. To make the solution, mix 2 quarts of water, 3/4 cup liquid soap and 1/4 cup glycerine (available from a local druggist). Dip plastic berry baskets and plastic six-pack holders into the solution. Wave to produce bubbles.

10. Show the children how to feel their **heart beat** after a vigorous activity.

11. Observe **popcorn** popping.

12. Record **body weights and heights**.

13. Prepare **hair and eye color charts**. This information can be made into bar graphs.

14. If climate permits, **freeze water outdoors**. Return it to the class and observe the effects of heat.

15. **Introduce water absorption** by providing containers with water. Allow the children to experiment with coffee filters, paper towels, newspaper, sponges, dish clothes, waxed paper, aluminum foil, and plastic wrap.

16. Explore **magnets**. Provide magnets of assorted sizes, shapes and strengths. With magnets, place paper clips, nuts, bolts, aluminum foil, copper pennies, metal spoons, jar lids, feathers, etc.

17. Plan a **seed party**. Provide the children with peanuts, walnuts, pecans and coconuts. Observe the different sizes, shapes, textures and flavors.

18. Make a **desk garden**. Cut carrots, turnips and a pineapple 1 1/2 inches from the stem. Place the stem in a shallow pan of water.

19. Create a **worm farm**. Place gravel and soil in a clear large-mouth jar. Add worms and keep soil moist. Place lettuce, corn or cereal on top of the soil. Tape

black construction paper around the outside of the jar. Remove the paper temporarily and see the tunnels.

20. Place a **celery stalk** with leaves in a clear container of water. Add blue or red food coloring. Observe the plant's absorption of the colored water. A similar experiment can be introduced with a white carnation.

21. Make a **rainbow** with a garden hose on a sunny day. Spray water across the sun rays. The rays of the sun contain all of the colors, but the water, acting as a prism, separates the colors.

22. Make **shadows**. In a darkened room, use a flashlight. Place a hand or object in front of the light source, making a shadow.

23. Produce **static electricity** by rubbing wool fabric over inflated balloons.

24. Install a **birdfeeder** outside the classroom window.

25. During large group, play the **What's missing game**. Provide children with a variety of small familiar items. Tell them to cover their eyes or put their heads down. Remove one item. Then tell the children to uncover. Ask them what is missing. As children gain skill, remove a second and a third item.

Records:

The following records can be found in preschool educational catalogs:

1. **Seasons for Singing.** Ella Jenkins.

2. **Springtime Walk.** Lucille Wood.

3. **All About Spring.** Lyons Publishers.

4. **Modern Tunes for Rhythm and Instruments.** "Sunshine" Hap Palmer.

5. **Raindrops.** Melody House Records.

Books and Stories:

The following books and stories can be used to complement the theme:

1. **Really Spring.** Gene Zion. (New York: Harper and Row, 1956).

2. **The Happy Day.** Ruth Krauss. (New York: Harper and Row, 1949).

3. **The Nicest Time of the Year.** Gay Zhemya. (New York: Viking Press, 1963).

4. **The Story of a Seed and How It Grew.** Mary Louise Downer. (New York: William R. Scott, Inc., 1955).

5. **Spring is a New Beginning.** Joan Anglund. (New York: Harcourt, Brace and World, Inc., 1963).

6. **Seeds and More Seeds.** Millicent E. Selsam. (New York: Harper and Row, 1959).

7. **Spring is Here.** Jane Moncure. (Elgin, IL: Child's World, 1975).

8. **Who Will Wake Up Spring?** Sharon Lerner. (Minneapolis, MN: Lerner Publications, 1967).

9. **The Very Hungry Caterpillar.** Eric Carle. (New York: Philomel Books, 1981).

10. **A Rainbow of My Own.** Freeman. (New York: The Viking Press, 1966).

11. **The Seed the Squirrel Dropped.** Haris Petie. (New York: Prentice-Hall, 1976).

12. **Spring Cleaning.** Pat Thornburg. (Racine, WI: Western Publishing Company, 1980).

13. **How Kittens Grow.** Millicent E. Selsam. (New York: Scholastic Book Services, 1973).

14. **Close Looks in a Spring Woods.** Martha McKeen Welch. (New York: Dodd, Mead, and Company, 1981).

15. **The Boy Who Didn't Believe in Spring.** Lucille Clifton. (New York: Dutton, 1973).

16. **Time For Spring.** Crockett Johnson. (New York: Harper and Brothers, 1979).

Puzzles:

The following puzzles can be found in preschool educational catalogs:

1. **"Butterfly"** Lauri.

2. **"Bug"** Lauri.

3. **"Rain"** 4 pieces. Judy/Instructo.

4. **"Robin"** 4 pieces. Judy/Instructo.

5. **"Ladybug"** 5 pieces. Judy/Instructo.

6. **"Sheep and Lambs"** 10 pieces. Judy/Instructo.

7. **"Chickens and Chicks"** 9 pieces. Judy/Instructo.

8. **"Tulip"** 9 pieces. Judy/Instructo.

9. **"Butterflies"** Lauri.

10. **"Flower"** Lauri.

50

SUMMER

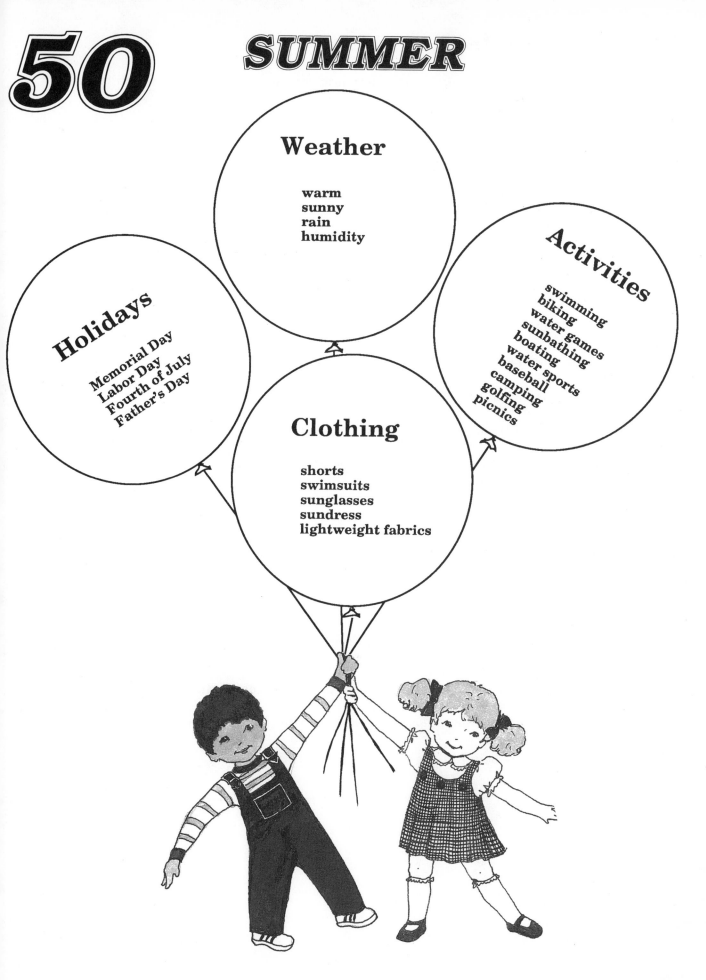

Weather

warm
sunny
rain
humidity

Activities

swimming
biking
water games
sunbathing
boating
water sports
baseball
camping
golfing
picnics

Holidays

Memorial Day
Labor Day
Fourth of July
Father's Day

Clothing

shorts
swimsuits
sunglasses
sundress
lightweight fabrics

Theme Goals:

Through participating in the experiences provided by this theme, the children may learn:

1. Summer holidays.

2. Types of summer clothing.

3. Summer clothing needs.

4. Summer activities.

Concepts for the Children to Learn:

1. Summer is usually the warmest season.

2. Summer months are usually warm and sunny.

3. Lightweight clothing is worn in the summer.

4. Shade trees protect us from the sun during the summer.

5. Memorial Day, Father's Day, the Fourth of July and Labor Day are all summer holidays.

6. Swimming, biking and camping are all summer activities.

Vocabulary:

1. **shorts**—short pants worn in warm weather.

2. **swimming**—a water sport usually enjoyed by many people during the summer months.

3. **hot**—a warm temperature experienced during summer months.

4. **beach**—a sandy place used for sunbathing and playing.

5. **shade**—being in the shadow of something.

Bulletin Board

The purpose of this bulletin board is to promote the identification of written numerals as well as matching sets of objects to a written numeral. Pairs of pails are constructed out of various scraps of tagboard. Using a black marker print a different numeral on each pail. The number of pairs made and numerals used should depend upon the developmental level of the children. Cut seashells out of tagboard and decorate as desired. Laminate all pieces. Attach pails to the bulletin board by stapling them along the side and bottom edges, leaving the tops of the pails open. The children should place the corresponding sets of shells in each pail.

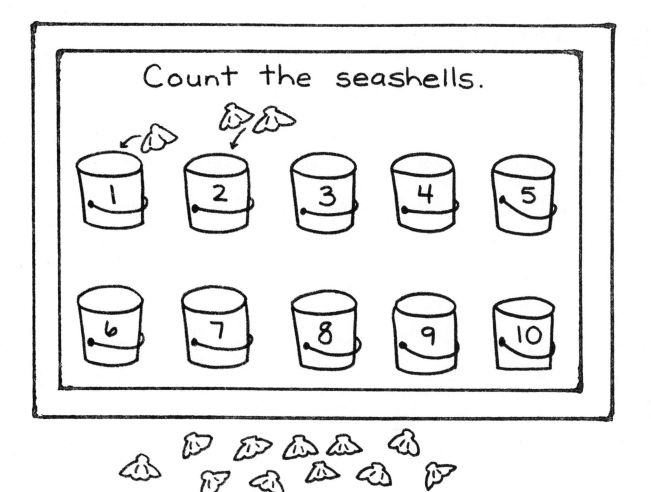

Parent Letter

Dear Parents,

Summer is the favorite season of most children. As summer approaches, we will be starting a week-long unit on the season. Through this unit, the children will become more aware of summer weather activities, food and clothing.

At School This Week

Learning experiences planned to highlight summer concepts include:

* exploring the outside and inside of a watermelon and then eating it!
* trying on shorts, sunglasses and sandals in the dramatic play area.
* preparing fruit juice popsicles.
* eating a picnic lunch on Wednesday. We will be walking to Wilson Park at 11:45. Please feel free to pack a sack lunch and meet us there!

At Home

To reinforce summer concepts at home, try the following:

* Plan a family picnic and allow your child to help plan what food and items will be needed.
* Take part in or observe any summer activity such as boating, fishing, biking, camping or taking a bike ride.

Have a good summer!

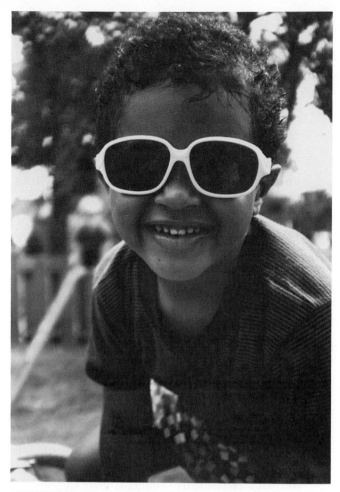

FIGURE 50 Summer is the time of year when the sun shines brightest.

Music:

1. This song can be used during transition times to point out children's summer clothing. Sing to the tune of "The Farmer in the Dell."

"Summer Clothing"

Oh, if you are wearing shorts,
If you are wearing shorts,
You may walk right to the door,
If you are wearing shorts.

Also include: stripes, sandals, tennis shoes, flowers, a sundress, blue jeans, belt, barrettes, etc.

2. Use this song as a transition song to introduce summer activities. Sing to the tune of "Skip to My Lou."

"Summer Activities"

Swim, swim, swim in a circle.
Swim, swim, swim in a circle.
Swim, swim, swim in a circle.
Swim in a circle now.

Also include: jump, hop, skip, run, walk, etc.

Fingerplays:

HERE IS THE BEE HIVE

Here is the bee hive. Where are the bees?
  (make a fist)
They're hiding away so nobody sees.
Soon they're coming creeping out of their hive,
1, 2, 3, 4, 5. Buzz-z-z-z-z.
  (draw fingers out of fist on each count)

GREEN LEAF

Here's a geen leaf
  (show hand)
And here's a green leaf.
  (show other hand)
That you see, makes two.

Here's a bud.
  (cup hands together)
That makes a flower;
Watch it bloom for you!
  (open cupped hands gradually)

A ROLY-POLY CATERPILLAR

Roly-poly caterpillar
Into a corner crept.
Spun around himself a blanket
  (spin around)
Then for a long time slept.
  (place head on folded hands)

Roly-poly caterpillar
Wakened by and by.
  (stretch)
Found himself with beautiful wings
Changed into a butterfly.
  (flutter arms like wings)

Science:

1. Science Table

Add the following items to the science table:

* all kinds of sunglasses with different colored shades
* plant grass seeds in small cups of dirt, water daily
* dirt and grass with magnifying glasses
* sand with scales and magnifying glasses
* pinwheels (children use their own wind to make them move)
* blow bubbles outdoors

2. Water and Air Make Bubbles

Bubble Solution Recipe

3/4 cup liquid soap
1/4 cup glycerine (obtain at a drugstore)
2 quarts water

Place mixed solution in a shallow pan and let children place the bubble makers in. Bubble makers can be successfully made from the following:

* plastic six-pack holder
* straws
* bent wire with no sharp edges
* funnels

3. Flying Kites

On a windy day, make and fly kites.

4. Making Rainbows

If you have a hose available the children can spray the hose into the sun. The rays of the sun contain all the colors mixed together. The water acts as a prism and separates the water into colors creating a rainbow.

Dramatic Play:

1. Juice Stand

Set up a lemonade or orange juice stand. To prepare use real oranges and lemons and let the children squeeze them and make the juice. The juice can be served at snack time.

2. Ice Cream Stand

Trace and cut ice cream cones from brown construction paper. Cottonballs or small yarn pompoms can be used to represent ice cream. The addition of ice cream buckets and ice cream scoopers can make this activity more inviting during self-selected play periods.

3. Indoors or Outdoors Picnic

A blanket, picnic basket, plastic foods, purses, small cooler, paper plates, plastic silverware, napkins, etc. can be placed in the classroom to stimulate play.

4. The Beach

In the dramatic play area place beach blankets, lawn chairs, buckets, sunglasses, beach balls, magazines and books. If the activity is used outdoors, a sun umbrella can be added to stimulate interest in play.

5. Camping Fun

A small freestanding tent can be set up indoors, if room permits, or outdoors. Sleeping bags can also be provided. Blocks or logs could represent a campfire.

6. Traveling by Air

Place a telephone, tickets, travel brochures and suitcases in the dramatic play area.

Arts and Crafts:

1. Outdoor Painting

An easel can be placed outside. The children choose to use the easel during outdoor playtime. If the sun is shining, encourage the children to observe how quickly the paint dries.

2. Chalk Drawings

Large pieces of chalk should be provided for the children to draw on the sidewalks outdoors. Small plastic berry baskets make handy chalk containers.

3. Foot Painting

This may be used as an outdoor activity. The children can dip their feet in a thick tempera paint mixture and make prints by stepping on large sheets of paper. Sponges and pans of soapy water should be available for cleanup.

4. Shake Painting

Tape a large piece of butcher block paper on a fence or wall outdoors. Let the children dip their brushes in paint and stand two feet from the paper. Then show them how to shake the brush, allowing the paint to fly onto the paper.

5. Sailboats

Color styrofoam meat trays with markers. Stick a pipe cleaner in the center of the tray and secure by bending the end underneath the carton. Prepare a sail and glue to the pipe cleaner.

Sensory:

Sensory Table

The following items can be added to the sensory table:

* sand with toys
* colored sand
* sand and water
* water with toy boats
* shells
* small rocks and pebbles
* grass and hay

Large Muscle:

1. Barefoot Walk

Check the playground to ensure that it is free of debris. Then sprinkle part of the grass and sandbox with water. Go on a barefoot walk.

2. Balls

On the outdoor play yard place a variety of large balls.

3. Catching Balloons

Balloons can be used indoors and outdoors. Close supervision is required. If a balloon breaks it should be immediately removed.

4. Parachute Play

Use a real parachute or a sheet to respresent one. The children should hold onto the edges. Say a number and then have the children count and wave the parachute in the air that number of times.

5. Balloon Racket Ball

Bend coat hangers into diamond shapes. Bend the handles closed and tape for safety. Then pull nylon stockings over the diamond shapes to form swatters. The children can use the swatters to keep the balloons up in the air by hitting them.

Field Trips/Resource People:

1. Picnic at the Park

A picnic lunch can be prepared and eaten at a park or on the play yard.

2. Resource People

The following resource people may be invited to the classroom:

* A lifeguard to talk about water safety.
* A camp counselor can talk to the children about camping and sing some camp songs with the children.

Math:

Sand Numbers and Shapes

During outdoor play informally make shapes and numbers in the sand and let children identify the shape or number.

Social Studies:

1. Making Floats

To celebrate the Fourth of July, decorate the trikes, wagons and scooters with crepe paper, streamers, balloons etc. Parade around the school or neighborhood.

2. Summer at School

Take pictures or slides of community summer activities. Construction workers, parades, children playing, sports activities, people swimming, library hours, picnics, band concerts and people driving are examples. Show the slides and discuss them during group time.

3. Summer Fun Book

Magazines should be provided for the children to find pictures of summer activites. The pictures can be pasted on a sheet of paper. Bind the pages by stapling them together to make a book.

Group Time (games, language):

1. Exploring a Watermelon

Serve watermelon for snack. Talk about the color of the outside which is called the rind. Next cut the watermelon into pieces. Give each child a piece to look at. Examine it carefully. "What color is the inside? Are there seeds? Do we eat the seeds? What can we do with them?" The children can remove all the seeds from their piece of watermelon. Then eat the watermelon. Collect all of the seeds. After circle time, wash the seeds. When dry, they can be used for a collage.

2. Puppet Show

Weather permitting, bring puppets and a puppet stage outdoors and have an outdoor puppet show.

Cooking:

1. Popsicles

pineapple juice
grape juice
cranapple juice
popsicle sticks
small paper cups

If frozen juice is used, mix according to the directions on the can. Fill the paper cups 3/4 full of juice. Place the cups in the freezer. When the juice begins to freeze, insert a popsicle stick in the middle of each cup. When frozen, peel the cup away and serve.

2. Watermelon Popsicles

Remove the seeds and rind from watermelon. Puree the melon in a blender. Follow the recipe for popsicles.

3. Zippy Drink

2 ripe bananas
2 cups orange juice
2 cups orange sherbet
ice cubes
orange slices

Peel the bananas, place in a bowl and mash with a fork. Add orange juice and sherbet and beat with a rotary beater until smooth. Pour into pitcher. Add ice cubes and orange slices.

4. Kulfi (Indian Ice Cream)

1 quart milk
1/2 pint heavy cream
1/4 cup sugar
1/2 cup chopped pistachio nuts
1/2 cup chopped almonds
1 tablespoon vanilla
2 drops red food coloring

Combine milk and heavy cream in a saucepan. Simmer over medium heat for about 20 minutes until thick. Add sugar, pistachio nuts, almonds, vanilla and food coloring. Mix thoroughly. Let cool. Fill small paper cups halfway with kulfi and place in a freezer for 1 hour until the kulfi has the consistency of soft sherbet. Makes 10 servings.

Source: *Wonderful World Macmillan Early Skills Program.* (New York: Macmillan Educational Company, 1985).

Records:

The following records can be found in preschool educational catalogs:

1. **Action Songs for Indoor Days.** Tom Thumb series.

2. **Children's Games.** Kimbo Records.

3. **Modern Marches.** Hap Palmer.

4. **Pretend to Be Me.** Melody House Records.

5. **Adventures in Sounds.** Melody House Records.

6. **Patriotic Songs of the U.S.** Melody House Records.

Books and Stories:

The following books and stories can be used to complement the theme:

1. **Mary Ann's Mud Day.** Janice May Urdy. (New York: Harper and Row Publishers, 1956).

2. **Swimmy.** Leo Lionni. (New York: Pantheon Publishers, 1968).

3. **The Biggest House in the World.** Leo Lionni. (New York: Pantheon Publishers, 1968).

4. **Over in the Meadow.** Ezra Jack Keats. (New York: Macmillan Publishers, 1973).

5. **Once We Went on a Picnic.** Arlien Fisher. (New York: Thomas Y. Crowell, 1963).

6. **I Saw the Sea Come In.** Alvin Tresselt. (New York: Lothrop, Lee and Shepard Company, 1970).

7. **A City in the Summer.** Eleanor Schich. (New York: Macmillan, 1970).

8. **The Summer Snowman.** Gene Zion. (New York: Harper and Row Publishers, 1955).

9. **Alex's Adventures at the Beach.** Edward Delgado. (New York: Derrydale Books, 1986).

10. **Summer Is. . .** Charolotte Zolotow. (New York: Thomas Y. Crowell, 1967).

Puzzles:

The following puzzles can be found in preschool educational catalogs:

1. **"Rainbow"** Lauri.

2. **"Volleyball"** Lauri.

3. **"Air Balloon"** Lauri.

4. **"Playground"** Lauri.

5. **"Tree"** Lauri.

6. **"Holiday Parade"** Judy/Instructo.

7. **"The Park"** Judy/Instructo.

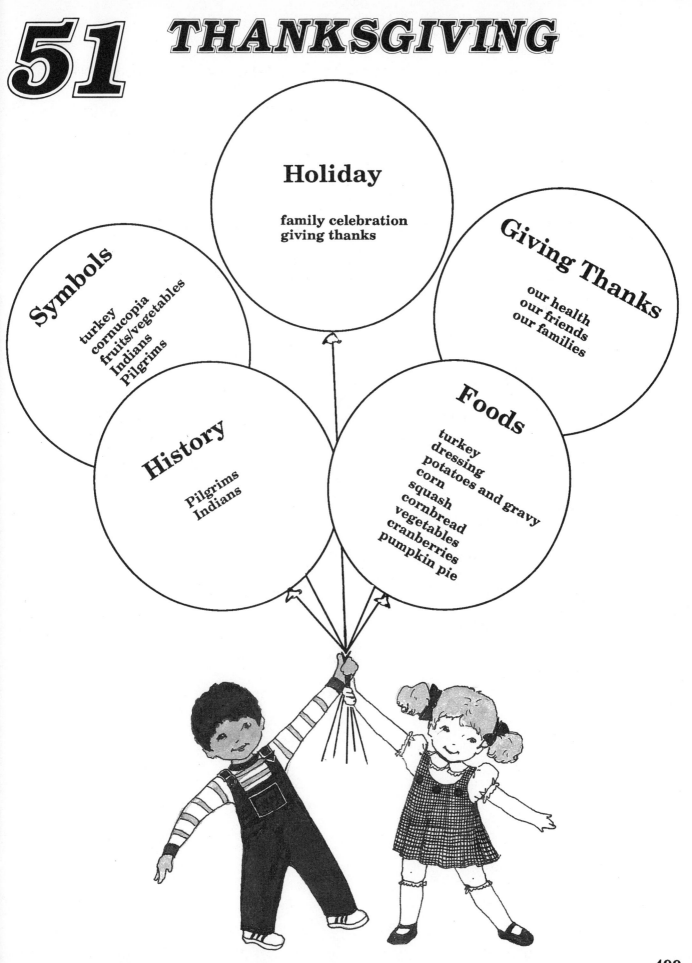

Holiday

family celebration
giving thanks

Giving Thanks

our health
our friends
our families

Symbols

turkey
cornucopia
fruits/vegetables
Indians
Pilgrims

Foods

turkey
dressing
potatoes and gravy
corn
squash
cornbread
vegetables
cranberries
pumpkin pie

History

Pilgrims
Indians

Theme Goals:

Through participating in the experiences provided by this theme, the children may learn:

1. Purpose of Thanksgiving.

2. Thanksgiving celebration.

3. Thanksgiving foods.

4. Thanksgiving symbols.

Concepts for the Children to Learn:

1. Thanksgiving is a holiday.

2. Thanksgiving is a time for giving thanks.

3. Families celebrate together on Thanksgiving.

4. Turkey, dressing, potatoes, vegetables, cranberries and pumpkin pie are often eaten on Thanksgiving.

5. A turkey and cranberries are Thanksgiving symbols.

Vocabulary:

1. **Thanksgiving**—a holiday in November.

2. **Pilgrims**—early settlers who sailed to our country (America).

3. **thankful**—expressing thanks.

4. **turkey**—large bird that is cooked for Thanksgiving.

5. **Indians**—natives who lived in America when the Pilgrims first arrived.

Bulletin Board

The purpose of this bulletin board is to have the children hang the color-coded card onto the corresponding colored feather. Construct a large turkey out of tagboard. Color each feather a different color. Hang the turkey on the bulletin board. Hang push pins in each feather. On small index cards, make a circle of each color and write the color name above it. Use a paper punch to make a hole in each card.

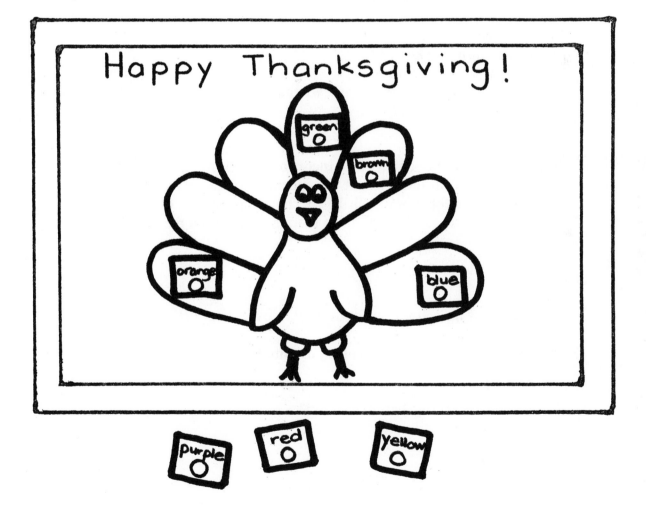

Parent Letter

Dear Parents,

During the month of November each year, we celebrate Thanksgiving. To coincide with this holiday at school, we will be focusing our curriculum on Thanksgiving. Through activities provided, the children will develop an understanding of the foods of Thanksgiving, as well as become more aware of the many people and things for which we are thankful.

At School This Week

Planned learning experiences for the week related to Thanksgiving include:

* popping corn.
* creating hand turkeys.
* visiting a turkey farm.
* exploring various types of corn with scales and magnifying glasses.

At Home

There are many ways for you to incorporate Thanksgiving concepts at home. Talk with your child about the special ways your family celebrates Thanksgiving. Involve your child in the preparation of a traditional Thanksgiving dish. Also emphasize things and people for which you are thankful.

Reminder

There will be no school on Thursday, November 27th.

For those of you who are traveling during the Thanksgiving weekend, drive safely!

Happy Thanksgiving from the staff!

Music:

1. "Popcorn Song"
(Sing to the tune of "I'm a Little Teapot")

I'm a little popcorn in a pot.
Heat me up and watch me pop.
When I get all fat and white, then I'm done.
Popping corn is lots of fun.

2. "If You're Thankful"
(Sing to the tune of "If You're Happy")

If you're thankful and you know it clap
your hands.
If you're thankful and you know it clap
your hands.
If you're thankful and you know it, then
you're face will surely show it,
If you're thankful and you know it, clap
your hands.

Additional verses could include, stomp
your feet, tap your head, turn around,
shout hooray, etc.

Fingerplays:

THANKSGIVING DINNER

Everyday we eat our dinner.
Our table is very small.
  (palms of hands close together)
There's room for father, mother, sister,
brother and me—that's all.
  (point to each finger)
But when it's Thanksgiving Day and the
company comes,
You'd scarcely believe your eyes.
  (rub eyes)
For that very same reason, the table
stretches until it is just this size!
  (stetch arms wide)

THE BIG TURKEY

The big turkey on the farm is so very proud.
  (form fist)
He spreads his tail like a fan
  (spread fingers of other hand being fist)
And struts through the animal crowd.
  (move two fingers of fist as walking)

If you talk to him as he wobbles along;
He'll answer back with a gobbling song.
"Gobble, gobble, gobble."
  (open and close hand)

Science:

1. Corn

Display several types of corn on the
science table. Indian corn, field corn, popcorn and popped popcorn.

2. Wishbone

Bring in a wishbone from a turkey and
place it in a bottle. Pour some vinegar in
the bottle covering the wishbone. Leave
the wishbone in the bottle for 24 hours.
Remove it and feel it. It will feel and bend
like rubber.

Sensory:

The following items can be placed in the
sensory area for the children to discover:

* unpopped or popped popcorn
* pinecones
* cornmeal and measuring cups

Dramatic Play:

Shopping

Set up a grocery store in the dramatic
play area. To stimulate play, provide a
cash register, shopping bags, as well as
empty food containers including boxes,
packages and plastic bottles.

Arts and Crafts:

1. Thanksgiving Collage

Place magazines on the art table for the
children to cut out things they are
thankful for. After the pictures are cut,
they can be pasted on paper to form a
collage.

2. Thanksgiving Feast

Place food items cut from magazines and the newspaper on a table along with paste and paper plates. Let the children select the foods they would like to eat for their Thanksgiving feast.

3. Cornmeal Playdough

Make cornmeal playdough. Mix 2 1/2 cups flour with 1 cup cornmeal. Add 1 tablespoon oil and 1 cup water. Additional water can be added to make desired texture. The dough should have a grainy texture. Cooky cutters and rolling pins can extend this activity.

4. Popcorn Collage

Place popped popcorn and dried tempera paint into small sealable bags. Have children shake bags to color the popcorn. Then have them create designs and pictures by gluing the popcorn onto the paper. You can also use unpopped colored popcorn. Make sure the children do not eat any of the popcorn after it has been mixed with paint.

5. Hand Turkey

Paper, crayons or pencils are needed. Begin by instructing the child to place a hand on a piece of paper. Then tell them to spread their fingers. If possible, have the child trace his own fingers. Otherwise, you need to trace them. The hand can be decorated to create a turkey. Eyes, a beak and a waddle can be added to the outline of the thumb. The fingers can be colored to represent the turkey's feathers. Then legs can be added below the outline of the palm.

Large Muscle:

Popping Corn

Pretend to be popping corn. Begin by demonstrating how to curl down on the floor, explaining that everyone is a kernel of corn. Then plug in popcorn popper and listen to the sounds. Upon hearing popping sounds, jump up and down to the sounds.

Field Trip/Resource Person:

Turkey Farm

Visit a turkey farm. The children can observe the behavior of the turkeys as well as the food they eat.

Math:

1. Turkey Shapes

Give children several geometric shapes to create their own turkeys with circles, squares and triangles. Have children identify the shapes and colors as they create their turkeys.

2. Colored Popcorn

Provide the children with colored popcorn seeds. Place corresponding colored circles in the bottom of muffin tins or egg cartons. Encourage the children to sort the seeds by color.

Group Time (games, language):

1. Turkey Chase

Have the children sit in a circle formation. The game requires two balls of different colors. Vary the size, depending on the age of the children. Generally the younger the child, the larger the ball size. Begin by explaining that the first ball passed is the "turkey." The second ball is the "turkey farmer." The first ball should be passed from child to child around the circle. Shortly after, pass the second ball in the same direction. The game ends when the turkey farmer, the second ball, catches up to the turkey, the first ball. This game is played like hot potato.

2. Feast

Place several kinds of food on a plate in the middle of the circle. Tell the children to cover their eyes. Choose one child to take something from the plate to eat. The child hides one item, and the others open their eyes and try to guess which food item the child has eaten! The number of items included in this activity should be determined by the children's developmental age. Even to begin the activity, it may be advisable to begin with only two food items.

3. Turkey Keeper

To play this game, a turkey cut from cardboard or even a small plastic replica is needed. Instruct one child to cover his eyes. Then quietly hide the turkey in the classroom. After this, instruct the child to open his eyes and begin to look for the turkey. When the child begins walking in the direction of the turkey, the rest of the children quietly provide a clue by saying "Gobble Gobble." As the child approaches the turkey, the children's voices serve as a clue by becoming louder. Once the turkey is located, another child becomes the turkey keeper.

4. Drop the Wishbone

Tell the children to sit in a circle formation. Choose one child to walk around the outside of the circle and drop a wishbone behind another child. (If a real wishbone is unavailable, a wishbone can be cut from cardboard.) The child who had the wishbone dropped behind him must pick it up and chase the first child. If the first child is tagged before he runs around the circle and sits in the second child's place, he is "it" again. If not, the second child is "it." This is a variation of Drop the Handkerchief.

5. Turkey Waddle

Provide the children with verbal and visual clues to waddle like turkeys. The following terms may be used:

* fat turkey
* little turkey
* fast turkey
* slow turkey
* tired turkey
* happy turkey
* proud turkey
* sad turkey
* hungry turkey
* full turkey

Cooking:

1. Fu Fu—West Africa

3 or 4 yams
water
1/2 teaspoon salt
1/8 teaspoon pepper

Optional: 3 tablespoons honey or sugar

Wash and peel yams and cut into 1/2 inch slices. Place slices in a large saucepan and add water to cover them. Bring to a boil over a hot plate or stove. Reduce heat, cover saucepan and simmer for 20 to 25 minutes, until yams are soft enough to mash. Remove saucepan from stove and drain off liquid into a small bowl. Let yams cool for 15 minutes. Place yam slices in a medium-sized mixing bowl, mash with a fork, add salt and pepper, and mash again until smooth. Roll mixture into small, walnut-sized balls. If mixture is too dry, moisten it with a tablespoon of the reserved yam liquid. For sweeter Fu Fu, roll yam balls in a dish of honey or sugar. Makes 24 balls.

2. Muffins

1 egg
3/4 cup milk
1/2 cup vegetable oil
2 cups all purpose flour
1/3 cup sugar
3 tablespoons baking powder
1 teaspoon salt

Heat oven to 400 degrees. Grease bottoms only of 12 medium muffin cups. Beat egg.

Stir in milk and oil. Stir in remaining ingredients all at once just until flour is moistened. Batter will be lumpy. Fill muffin cups about 3/4 full. Bake until golden brown about 20 minutes. For pumpkin muffins: Stir in 1/2 cup pumpkin and 1/2 cup raisins with the milk and 2 teaspoons pumpkin pie spice with the flour.

For cranberry-orange muffins: Stir in 1 cup cranberry halves and 1 tablespoon grated orange peel with milk.

3. Cranberry Freeze

16-ounce can (2 cups) whole cranberry sauce
8-ounce can (1 cup) crushed pineapple, drained
1 cup sour cream or yogurt

In a medium bowl, combine all the ingredients and mix well. Pour the mixture into an 8-inch square pan or an ice cube tray. Freeze 2 hours or until firm. To serve cut into squares or pop out of the ice cube tray.

Record:

The following record can be found in preschool educational catalogs:

Holiday Songs and Rhymes. "Things I am Thankful For." Hap Palmer.

Books and Stories:

The following books and stories can be used to complement the theme:

1. **An Old-Fashioned Thanksgiving.** Louisa Alcott. (Philadelphia: J. B. Lippincott, 1974).

2. **Thanksgiving Day.** Robert Merrill Bartlett. (New York: Thomas Y. Crowell, 1965).

3. **Little Bear's Thanksgiving.** Janice Brustlein. (New York: Lothrop, Lee and Shepard, 1967).

4. **Cranberry Thanksgiving.** Wende Devlin. (New York: Parents Magazine Press, 1971).

5. **It's Thanksgiving.** Jack Prelutsky. (New York: Greenwillow Books, 1982).

6. **The Thanksgiving Story.** Alice Dalgliesh. (New York: Charles Scribner's Sons, 1954).

7. **If You Sailed on the Mayflower.** Ann McGovern. (New York: Four Winds Press, 1969).

8. **The Coming of the Pilgrims.** Brooks Smith. (Boston: Little, Brown and Company, 1964).

9. **Turkeys, Pilgrims and Indian Corn.** Edna Barth. (New York: Seabury Press, 1975).

10. **Feast of Thanksgiving.** June Behrens. (Chicago: Childrens Press, 1976).

11. **The Thanksgiving Treasure.** Gail Rock. (New York: Knopf, 1974).

12. **Our Thanksgiving Book.** Jane Beek Moncure. (Chicago: Child's World, Inc., 1976).

13. **Gobble, Gobble, Gobble.** Mary Jackson Ellis. (Minneapolis, MN: Denison and Company, 1956).

14. **The Pilgrims' Party.** S. and Anson Lowitz. (Minneapolis, MN: Lerner Publishing Company, 1969).

15. **Hard Scrabble Harvest.** Apcar Dahlor. (New York: Doubleday and Company, Inc., 1976).

16. **My First Thanksgiving Book.** Jane Belk Moncure. (Chicago: Childrens Press, 1984).

Puzzles:

The following puzzles can be found in preschool educational catalogs:

1. **"Fruits"** 5 pieces. Puzzle People.

2. **"Thanksgiving"** 20 pieces. Judy/Instructo.

3. **"Vegetables"** 5 pieces. Puzzle People.

4. **"Table Setting"** 10 pieces. Judy/Instructo.

5. **"Thanksgiving Turkey"** 15 knobbed pieces. Puzzle People.

6. **"Thanksgiving"** 15 knobbed pieces. Puzzle People.

52 VALENTINE'S DAY

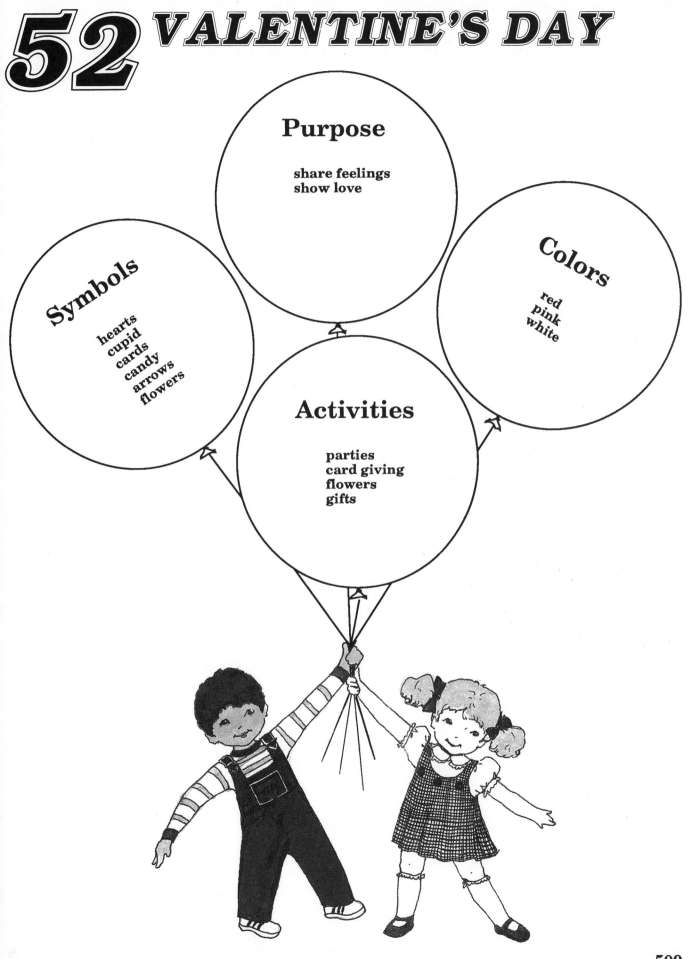

Purpose

share feelings
show love

Symbols

hearts
cupid
cards
candy
arrows
flowers

Colors

red
pink
white

Activities

parties
card giving
flowers
gifts

Theme Goals:

Through participating in the experiences provided by this theme, the children may learn:

1. Valentine's Day colors.

2. Valentine's Day activities.

3. Symbols of Valentine's Day.

4. Purpose of Valentine's Day.

Concepts for the Children to Learn:

1. Red, pink and white are Valentine's Day colors.

2. On Valentine's Day we share our love with others.

3. Hearts, cupids and flowers are symbols of Valentine's Day.

4. People send cards on Valentine's Day.

Vocabulary:

1. **heart**—a symbol of love.

2. **Valentine**—a card designed for someone special.

3. **cupid**—a symbol of Valentine's Day, usually a baby boy with a bow and arrows.

4. **card**—a decorative paper with a written message.

Bulletin Board

The purpose of this bulletin board is to have the children place the correct number of hearts in the corresponding numbered box. Using boxes as illustrated, a Valentine's Day bulletin board can be made. The bottom of each box should be cut, so it can be taped shut while putting hearts in and easily opened to release the hearts. Mark each box with a numeral and a corresponding number of hearts. The number of numerals will depend upon developmental appropriateness. Attach the boxes to the bulletin board using push pins or staples. Next, construct many small hearts.

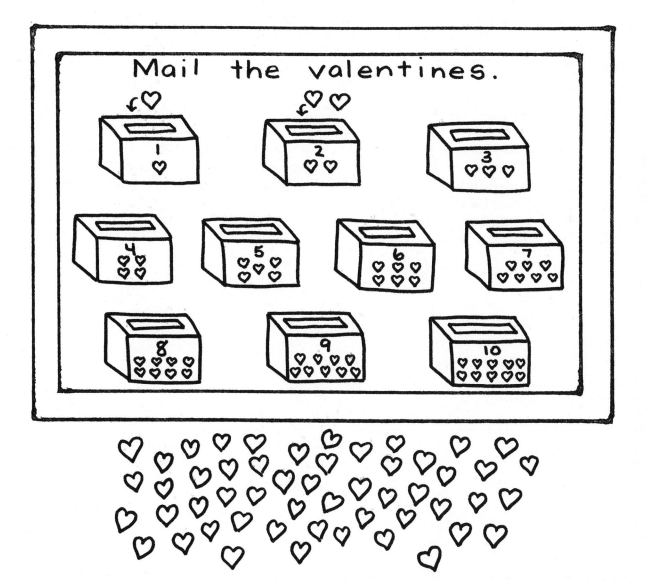

Parent Letter

Dear Parents,

   Valentine's Day is a special day, so this week we will be celebrating Valentine's Day. It is a day when we share our good feelings about special people. This day is also an opportunity to talk about the importance of sharing, giving, loving and friendship.

At School This Week

   Some of the activities this week will include:

* having a post office in dramatic play to mail valentines to friends.
* constructing valentine mobiles to decorate our room.
* constructing a "What a Friend is..." chart to hang in our room.
* Sending and receiving valentines.

At Home

   Try to set aside time to have a heart to heart chat with your child. To develop self esteem talk to your child about feelings and why you are proud of him. Also, help your child make a valentine for a grandparent, aunt, uncle or other person. A special note could be dictated by your child and written by you.

   Have a hearty good week!

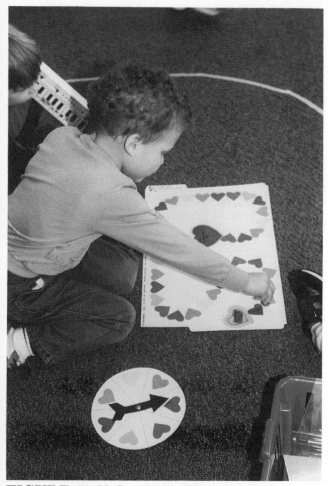

FIGURE 52 Valentine's Day is when everyone says "I Love You!"

Music:

1. **"My Valentine"**
(Sing to the tune of "The Muffin Man")

Oh, do you know my valentine,
My valentine, my valentine?
Oh, do you know my valentine?
His name is _____.

Chosen valentine then picks another child.

2. **"Ten Little Valentines"**
(Sing to the tune of "Ten Little Indians")

One little, two little, three little valentines.
Four little, five little, six little valentines.
Seven little, eight little, nine little valentines.
Ten little valentines here!

3. **"Two Little Cupids"**
(Sing to the tune of "Two Little Blackbirds")

Two little cupids sitting on a heart.
(hold hands behind back)
One named _____. One named _____.
(bring out one pointer for each name)
Fly away _____. Fly away _____.
(place one pointer behind back for each name)
Come back _____. Come back _____.
(bring out pointers one at a time again)
Two little cupids sitting on a heart.
(hold up 2 fingers)
One named _____. One named _____.
(wiggle each pointer separately.)

For each _____ insert a child's name.

Fingerplay:

FIVE LITTLE VALENTINES

Five little valentines were having a race.
The first little valentine was frilly with lace.
(hold up one finger)
The second little valentine had a funny face.
(hold up two fingers)
The third little valentine said, "I love you."
(hold up three fingers)
The fourth little valentine said, "I do too."
(hold up four fingers)
The fifth little valentine was sly as a fox.
He ran the fastest to the valentine box.
(make five fingers run behind back.)

Science:

1. **Valentine's Day Flowers**

In the science area, place various flowers and magnifying glasses. The children can observe and explore the various parts of the flowers.

2. **Valentine's Day Colors**

Mixing red and white tempera paint, the children can make various shades of red or pink.

Dramatic Play:

1. Mailboxes

Construct an individual mailbox for each child using shoeboxes, empty milk cartons, paper bags or partitioned boxes. Print each child's name on the box or encourage the child to do so. The children can sort mail, letters and small packages into the boxes.

2. Florist

Plastic flowers, vases, styrofoam pieces, tissue paper, ribbons, candy boxes, a cash register and play money can be used to make a flower shop.

3. Card Shop

Stencils, paper, markers, scraps, stickers, etc. can be provided to make a card making shop.

Arts and Crafts:

1. Easel Painting

Mix red, white and pink paint and place at the easel.

2. Chalk Drawings

White chalk and red and pink construction paper can be used to make chalk drawings.

3. Classroom Valentine

Cut out one large paper heart. Encourage all children decorate and sign it. The valentine can be hung in the classroom or be given to a classroom friend. The classroom friend may be the cook, janitor, center director or principal.

4. Heart Prints

On the art table place white paper and various heart-shaped cookie cutters. Mix pink and red tempera paint and pour into shallow pans. The children can print hearts on white construction paper by using the cookie cutters as a tool and then paint them.

5. Heart Materials

The children can cut hearts out of construction paper and decorate them with lace scraps, yarn and glitter to make original Valentine's Day cards. Precut hearts should be available for children who have not mastered the skill. For other children who have cutting skills, a heart shape can be traced on paper for them to cut.

Sensory:

Soap

Mix dish soap, water and red food coloring in the sensory table. Provide egg beaters for children to make bubbles.

Large Muscle:

1. Hug Tag

One child is "it" and tries to tag another child. Once tagged, the child is "frozen" until another child gently hugs him to "unfreeze" them.

2. Balloon Ball

Blow up two or three red, pink or white balloons. Using nylon paddles made by stretching nylon pantyhose over bent coat hangers, the children can hit the balloons to each other. The objective is to try to keep the balloon up off the floor or ground. This activity needs to be carefully supervised. If a balloon breaks, it needs to be immediately removed.

Field Trips/Resource People:

1. Visit a Post Office

Visit the local post office. Valentine's Day cards made in the classroom can be mailed.

2. Visit a Floral Shop

Visit a flower store. Observe the different valentine arrangements. Call attention to the beautiful color of the flowers, arrangements and containers.

Math:

1. Broken Hearts

Cut heart shapes out of red and pink tagboard. Print a numeral on one side and a number set of heart stickers or drawings on the other side. Cut the hearts in half as a puzzle. The children can match the puzzle pieces.

2. Heart Seriation

Cut various sized hearts from pink, red and white construction paper. The children can sequence the heart shapes from small to big or vice versa.

Social Studies:

1. Sorting Feelings

Cut pictures of happy and sad people out of magazines. On the outside of two boxes, draw a smiling face on one and a sad face on the other. The children can sort the pictures into the corresponding boxes.

2. Sign Language

Show the children how to say "I love you" in sign language. They can practice with each other. When the parents arrive, the children can share with them.

I	Point to self
love	Cross arms over chest
you	Point outwards

Group Time (games, language):

Valentine March

Place large material hearts with numerals on them on the floor. Include one valentine per child. Play a marching song and encourage children to march from heart to heart. When music stops, so do children. Each child then tells the numeral he is standing on. To make the activity developmentally appropriate for young children, use symbols. Examples might include a ball, car, truck, glass, cup, door, etc.

Cooking:

1. Valentine Cookies

2/3 cup shortening
1 egg
3/4 cup sugar
1 teaspoon vanilla
1 1/2 cups flour
1 1/2 teaspoons baking powder
4 teaspoons milk
1/4 teaspoon salt

Mix all of the ingredients together. If time permits, refrigerate the dough. Roll out dough. Use heart-shaped cookie cutters. Bake at 375 degrees for 12 minutes. Frost. The children can make two cookies, one for themselves and one to give a friend.

2. Heart-shaped Sandwiches

1 loaf bread
heart-shaped cookie cutters
strawberry jam or jelly

Give each child 1 or 2 pieces of bread (depending on size of cutter). Cut out 2 heart shapes from bread. Spread on jam or jelly to make a sandwich. Eat at snack time.

MATERIALS TO COLLECT FOR THE ART CENTER

aluminum foil
ball bearings
barrel hoops
beads
belts
bottles
bracelets
braiding
brass
buckles
burlap
buttons
candles
cartons
canvas
cellophane
chains
chalk
chamois
clay
cloth
colored pictures
confetti
containers
copper foil
cord
corn husks
corn stalks
costume jewelry
crayon pieces
crystals
emery cloth
eyelets
fabrics
felt
felt hats
flannel
floor covering
glass
gourds
hat boxes
hooks
inner tubes
jars

jugs
lacing
lampshades
leather remnants
linoleum
marbles
masonite
metal foil
mirrors
muslin
nails
necklaces
neckties
oilcloth
ornaments
pans
paper bags
paper boxes
paper cardboard
paper corregated
paper dishes
paper doilies
paper napkins
paper newspaper
paper tissue
paper towels
paper tubes
paper wrapping
phonograph records
photographs
picture frames
pinecones
pins
pipe cleaners
plastic bags
plastic board
plastic paint
pocket books
reeds
ribbon
rings
rope
rubber bands

rug yarn
safety pins
sand
sandpaper
seashells
seeds
sheepskin
shoelaces
shoe polich
snaps
soap
sponges
spools
stockings
sweaters
tacks
tape
thread
tiles
tin cans
tin foil
tongue depressors
towels
tubes
twine
wallpaper
wax
window blinds
wire
wire eyelets
wire hairpins
wire hooks
wire mesh
wire paper clips
wire screen
wire staples
wooden beads
wooden blocks
wooden clothespins
wooden sticks
wool
yarn
zippers

Records:

The following records can be found in preschool educational catalogs:

1. **The Singing Calendar.** Kimbo Records.

2. **Holiday Songs and Rhythms.** Hap Palmer.

Books and Stories:

The following books and stories can be used to complement the theme:

1. **The Great Valentine's Day Balloon Race.** Adrienne Adams. (New York: Charles Scribner's Sons, 1980).

2. **Four Valentines in a Rainstorm.** Felicia Bond. (New York: Thomas Y. Crowell, 1983).

3. **Arthur's Valentines.** Mark Brown. (Boston: Little, Brown, 1980).

4. **The Valentine Bears.** Eve Bunting. (New York: Clarion Books, 1983).

5. **Bee My Valentine.** Miriam Cohen. (New York: William Morrow and Company, Inc., 1978).

6. **One Zillion Valentines.** Frank Modell. (New York: William Morrow and Company, Inc., 1981).

7. **The Best Valentine in the World.** Marjorie Shermat. (New York: Holiday House, 1982).

8. **My First Valentine's Day Book.** Marion Bennett. (Chicago: Childrens Press, 1985).

Puzzles:

The following puzzles can be found in preschool educational catalogs:

1. **"Valentine's Day"** 19 pieces. Judy/Instructo.

2. **"Valentine Heart"** 16 pieces. Puzzle People.

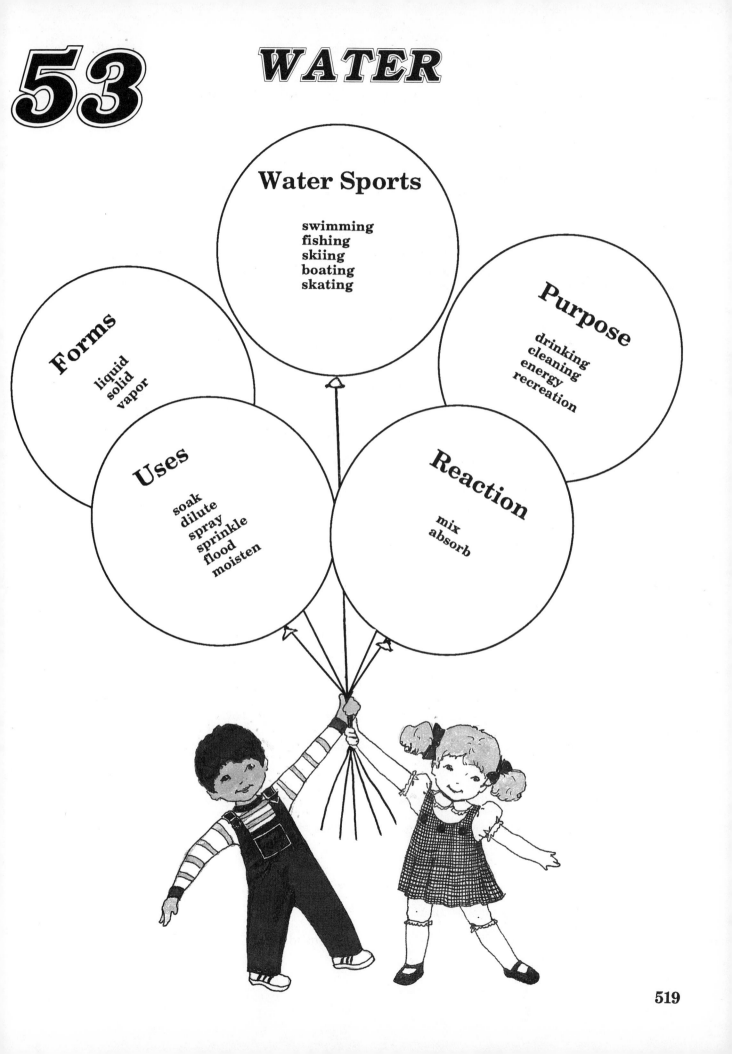

53 WATER

Water Sports

swimming
fishing
skiing
boating
skating

Purpose

drinking
cleaning
energy
recreation

Forms

liquid
solid
vapor

Uses

soak
dilute
spray
sprinkle
flood
moisten

Reaction

mix
absorb

Theme Goals:

Through participating in the experiences provided by this theme, the children may learn:

1. Uses of water.
2. Forms of water.
3. Water sports.
4. Purposes of water.

Concepts for the Children to Learn:

1. All living things need water.
2. Water takes three forms: liquid, vapor and solid.
3. Ice is a solid form of water.
4. Steam is a vapor form of water.
5. Some things mix with water, others do not.
6. Some things absorb water, others do not.
7. Some things float when placed on water.
8. Some animals and plants live in bodies of water.
9. Water can be used to soak, dilute, spray, sprinkle, flood and moisten.

Vocabulary:

1. **water**—a clear, colorless, odorless, tasteless liquid.
2. **lake**—a large body of water surrounded by land.
3. **ocean**—body of salt water.
4. **swimming**—moving yourself through water with body movements.
5. **cloud**—water droplets formed in the sky.
6. **rain**—water that falls from clouds.
7. **snow**—water that freezes and falls from the sky.
8. **liquid**—substance that can be poured.
9. **freeze**—hardened liquid.
10. **melt**—to change from a solid to a liquid.
11. **ice**—water that has frozen.
12. **sink**—to drop to the bottom of a liquid.
13. **float**—to rest on top of a liquid.

Bulletin Board

The purpose of this bulletin board is to develop visual discrimination and matching skills. Construct and color four or five pictures of swimming and water-related items from tagboard. Laminate. Trace these pictures on black construction paper to make shadows. Staple the shadows on the bulletin board. Encourage the children to hang the colored picture over the correct shadow.

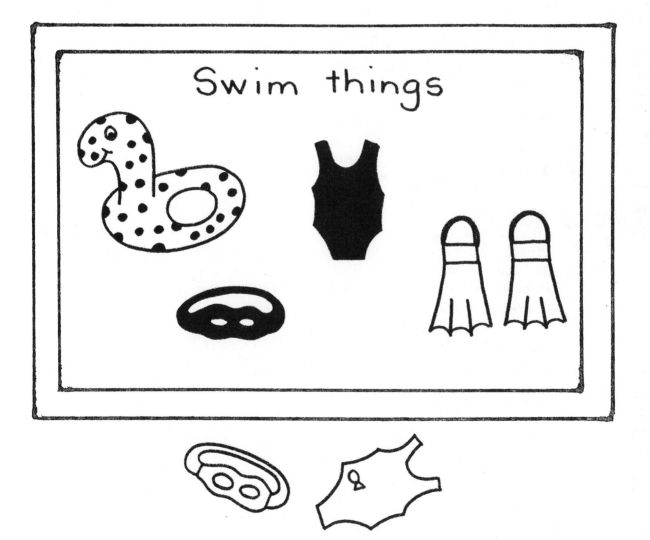

Parent Letter

Dear Parents,

Did you know all living things have something in common? All living things need water to survive. Water will be the subject that we will explore this week. The children will become familiar with the forms, uses and bodies of water, as well as sports that require water to be played.

At School This Week

Some of the learning experiences planned to include water concepts are:

* placing celery stalks in colored water to observe plants' use of water.
* experimenting with objects that sink or float when placed in water.
* washing doll clothes in the sensory table.
* observing ice with magnifying glasses and watching it change from a solid to a liquid.

At Home

There are many ways that you can reinforce water concepts at home. Try any of the following with your child.

* Allow your child to assist in washing dishes after a meal. This will give your child a sense of responsibility and will develop self-esteem.
* Provide water and large paintbrushes for your child to paint sidewalks and fences outdoors.
* Bubbles made with an eggbeater in a container of soapy water are fun for children of all ages!

Enjoy the week!

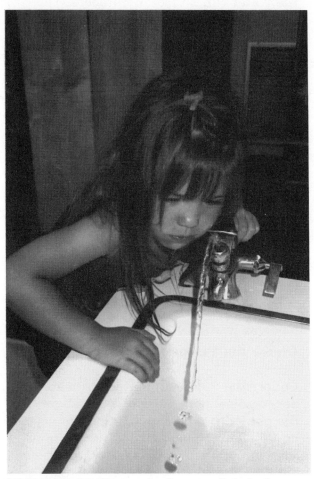

FIGURE 53 Water is fun to drink from the fountain.

Music:

"Raindrops"
(Sing to the tune of "London Bridges")

Raindrops falling from the sky,
From the sky, from the sky.
Raindrops falling from the sky
On my umbrella.

Fingerplays:

FIVE LITTLE DUCKS

Five little ducks
   (hold up five fingers)
Swimming in the lake.
   (make swimming motions)
The first duck said,
   (hold up one finger)
"Watch the waves I make."

   (make waves motions)
The second duck said,
   (hold up two fingers)
"Swimming is such fun."
   (smile)
The third duck said,
   hold up three fingers)
"I'd rather sit in the sun."
   (turn face to sun)
The fourth duck said,
   (hold up four fingers)
"Let's swim away."
   (swimming motions)
The fifth duck said,
   (hold up five fingers)
"Oh, let's stay."
Then along came a motorboat.
With a Pop! Pop! Pop!
   (clap three times)
And five little ducks
Swam away from the spot.
   (put five fingers behind back)

SWIMMING

I can dive.
   (make diving motion with hands)
I can swim.
   (swimming motion)
I can float.
   (hands outstretched with head back)
I can fetch.
But dog paddle
   (paddle like dog)
Is the stroke I do best.

FIVE LITTLE FISHES

Five little fishes swimming in a pond.
   (wiggle five fingers)
The first one said, "I'm tired," as he yawned.
   (yawn)
The second one said, "Well, let's take a nap."
   (put hands together on side of face)
The third one said, "Put on your sleeping cap."
   (pretend to pull on hat)
The fourth one said, "Wake up! Don't sleep."
   (shake finger)
The fifth one said, "Let's swim where it's deep."
   (point down and say with a low voice)
So, the five little fishes swam away.
   (wiggle fingers and put behind back)

But they came back the very next day.
   (wiggle fingers out front again)

THE RAIN

I sit before the window now
   (sit down)
And look out at the rain.
   (shade eyes and look around)
It means no play outside today,
   (shake head)
So inside I remain.
   (rest chin on fist; look sad)

I watch the water dribble down
   (look up and down)
As it turns the brown grass green.
And after a while I start to smile
At nature's washing machine.
   (smile and lean back)

Science:

1. Painting Sidewalks

On a sunny day, allow children to paint
sidewalks with water. To do this, provide
with various paintbrushes and buckets of
water. Call attention to the water
evaporation.

2. Measuring Rainfall

During spring, place a bucket outside with
a plastic ruler set vertically by securing to
the bottom. Check the height of the water
after each rainfall. With older children,
make a chart to record rainfalls.

3. Testing Volume

Containers that hold the same amounts of
liquid are needed. Try to include containers that are tall, skinny, short and
flat. Ask the children, "Do they hold the
same amount?" Encourage them to experiment by pouring liquids from one container to another.

4. Freezing Water

Freeze a container of water. Periodically
observe the changes. In colder climates,
the water can be frozen outdoors. The
addition of food coloring may add interest.

5. Musical Scale

Make unique musical tone jars by pouring
various levels of water into glass soda bottles. Color each bottle of water differently.
Provide the children with spoons, encouraging them to experiment with sounds
by tapping each bottle.

6. Plants Use Water

Place celery stalks in colored water.
Observe how water is absorbed in its
veins.

7. Chase the Pepper

Collect the following materials: water, pepper, shallow pan, piece of soap, sugar. Fill
the pan with water and shake the pepper
on the water. Then take a piece of wet
soap and dip it into the water. What happens? (The pepper moves away from the
soapy water to the clear water.) The skin
on water pulls and on soapy water the pull
is weak. On clear water it is strong and
pulls the pepper along. Now take some
sugar and shake it into the soapy water.
What happens? Sugar gives the skin a
stronger pull.

8. Warm Water/Cold Water

Collect the following materials: a small
aquarium, a small bottle, food coloring,
water. First fill the aquarium with very
warm water. Fill the small bottle with colored cold water. Put your thumb on the
mouth of the bottle. Hold the bottle
sideways and lower it into the warm
water. Take away your thumb. What
happens? (The cold water will sink to the
bottom of the tank. The cold water is
heavier than the warm water.) Now fill
the tank with cold water and fill the small
bottle with colored warm water. What do
you predict will happen when you repeat
the procedure?

9. Wave Machine

Collect the following materials: mineral oil, water, food coloring, transparent jar. Fill the jar 1/2 to 2/3 full with water. Add a few drops of food coloring. Then add mineral oil to completely fill the jar. Secure the lid on the jar. Tilt the jar slowly from side to side to make waves. Notice that the oil and water have separate layers and do not stay mixed after the jar is shaken.

10. Water and Vinegar Fun

Collect the following materials: two small jars with lids, water and white vinegar. Pour water into one jar and an equal amount of vinegar into the other jar. Replace caps. Then let the children explore the jars of liquids and discuss the similarities. Then let the children smell each jar.

Dramatic Play:

1. Firefighter

Place hoses, hats, coats and boots in the dramatic play area.

2. Doll Baths

Fill the dramatic play sink with water. Children can wash dishes or give dolls baths.

3. The Beach

Provide towels, sunglasses, umbrellas, pails, shovels and beach toys for the children to use indoors or outdoors.

4. Canoeing

Bring a canoe into the classroom or onto the play yard. Provide paddles and life vests for the children to wear.

Arts and Crafts:

1. Liquid Painting

Paper, straws, thin tempera and spoons can be placed on the art table. Spoon a small amount of paint onto paper. Using a straw, blow paint on the paper to make a design.

2. Bubble Prints

Collect the following materials: 1/2 cup water, 1/2 cup liquid soap, food coloring, straws and light-colored construction paper. Mix together the water, soap and food coloring in a container. Place a straw in the solution and blow until the bubbles reach about one to two inches over the top of the container. Remove the straw and place a piece of paper over the jar. The bubbles will pop as they touch the paper, leaving a print.

3. Wet Chalk Drawings

Chalk, paper and water in a shallow pan are needed for this activity. The children can dip chalk into water and then draw on paper. Encourage children to note the difference between wet and dry chalk.

Sensory:

1. Colored Ice

Fill the sensory table with colored ice cubes for the children to explore.

2. Sink and Float

Fill sensory table with water. Provide the children with a variety of items that will sink and float. Let them experiment. A chart may be prepared listing items that sink and float.

3. Boating

Fill the water table. Let the children add blue food coloring. Provide a variety of boats for them to play with.

4. Moving Water

Provide the children with a variety of materials that move water. Include the following:

* sponges
* basters
* eye droppers
* squeeze bottles
* funnels
* measuring cups
* pitchers
* empty film canisters
* plastic tubing

Large Muscle:

Catch Me

Children form a circle with one child in the middle. While walking in a circle they chant:

_____ over the water.
_____ over the sea.
_____ caught a tunafish.
But he can't catch me!

(Insert child's name.)

On "me" all the children stoop quickly. If the child in the middle touches another child, the fish, before he stoops, that child is it. Likewise, he now goes into the middle. This game is for older children.

Math:

Measuring

Assorted measuring cups of a variety of sizes can be added to the sensory table or sand box.

Group Time (games, language):

Water Fun

Discuss the various recreational uses of water. Included may be swimming, boating, ice fishing, ice skating, fishing and canoeing. Encourage the children to name their favorite water activities. Prepare a chart using each child's name and favorite water activity along with a small picture of that activity. Display in the room.

Cooking:

1. Fruit Ice

Mix 1/2 can partially thawed juice concentrate with 2 cups of crushed ice in the blender. Liquify until the contents become snowy. Serve immediately.

2. Floating Cake—Philippines

2 cups sweet rice flour
1 cup water
1/2 to 3/4 cup sugar
1/2 cup toasted sesame seeds, hulled
1 cup grated coconut

Mix rice flour and water. Form into 10 to 20 small balls. Flatten each ball into a round or elongated shape and drop into 8 to 10 cups boiling water. As each cake floats to the surface, remove from water with a slotted spoon. Roll in grated coconut and coat with sugar and sesame seeds. Adult supervision is required. Makes 4 servings.

Sensory experiences are especially appealing to young children. They delight in feeling, listening, smelling, tasting and seeing. They also love to manipulate objects by pulling, placing, pouring, tipping, shoving, as well as dipping. As they interact, they learn new concepts and solutions to old problems. When accompanied by other children, these experiences lead to cooperative, social interactions. As a result, the child's egocentricity is reduced, allowing him to become less self-centered.

Containers

Begin planning sensory experiences by choosing an appropriate container. Remember that it should be large enough so that several children may participate at any given time. If you select a dishpan, due to its size, you may want to use several. Other containers that may be used include a commercially-made sensory/water table, baby bathtub, wash tub, pail, wading pool, sink or bath tub.

Things to Add to Water

A variety of substances can be added to water to make it more inviting. Food coloring is one example. Start by individually choosing and adding one primary color. Later soaps can be added. These may be in liquid or flake form. Baking soda, cornstarch and salt will affect the feel of the water. Whereas, baby and vegetable oil may leave a residue on the child's hand. Extracts add another dimension. Lemon, almond, pine oil, peppermint, anise and orange all permit a variety for the child. On the other hand, ice cubes allow the child to experience an extreme touch.

Tools and Utensils

A wide variety of household tools can be used in the water play table. Measuring cups, small pitchers, small pots and pans and film canisters can all be used for pouring. Scoops, spoons, turkey basters, small squeeze bottles and funnels can be used for transferring the liquid from one container to another. Pipes, rubber hoses, sponges, wire whips and eggbeaters all can be used for observing water in motion. Plastic toys, corks, spools, strainers, boots, etc. also encourage exploration.

Other Sensory Experiences

There are wide varieties of other materials that can be used in the sensory table. Natural materials such as sand, gravel, rocks, grain, mud, wood chips, clay, corn and birdseed can be used. Children also enjoy having minnows and worms in the table. They delight in visually tracking the minnow and worm movement. As they attempt to pick them up, eye-hand coordination skills are practiced. Styrofoam pieces and shavings are attractive materials that can lend variety.

A strange mixture called goop is a fun material to play with. To prepare goop empty 1 box of cornstarch into a dishpan or similar container. Sprinkle a few drops of food coloring on the cornstarch. Add small amounts of water (about 1/2 cup) at a time and mix with a spoon or with fingers. (This is a unique sensory experience!) The mixture feels hard when you touch it on the surface, yet melts in your hands when you pick some up! (This will keep for up to one week if kept covered when not in use. You will probably need to add water the next time you use it.)

Silly putty is just as easy to prepare as goop. This mixture is prepared by combining

1 part of liquid starch, 2 parts of white glue and dry tempera paint for color. Begin by measuring the liquid starch first, as it will prevent the glue from sticking to the measuring cup. Mix with a spoon adding single tablespoons of liquid starch to get the right consistency.

Then knead with hands. Store in an air-tight container (such as a zip-lock bag) in the refrigerator. You will be thrilled to find that it will keep for several weeks.

Enjoy yourself with the children, but always change the sensory experiences on a daily basis. In doing so, you stimulate the child's curiosity as well as provide a meaningful curriculum.

For health purposes, children should be encouraged to wash their hands after sensory play.

Records:

The following record can be found in preschool educational catalogs:

Rhythms of Childhood with Ella Jenkins. Folkway Records.

Books and Stories:

The following books and stories can be used to complement the theme:

1. **Fish Is Fish.** Lee Lionni. (New York: Pantheon, 1970).

2. **Umbrella.** Taro Yaṣhima. (New York: Viking Press, 1958).

3. **Water All Around.** Tillie Pine. (New York: McGraw-Hill, 1959).

4. **Wonders Of The Pond.** Francene Sabin. (New York: Troll Associates, 1982).

5. **Walk In The Snow.** Phyllis Busch. (New York: J. B. Lippincott, 1971).

6. **Fog In The Meadow.** Joanne Ryder. (New York: Harper and Row, 1979).

7. **Follow The Brook.** Howard Knotts. (New York: Harper and Row, 1975).

8. **Water For Dinosaurs and You.** Roma Gans. (New York: Thomas Y. Crowell, 1972).

9. **Do You Know About Water?** Mae Freeman. (New York: Random House, 1970).

10. **Rain.** Robert Kalan. (New York: Greenwillow Books, 1978).

11. **Rain Rain River.** Uri Schulevitz. (New York: Farrar and Straus, 1969).

12. **Davey's First Boat.** Leonard Shartall. (New York: William Morrow, 1963).

13. **Peter Spier's Rain.** Peter Spier. (New York: Doubleday, 1982).

14. **The Water We Drink!** Enid Bloome. (Garden City, NY: Doubleday, 1971).

15. **Down By the Bay.** Raffi. (New York: Crown Publishers, Inc., 1987).

16. **Alex's Adventures at the Beach.** Edward Delgado. (New York: Derrydale Books, 1986).

17. **Splish, Splash!** Yvonne Hooker. (New York: Gossset and Dunlap, 1981).

18. **Life in Ponds and Streams.** William H. Amos. (Washington, DC: National Geographic Society, 1981).

19. **Exploring the Seashore.** William H. Amos. (Washington, DC: National Geographic Society, 1984).

20. **Pond Life.** Lynn M. Stone. (Chicago: Childrens Press, 1983).

21. **A Salmon For Simon.** Betty Waterton. (New York: Antheneum, 1980).

22. **Rub-A-Dub-Dub-What's In the Tub?** Mary Blocksma. (Chicago: Childrens Press, 1987).

23. **My Favorite Place.** Susan Sargent and Donna Aaron Wirl. (Nashville: Abingdon Press, 1983).

24. **From Ice to Rain.** Marlene Reidel. (Minneapolis, MN: Carolrhoda, 1981).

Puzzles:

The following puzzles can be found in preschool educational catalogs:

1. **"Fish"** 6 pieces. Judy/Instructo.

2. **"Fish"** 12 pieces. Lauri.

3. **"Tug"** 12 pieces. Judy/Instructo.

4. **"Sea Horse"** 5 pieces. Childcraft.

5. **"Frog"** 5 pieces. Childcraft.

6. **"Lobster"** 9 pieces. Childcraft.

7. **"Goldfish"** 7 pieces. Childcraft.

8. **"Rain"** 4 pieces. Judy/Instructo.

9. **"Fishing Hole"** 16 pieces. Judy/Instructo.

54 WHEELS

Sizes

many

Functions

movement
transportation

Materials

rubber
plastic
wood
metal

Uses

bicycles
motorcycles
trikes
scooters
cars/trucks
buses
planes
unicycles
wagons
wheelbarrows
carts
chairs
trailers
rollerskates
pulleys
gears
trains
wheelchairs

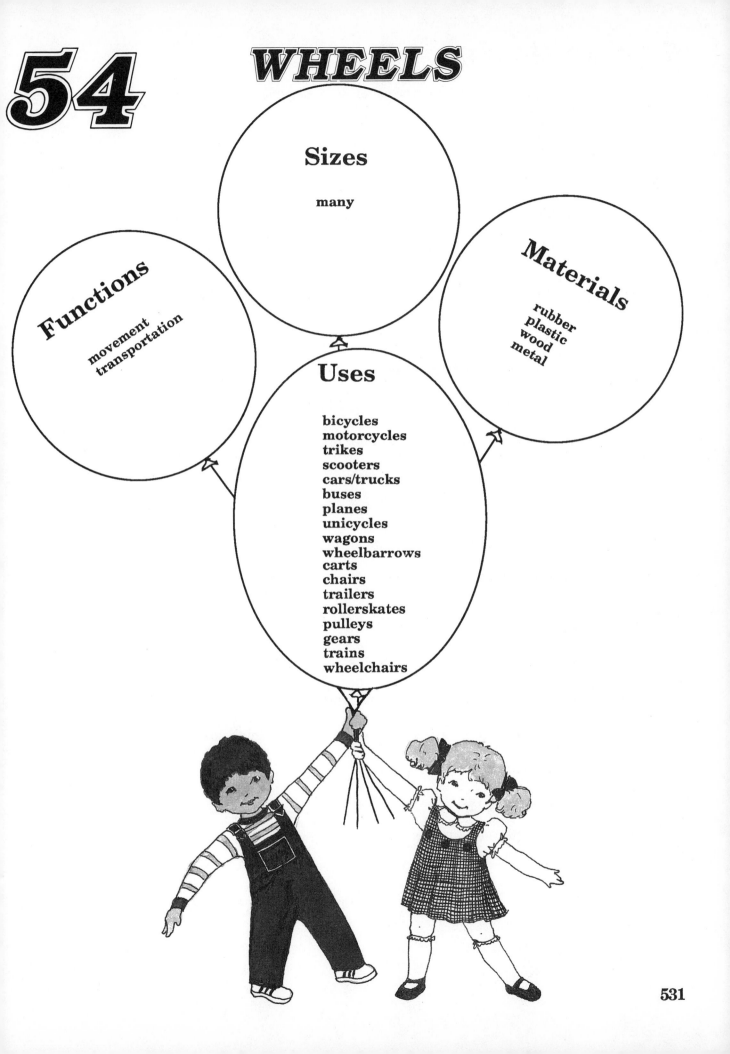

Theme Goals:

Through participating in the experiences provided by this theme, the children may learn:

1. Sizes of wheels.

2. Purposes of wheels.

3. Materials used to make wheels.

4. Movement of wheels.

Concepts for the Children to Learn:

1. Wheels are round.

2. Wheels can help us to do our work.

3. Wheels help move people and things.

4. Cars, buses, motorcycles and bicycles have wheels.

5. Wheels can be different sizes.

6. A unicycle is a one-wheeled cycle.

7. Wheels can be made of rubber, plastic, metal or wood.

8. Wheels can be connected by an axle.

Vocabulary:

1. **wheel**—a form in the shape of a circle.

2. **unicycle**—a vehicle with one wheel.

3. **wheelbarrow**—a vehicle used for moving small loads.

4. **wheelchair**—a chair on wheels.

5. **bicycle**—a two-wheeled vehicle.

6. **pulley**—a wheel that can be connected to a rope to move things.

Bulletin Board

The purpose of this bulletin board is to encourage the development of mathematical concepts. To prepare the bulletin board, draw pictures of a unicycle, bicycle and tricycle on tagboard. Color, cut out and post on the bulletin board. Next, construct the numerals 1, 2 and 3 out of tagboard. Hang the numerals on the top of the bulletin board. A corresponding set of dots can be placed below the numeral to assist children in counting. A string can be attached to each numeral by using a stapler. Have the children wind the string around a push pin connected to the vehicle with the corresponding number of wheels.

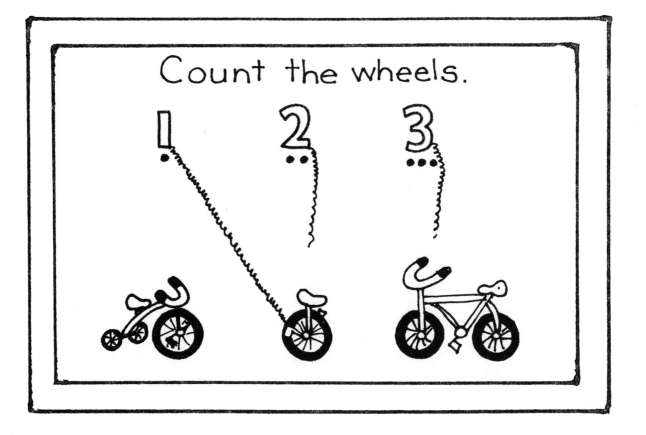

Parent Letter

Dear Parents,

Wheels! Wheelchairs, wheelbarrows, bicycle wheels and car wheels! Children see wheels almost every day of their lives. We will be studying wheels this week in our center. Through participating in the activities planned for this unit, the children will discover that wheels can be made from many different materials and that there are many different uses and sizes of wheels.

At School This Week

We have many learning experiences planned for this week which include:

* examining tire rubber at the science table.
* painting with toy cars at the art table.
* singing a song called "The Wheels on the Bus."

At Home

There are many ways that you can incorporate this unit in your own home. Try any of these activities with your child.

* Walk around the neighborhood with your child. To develop observation skills look for different wheels.
* Count the wheels on the different types of transportation. Semi-trucks have several, while a unicycle has only one.
* Recite the following fingerplay with your child to foster language and memory skills. We will be learning it this week.

Wheels

Wheels big.
  (form big circles with fingers)
Wheels small.
  (form little circles with fingers)
Count them one by one.
Turning as they're pedaled
  (make pedaling motion with hands)
In the springtime sun!
1-2-3-4-5
  (count fingers)

Have a great week!

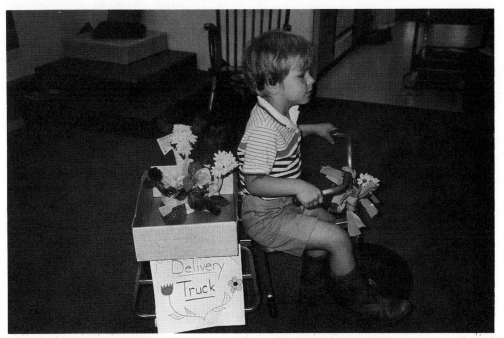

FIGURE 54 Wheels are important for transportation.

Music:

"The Wheels on the Bus"

The wheels on the bus go round and
round,
Round and round, round and round.
The wheels on the bus go round and round
All through the town.

Other verses:
The wipers on the bus go swish, swish, swish.
The doors on the bus go open and shut.
The horn on the bus goes beep, beep, beep.
The driver on the bus says, "Move on back."
The people on the bus go up and down.

Fingerplays:

MY BICYCLE

One wheel, two wheels on the ground.
  (revolve hand in forward circle to form
  each wheel)
My feet make the pedals go round and
round.
  (move feet in pedaling motion)
Handle bars help me steer so straight
  (pretend to steer bicycle)
Down the sidewalk, through the gate.

WHEELS

Wheels big.
  (form big circles with fingers)
Wheels small.
  (form little circles with fingers)
Count them one by one
Turning as they're pedaled
  make pedaling motion with hands)
In the springtime sun.
1-2-3-4-5
  (count fingers)

Science:

1. **Tire Rubber**

   Cut off several pieces of rubber from old
   tires. Provide magnifying glasses.
   Encourage the children to observe
   similarities and differences.

2. **Pulley**

   Set up a pulley. Provide the children with
   blocks so they may lift a heavy load with
   the help of a wheel. Supervision may be
   necessary for this activity.

3. Gears

Collect gears and place on the science table. The children can experiment, observing how the gears move. When appropriate, discuss their similar and different characterisitics.

4. Wheels and Axles

Set out a few wheels and axles. Discuss how they work as a lever to help lift heavy loads. Encourage the children to think about where they might find wheels and axles.

Dramatic Play:

1. Car Mechanic

Outdoors, place various wheels, tires, tools, overalls and broken trikes. The children can experiment using tools.

2. Floats

Paper, tape, crepe paper and balloons can be provided to decorate the wheels on the tricycles, wagons and scooters.

Arts and Crafts:

1. Circle Templates

Cut out various sized circle templates from tagboard. Provide paper, pencils, and crayons for the children to trace the circles.

2. Car Painting

Provide small plastic cars, tempera paint and paper. Place the tempera paint in a shallow pan. Car tracks can be created by dipping the car wheels in the tempera paint and rolling them across paper.

3. Wheel Collage

Provide magazines for the children to cut out pictures of wheels. The pictures can be pasted or glued onto sheets of paper.

4. Tracing Wheels

Provide sewing tracing wheels, pizza cutters, pastry wheels, carbon paper and construction paper. The children can place the carbon paper on the construction paper and with one of the wheels run it over the carbon paper making a design on the construction paper.

Sensory:

Sensory Table

Add the following items to the sensory table:

* sand with wheel molds
* rubber from tires
* gravel and small toy cars and trucks

Large Muscle:

1. Wheelbarrow

Place wheelbarrows in the play yard. Provide materials of varying weights for the children to move.

2. Wagons

Place wagons in the playground. Provide objects for the children to move.

Field Trips/Resource People:

1. Cycle Shop

Visit a cycle shop. Observe the different sizes of wheels that are in the shop. Talk about the different materials that wheels can be made of.

2. Machine Shop

Visit a machine parts shop. Look at the different gears, pulleys and wheels. Discuss their sizes, shapes and possible uses.

3. Resource People

* cycle specialist
* mechanic
* machinist
* person who uses a wheelchair

Math:

1. Wheel Sequence

Cut out various sized circles from tagboard to represent wheels. The children can sequence the wheels from largest to smallest.

2. How Many Wheels?

Pictures of a unicycle, bicycle, tricycle, cars, scooters and trucks of all sizes can be cut from magazines and catalogs. Mount the pictures on tagboard. Laminate. Sort the pictures according to the number of wheels.

Social Studies:

Wheelchair

Borrow wheelchair (child-sized if possible) from a local hospital or pharmacy. During group time discuss how wheelchairs help some people to move. Children can experience moving and pushing a wheelchair.

Records:

The following records can be found in preschool educational catalogs:

1. Rise and Shine. "The Wheels on the Bus" Raffi.

2. Special Delivery. "Marvelous Toy" Fred Penner.

Books and Stories:

The following books and stories can be used to complement the theme:

1. Wings and Wheels. Cynthia Chapman. (Niles, IL: Albert Whitman & Co., 1967).

Group Time (games, language):

Who Took the Wheel?

(Variation of "Who Took the Cookie From the Cookie Jar")

Who took the wheel off the car today?
_____ took the wheel off the car today.
(fill _____ with a child's name)
Chosen child says, "Who me?"
Class responds, "Yes, you!"
Chosen child says, "Couldn't be!"
Class responds, "Well then, who?"

The chant continues as the chosen child picks another child. Continue repeating the chant using the children's names.

Cooking:

1. Cheese Wheels

Cut cheese slices using a cookie cutter into circle shapes to represent wheels. Top the pieces with raisins or serve with crackers.

2. Pizza Rounds

Provide each child with a half an English muffin. Demonstrate how to spread pizza sauce on a muffin. Then lay a few skinny strips of cheese across the top, making the cheese look like wheel spokes. Now let the children prepare their own. Bake in an oven at 350 degrees for 5 to 7 minutes or until the cheese melts. Cool slightly before serving.

2. **Cars, Trucks, Things that Go.** Richard Scarry. (New York: Golden Press, 1974).

3. **Wheels.** Byron Barton. (New York: Thomas Y. Crowell, 1979).

4. **Skates.** Ezra Jack Keats. (New York: Franklin Watts Inc., 1973).

5. **Curious George Rides a Bike.** H.A. Rey. (Boston: Houghton Mifflin, 1952).

6. **Willy and His Wagon Wheel.** Gail Gibbons. (Englewood Cliffs, NJ: Prentice Hall, 1975).

7. **Wheels.** Wilfred Owen. (New York: Time Inc., 1967).

8. **Round and Round and Round.** Tana Hoban. (New York: Greenwillow Books, 1983).

9. **Wheels: A Pictorial History.** Edwin Tunis. (New York: Thomas Y. Crowell, 1977).

10. **Monsters on Wheels.** George Ancona. (New York: E.P. Dutton and Company, Inc., 1974).

11. **Little Wheels, Big Wheels.** Frank Fitzgerald. (New York: Golden Press, 1980).

12. **David's First Bicycle.** Rosalie Silver. (New York: Golden Press, 1983).

13. **Wheels Go Round.** Yvonne Hooker. (New York: Gosset and Dunlap, 1978).

14. **Grandma's Wheelchair.** Lorraine Henroid. (Niles, IL: Albert Whitman and Company, 1982).

Puzzles:

The following puzzles can be found in preschool educational catalogs:

1. **"Transportation"** 20 pieces. Judy/Instructo.

2. **"Car Mechanic"** 16 pieces. Judy/Instructo.

3. **"Cycling Clown"** 8 pieces. Judy/Instructo.

4. **"Shape Disks"** 32 pieces. Lauri.

5. **"Transportation Roller Puzzles"** 6 pieces. Childcraft.

WINTER

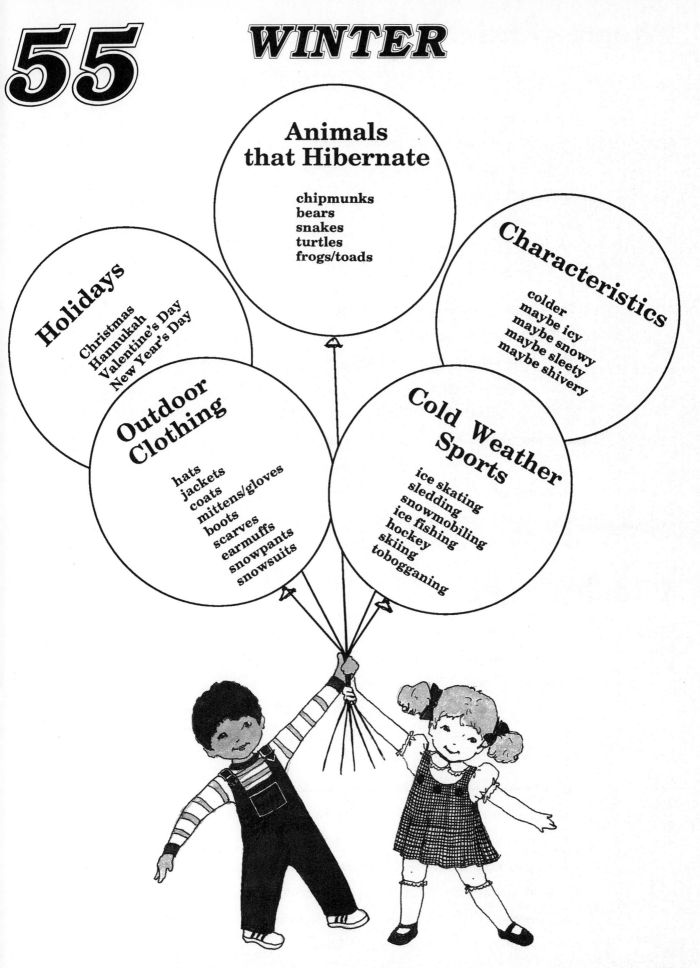

Animals that Hibernate

chipmunks
bears
snakes
turtles
frogs/toads

Characteristics

colder
maybe icy
maybe snowy
maybe sleety
maybe shivery

Holidays

Christmas
Hannukah
Valentine's Day
New Year's Day

Outdoor Clothing

hats
jackets
coats
mittens/gloves
boots
scarves
earmuffs
snowpants
snowsuits

Cold Weather Sports

ice skating
sledding
snowmobiling
ice fishing
hockey
skiing
tobogganing

Theme Goals:

Through participating in the experiences provided by this theme, the children may learn:

1. Winter holidays.
2. Characteristics of winter weather.
3. Winter sports.
4. Winter clothing.
5. Hibernating animals.

Concepts for the Children to Learn:

1. Winter is one of the four seasons.
2. Winter is usually the coldest season.
3. It snows in the winter in some areas.
4. People wear warmer clothes in the winter.
5. Some animals hibernate in the winter.
6. Trees may lose their leaves in the winter.
7. Lakes, ponds and water may freeze in the winter.
8. Sledding and ice skating are winter sports in colder areas.
9. To remove snow, people shovel and plow.
10. December, January and February are winter months.

Vocabulary:

1. **ice**—frozen water.
2. **cold**—not warm.
3. **frost**—very small ice pieces.
4. **snow**—frozen particles of water that fall to the ground.
5. **temperature**—how hot or cold something is.
6. **sleet**—mixture of rain and snow.
7. **hibernate**—to sleep during the winter.
8. **snowman**—snow shaped in the form of a person.
9. **ski**—a runner that moves over snow and ice.
10. **icicle**—a hanging piece of frozen ice.
11. **sled**—transportation for moving over snow and ice.
12. **boots**—clothing worn on feet to keep them dry and warm.
13. **shiver**—to shake from cold or fear.

Bulletin Board

The purpose of this bulletin board is to provide the children with an opportunity to match patterns. Construct several pairs of mittens out of tagboard, each with a different pattern, as illustrated. Laminate them. On the bulletin board, string one of each pair of the mittens through a rope or clothesline (one or two rows). Tie enough clothespins in place by putting the line through the wire spring to put up the matching mittens. (Tie the clothespins beside the first mitten.) Children can match the mittens by hanging the second next to the first with a clothespin. This is a good matching exercise for twos, who sometimes need help with the clothespins. It is mainly a small motor exercise for older children, unless you make the mittens fairly similar so that finding the correct pairs is not a difficult task.

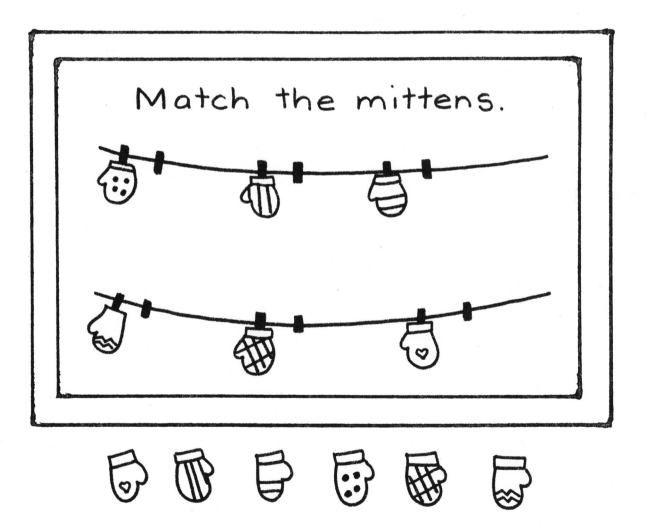

Parent Letter

Dear Parents,

This week at school we will begin a unit on winter. The children will be learning about the coldest season by taking a look at winter clothing, changes that occur during this season indoors and outdoors and winter sports. Throughout the week, the children will develop an awareness of winter activities.

At School This Week

Some of the weekly learning experiences include:

* creating cottonball snowmen.
* sorting mittens by size, shape and color.
* enjoying stories about winter.
* setting up an ice-skating rink in the dramatic play area.
* experiencing snow and ice in the sensory table.

At Home (Delete this paragraph if snow is unavailable.)

To experience winter at home, try this activity—snow in the bath tub! Bring in some snow from outside and place in your bath tub. Also place some measuring cups, spoons and scoops in the bath tub and let your child use mittens to play in the snow. In addition, a spray bottle filled with colored water (made with food coloring) will allow your child to make colorful sculptures. This is sure to keep your children busy and will develop an awareness of the senses.

From all of us!

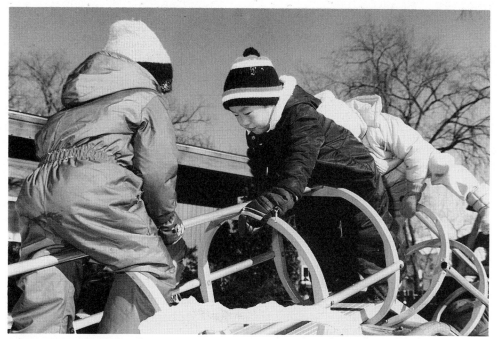

FIGURE 55 Bundle up for warmth in the winter.

Music:

1. **"Snowman"**
   (Sing to the tune of "Twinkle, Twinkle, Little Star")

   Snowman, snowman, where did you go?
   I built you yesterday out of snow.
   I built you high and I built you fat.
   I put on eyes and a nose and a hat.
   Now you're gone all melted away
   But it's sunny outside so I'll go and play.

2. **"Winter Clothes"**
   (Tune: "Did you Ever See a Lassie?")

   Children put your coats on, your coats on,
   your coats on.
   Children put your coats on, one, two and
   three.

   (hats, boots, mittens, etc.)

3. **"Mitten Song"**

   Thumbs in the thumb place, fingers all
   together.
   This is the song we sing in mitten
   weather.

Fingerplays:

FIVE LITTLE SNOWMEN

Five little snowmen standing in the door.
This one melted and then there were four.
   (hold up all five fingers, put down
   thumb)
Four little snowmen underneath a tree.
This one melted and then there were
three.
   (put down pointer finger)
Three little snowmen with hats and
mittens too.
This one melted and then there were two.
   (put down middle finger)
Two little snowmen outside in the sun.
This one melted and then there was one.
   (put down ring finger)
One little snowman trying hard to run.
He melted too, and then there were none.
   (put down pinky)

Variations:
* Make five little snowmen finger puppets
  and remove them one by one.
* Make five stick puppets for children to
  hold and sit down one by one at appropriate times during fingerplay.

MAKING A SNOWMAN

Roll it, roll it, get a pile of snow.
  (make rolling motions with hands)
Rolling, rolling, rolling, rolling, rolling
here we go.
Pat it, pat it, face it to the south.
  (patting motion)
Now my little snowman's done, eyes and
nose and mouth.
  (point to eyes, nose and mouth)

ZIPPERS

Three little zippers on my snowsuit,
  (hold up three fingers)
Fasten up as snug as snug can be
It's a very easy thing as you can see
Just zip, zip, zip!
  (do three zipping motions)
I work the zippers on my snowsuit.
Zippers really do save time for me
I can fasten them myself with one, two,
three.
Just zip, zip, zip!
  (do three zipping motions)

THE SNOWMAN AND THE BUNNY

A chubby little snowman
  (make a fist)
Had a carrot nose.
  (poke thumb out)
Along came a bunny
And what do you suppose?
  (other hand, make rabbit ears)
That hungry little bunny
Looking for his lunch
  (bunny hops around)
Ate that snowman's carrot nose.
  (bunny nibbles at thumb)
Crunch, crunch, crunch.

BUILD A SNOWMAN

First you make a snowball,
  (rolling motion)
Big and fat and round.
  (extend arms in large circle)
Then you roll the snowball,
  (rolling motion)
All along the ground.
Then you build the snowman

One-Two-Three!
  (place three pretend balls on top of each
  other)
Then you have a snowman,
Don't you see?
  (point to eyes)
Then the sun shines all around and
Melts the snowman to the ground.
  (drop to the ground in a melting motion)

Science:

1. Weather Doll

Make a felt weather doll. Encourage the
children to dress and undress the doll
according to the weather.

2. Make Frost

Changes in temperature cause dew. When
dew freezes it is called frost. Materials
needed are a tin can with no lid, rock salt
and crushed ice. Measure and pour 2 cups
of crushed ice and 1/2 cup rock salt in a
can. Stir rapidly. Let the mixture sit for
30 minutes. After 30 minutes, the outside
of can will have dew on it. Wait longer
and the dew will change to frost. To
hasten the process, place in a freezer.

3. Make Birdfeeders

Roll pinecones in peanut butter and then
birdseed. Attach a string to the pinecones
and hang them outside. Encourage the
children to check the birdfeeders
frequently.

A bird feeder can also be prepared from
suet. To do this, wrap suet in a netting.
Gather the edges up and tie together with
a long string. Another method is to place
suet in an oven bag.

4. Snow

Bring a large container of snow into the
classroom. After it is melted add colored
water and place the container outdoors.
When frozen, bring a colored block of ice
back into classroom and observe it melt.

5. Examine Snowflakes

Examine snowflakes with a magnifying glass. Each is unique. For classrooms located in warmer climates, make a snow-like substance by crushing ice.

6. Catching Snowflakes

Cover a piece of cardboard with dark felt. Place the cardboard piece in the freezer. Go outside and let snowflakes land on the board. Snowflakes will last longer for examination.

7. Coloring Snow

Provide children with spray bottles containing colored water, preferably red, yellow and blue. Allow them to spray the snow and mix colors.

8. Thermometers

Experiment with a thermometer. Begin introducing the concept by observing and discussing what happens when the thermometer is placed in a bowl of warm water and a bowl of cold water. Demonstrate to the children and encourage the children to experiment under supervision during the self-selected activity period.

9. Signs and Sounds of Winter

On a winter walk in colder climates have the children watch and listen for signs and sounds of winter. The signs of winter are weather: cold, ice, daylight is shorter, darkness is earlier; plants: all but evergreen trees are bare, and people: we wear warmer clothes, we play inside more, we shovel snow, we play in the snow. Some of the sounds of winter are: boots crunching, the snow, rain splashing, wind howling, etc. (Adapt this activity to the signs of winter in your climate.)

Dramatic Play:

1. Ice Skating Palace

Make a masking tape border on a carpeted floor. Give child 2 pieces of waxed paper.

Show children how to fasten waxed paper to their ankles with rubber bands. Play instrumental music and encourage the children to skate around on the carpeted floor.

2. Dress Up

If available, put outdoor winter clothing such as coats, boots, hats, mittens, scarves and ear muffs in the dramatic play area of the classroom with a large mirror. The children may enjoy trying on a variety of clothing items.

Arts and Crafts:

1. Whipped Soap Painting

Mix 1 cup Ivory Soap flakes with 1/2 cup warm water in bowl. The children can beat with a hand eggbeater until mixture is fluffy. Apply mixture to dark construction paper with various tools (toothbrushes, rollers, tongue depressors, brushes, etc.) To create variety, food coloring can be added to paint mixture also.

2. Cottonball Snowman

Cut a figure of a snowman figure from dark construction paper. Provide the children with cottonballs and glue. They can decorate the snowman by gluing on cottonballs.

3. Snowflakes

Cut different sized squares out of white construction paper. Fold the squares in half, and then in half again. Demonstrate and encourage the children to cut and open their own designs. The snowflakes can be hung in the entry or classroom for decoration.

4. Windowpane Frost

On a piece of construction paper, draw an outline of a window. Spread glue around and on the frame and sprinkle with glitter.

5. Winter Mobile

Cut out pictures of winter from magazines or have children create their own winter pictures. Attach several pictures with string or yarn to a branch, hanger (masking taped) or paper plate. Glitter can be added.

6. Ice Cube Art

Place a popsicle stick on each ice compartment of a tray and fill with water. Freeze. Sprinkle dry tempera paint on paper. Then to make their own design, the children can move an ice cube on the paper.

7. Frosted Pictures

Mix 1 part Epsom salts with 1 part boiling water. Let the mixture cool. Encourage the children to make a crayon design on paper. The mixture can be brushed over the picture. Observe how the crystals form as the mixture dries.

8. Winter Shape Printing

Cut sponges into various winter shapes such as boots, snowmen, mittens, snowflakes, fir trees and stars. The children can use the sponges as a tool to print on different pieces of colored construction paper.

9. Easel Ideas

Feature white paint at the easel for snow pictures on colored paper. Or, cut easel paper into winter shapes: snowmen, hats, mittens, scarves, snowflakes, etc.

10. Snow Drawings

White chalk and dark construction paper can be placed in the art area.

11. Snow Painting

Using old spray bottles filled with colored water, let the children make pictures in the snow outside. This activity is limited to areas where snow is available.

Sensory:

The following items can be placed in the sensory table.

* snow and ice (plain or colored with drops of food coloring)
* cottonballs with measuring/balancing scale
* pinecones
* ice cubes (colored or plain)
* snow and magnifying glasses

Large Muscle:

1. Freeze

Play music and have children walk around in a circle. When music stops, the children freeze by stooping still. Vary the activity by substituting other actions such as hopping, skipping, galloping, sliding, etc.

2. Snowman

During outdoor play make a snowman. Decorate with radish eyes, carrot nose, scarf, hat and holding a stick. Other novel accessories can be substituted by using the children's ideas.

3. Snow People

After a snowfall, have the children lay down in the snow and move their arms and legs to make shapes.

4. Snowball Target

Since children love throwing snowballs, set up a target outside for children to throw at.

5. Shovel

Provide child-sized shovels for the children to help shovel a walk.

6. Balance

Make various tracks in the snow, such as a straight line, a zig-zag line, a circle, square, triangle and rectangle.

Field Trips/Resource People:

1. Visit an ice skating rink. Observe the ice and watch how it is cleaned.

2. Visit a sledding hill. Bring sleds along and go sledding.

3. Invite a snowplow operator to school to talk to the children. After a snowfall, the children can observe the plowing.

4. Take the children to a grocery store and view the freezer area. Also observe a refrigerated delivery truck.

Math:

1. **Shape Sequence**

   Cut three different round-sized white circles from construction paper for each child to make a snowman. Which is the largest? smallest? How many do you have? What shape? Then have children sequence the circles from largest to smallest and smallest to largest.

2. **Mitten Match**

   From construction paper or tagboard design and cut several pairs of mittens. On one pair of mittens write a numeral and on the other, the corresponding number of dots. The children can match the dots to the numerals locating the pairs of mittens.

3. **Winter Dominoes**

   Trace and cut 30 squares out of white tagboard. Section each square into four spaces diagonally. In each of the four spaces, draw different winter objects or stick winter stickers on. The children can match the pictures by playing dominoes.

4. **Dot to Dot**

   Make a dot-to-dot snowman. The children connect the dots in numerical order. Can also make dot-to-dot patterns of other winter objects such as hats, snowflakes,

mittens, etc. This activity requires numeral recognition and order so is restricted to the school-aged child.

5. **Puzzles**

   Mount winter pictures or posters on tagboard sheets. Cut into pieces. The number of pieces cut will be dependent upon the children's developmental age. Place in the small manipulative area of the classroom for use during self-selected activity periods.

Social Studies:

1. **Travel**

   Discuss ways which people travel in winter such as sled, toboggan, snowmobile, snowshoes, skis, etc.

2. **Winter Happenings**

   Display pictures of different winter happenings, sports, clothing, snow, etc. around the room at the children's eye level.

3. **Winter Book**

   Encourage the children to make a book about winter. Do one page a day. The following titles could be used:

   * What I wear in winter.
   * What I like to do outside in winter.
   * What I like to do inside in winter.
   * My favorite food during winter.
   * My favorite thing about winter.
   (This activity may be more appropriate for the school aged child.)

4. **Winter Clothing Match**

   Draw a large paper figure of a boy and of a girl. Design and cut winter clothing to fit each figure. The children can dress the figures for outdoor play.

Group Time (games, language):

1. **Who Has the Mitten?**

   Ask the children to sit in a circle. One child should sit in the middle. Make a very small mitten out of felt or construction paper. Tell the children to pass the mitten around the circle. All the children should imitate the passing actions even if they do not have the mitten in hand. When the verse starts the child in the middle tries to guess who has the mitten. Chant the following verse while passing a mitten.

I pass the mitten from me to you to you
I pass the mitten and that is what I do.

2. Hat Chart

Prepare a hat chart by listing all the types and colors of hats worn by the children in the classroom.

Cooking:

1. Banana Snowmen

2 cups raisins
2 bananas
shredded coconut

Chop the bananas and raisins in a blender. Then place them in a mixing bowl and refrigerate until mixture is cool enough to be handled. Roll the mixture into balls and into shredded coconut. Stack three balls and fasten with toothpicks.

2. Hot Chocolate

Add warm water or milk to instant hot chocolate and mix. Heat as needed.

3. Snow Cones

Crush ice and spoon into small paper cups. Pour a fruit juice over the ice. Serve.

4. Snowballs—China

1/4 cup walnuts, ground
1/4 cup almonds, ground
1/4 cup sesame seeds, toasted
1/2 cup sugar
1 tablespoon shortening
1 pound glutinous rice flour

In a bowl, mix nuts, sesame seeds, sugar and shortening. Form mixture into 1/2-inch balls. Fill a big mixing bowl with 1/2-inch layer of rice flour. Moisten the nut balls by dipping them into water. Place balls individually in floured bowl and shake bowl back and forth, coating the balls with flour. Redip coated balls in water and coat three times. Slip balls into boiling water and gently boil for about 5 minutes until balls float to the surface. Add a cup of cold water and boil for about 3 to 4 minutes. Serve about 4 to each person along with the hot liquid. This activity requires supervision.

Records:

The following records can be found in preschool educational catalogs:

1. **Seasons for Singing.** Ella Jenkins.

2. **Environment.** Alpine Blizzard. Side 1. Syntonic Research, Inc.

Books and Stories:

The following books and stories can be used to complement the theme:

1. **Snow is Falling.** Franklyn M. Branley. (New York: Thomas Y. Crowell Company, 1963).

2. **A Walk in the Snow.** Phyllis Busch. (New York: Viking Press Magazine, 1973).

3. **The First Sign of Winter.** Mary Blount Christian. (New York: Parents Press Magazine, 1973).

4. **When the Snow is Blue.** Marguerite Dorian. (New York: Lothrop, Lee and Shepard Company, Inc., 1962).

5. **When Winter Comes.** Charles Phillip Fox. (Chicago: Reilly and Lee Company, 1962).

6. **Winter's Birds.** May Garelick. (New York: Young Scott Book Company, 1965).

7. **I Like Winter.** Lois Lenski. (New York: Henry Z. Walck, 1950).

8. **When Peter was Lost in the Woods.** Peterson, Hans and Wiberg. (New York: Parents Press Magazine, 1968).

9. **White Snow, Bright Snow.** Alvin Tresselt. (New York: Lothrop, Lee and Shepard Co. Inc., 1947).

10. **It's Winter.** Sister Nomi Weygant. (Philadelphia: The Westmaster Press, 1965).

11. **All Ready for Winter.** Leone Adelson. (New York: David McKay Company, 1952).

12. **The Snowy Day.** Ezra Jack Keats. (New York: Viking Press, 1962).

13. **The Mystery of the Missing Red Mitten.** (New York: Doubleday Company, Inc., 1967).

14. **A Walk in the Snow.** Phyllis Busch. (New York: J. B. Lippincott, 1971).

15. **Slush, Slush.** Ethel and Leonard Kessler. (New York: Parents Magazine Press, 1973).

16. **Our Snowman.** M.B. Goffstein. (New York: Harper and Row, 1986).

17. **Snowy Day Stories and Poems.** Caroline Feller Bauer. (New York: J. B. Lippincott, 1986).

18. **Snow is Falling: A Let's Read and Find Out Science Book.** Franklyn M. Branley. (New York: Thomas Y. Crowell, 1986).

19. **Sadie and the Snowman.** Allen Morgan. (New York: Scholastic, Inc., 1985).

20. **Why Do Animals Sleep Through Winter?** Chris Arvetis. (Chicago: Childrens Press, 1987).

Puzzles:

The following puzzles can be found in preschool educational catalogs.

1. **"Building a Snowman"** 4 pieces. Puzzle People.

2. **"Sort the Seasons"** 16 pieces. Childcraft.

3. **"Apple Tree Seasons"** Story Sequence Board. Childcraft.

4. **"Snowy Day"** 9 pieces. Judy/Instructo.

5. **"Snowman"** 3 pieces. Judy/Instructo.

6. **"Snowman"** 5 pieces. Childcraft.

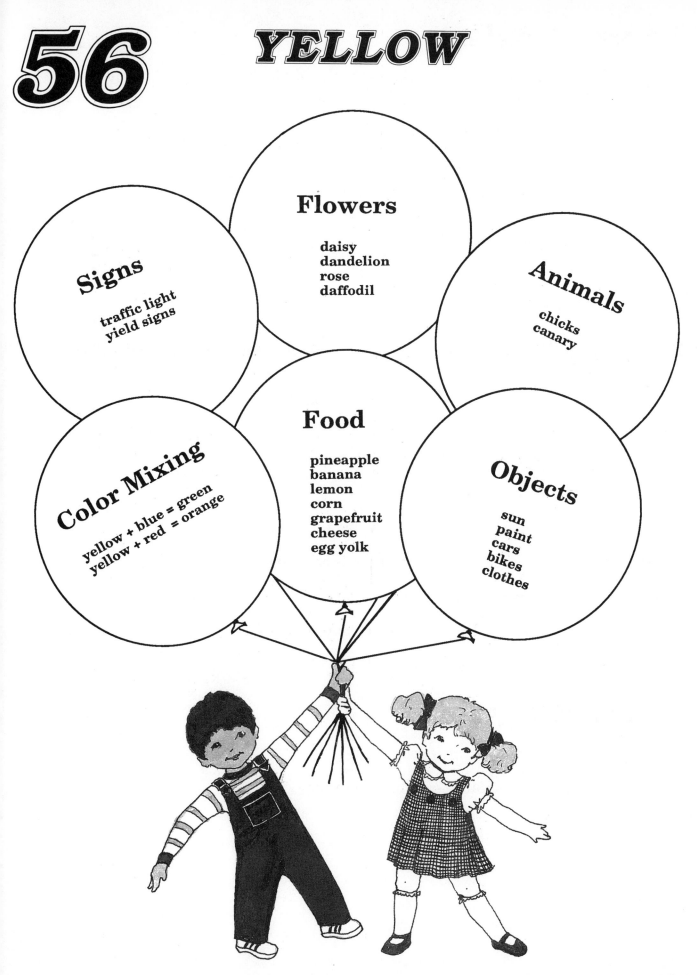

Flowers

daisy
dandelion
rose
daffodil

Signs

traffic light
yield signs

Animals

chicks
canary

Food

pineapple
banana
lemon
corn
grapefruit
cheese
egg yolk

Color Mixing

yellow + blue = green
yellow + red = orange

Objects

sun
paint
cars
bikes
clothes

Theme Goals:

Through participating in the experiences provided by this theme, the children may learn:

1. Yellow flowers.

2. Yellow traffic signs.

3. Yellow animals.

4. Yellow colored foods.

5. Colors formed by adding yellow.

6. Yellow objects.

Concepts for the Children to Learn:

1. Yellow is a primary color.

2. Yellow mixed with blue makes green.

3. Yellow mixed with red makes orange.

4. The sun is a yellow color.

5. The middle color on a traffic light is yellow.

6. Daisies, dandelions and daffodils are yellow flowers.

7. A canary is a yellow bird.

8. Pineapples, bananas and corn are yellow foods.

9. Bikes and cars can be yellow.

Vocabulary:

1. **yellow**—a primary color.

2. **primary colors**—red, blue and yellow.

Bulletin Board

The purpose of this bulletin board is to have the children match the shapes, providing practice in visual discrimination. To prepare the bulletin board, collect yellow tagboard, a black felt-tip marker, scissors, yellow string and push pins. Using yellow tagboard, draw sets of different shaped balloons as illustrated. Outline with a black felt-tip marker and cut out. Take one from each set and attach to the top of the bulletin board. Staple a yellow string to hang from each balloon. Next, attach the remaining balloons on the bottom of the bulletin board. A push pin can be fastened next to each balloon, and the children can match the balloons by shape.

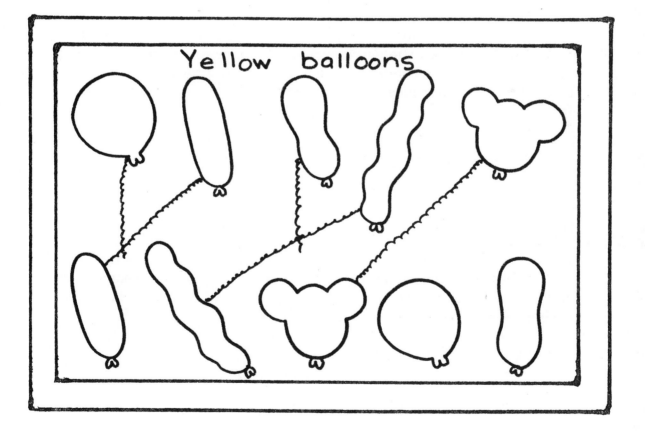

Parent Letter

Dear Parents,

Colors are such a big part of our world. Consequently, our theme this week will focus on the color yellow. Throughout this week, the children will become aware of the color in their environment. It should be a bright week discovering the color yellow!

At School This Week

Some learning experiences planned for the week include:

* making scrambled eggs.
* visiting a paint store.
* learning the fingerplay "Six Yellow Chickadees."
* making yellow soap crayons.
* playing with corn kernels in the sensory table.

At Home

This week at school we will be making yellow playdough. The children enjoy helping prepare the playdough and of course, playing with it! It would be great fun for them to make it at home and they will be exposed to the mathematical concepts of amounts, fractions and measurements. Here is the recipe.

2 cups flour
1 cup of salt
1 cup of water
2 tablespoons cooking oil
food coloring

Let your child assist in gathering and measuring the ingredients. Then mix all the ingredients together. To encourage play, provide some tools for your child to use: rolling pins, cookie cutters, spatulas or potato mashers. Have Fun!

Have a sunny yellow week!

Fingerplays:

SIX YELLOW CHICKADEES
(Suit the actions to the words.)

Six yellow chickadees sitting by a hive.
One flew away and then there were five.
Five yellow chickadees sitting by the door.
One flew away and then there were four.
Four yellow chickadees sitting in a tree.
One flew away and then there were three.
Three yellow chickadees sitting by my shoe.
One flew away and then there were two.
Two yellow chickadees sitting by my thumb.
One flew away and then there was one.
One yellow chickadee flying around the sun.
He flew away and then there was none.

TEN FLUFFY CHICKENS

Five eggs and five eggs
   (hold up two hands)
That makes ten.
Sitting on top is the mother hen
   (fold one hand over the other)
Crackle, crackle, crackle
   (clap hands three times)
What do I see?
Ten fluffy chickens
   (hold up ten fingers)
As yellow as can be!

Science:

1. Paper Towel Dip

Fold a paper towel in half several times.
Dip the towel into red water and then into
yellow water. Open the towel carefully and
allow it to dry. Orange designs will appear
on the paper towel.

2. Carnation Coloring

Put a carnation into a glass of water
which has been dyed yellow with food
coloring. Soon the carnation will show
yellow streaks. During the summer other
white garden flowers can be substituted.

3. Yellow Soap Crayons

Measure one cup of mild powdered laundry
soap. Add one tablespoon of food coloring.
Add water by the teaspoonful until the
soap is in liquid form. Stir well. Pour the
soap into ice cube trays. Set in a sunny,
dry place until hard. Soap crayons are
great for writing in the sink, tub or sensory table.

Dramatic Play:

Paint Store

Set up a paint store by including paint
caps, paintbrushes, pans, rollers, drop
cloths, paint clothes, a cash register and
play money.

Arts and Crafts:

1. Yellow Paint

Provide yellow fingerpaint and yellow
tempera paint in the art area.

2. Corn Cob Painting

Cover the bottom of a shallow pan with
thick yellow tempera paint. Using a corn
cob as an applicator, apply paint to paper.

3. Popsicle Stick Prints

Cover the bottom of a shallow pan with
thick yellow tempera paint. Apply the
paint to paper using a popsicle stick as an
applicator.

4. Yellow Playdough

Combine two parts flour, one part salt, one
part water and two tablespoons cooking
oil. Add yellow food coloring. Mix well. If
prepared dough becomes sticky add more
flour.

5. Baker's Clay

Combine 4 cups flour, 1 cup salt and 1½
cups water. Mix the ingredients. The

children can shape forms. Place the forms on a cookie sheet and bake at 350 degrees for about 1 hour. The next day the children can paint the objects yellow.

6. Yarn and Glue Designs

Provide yellow yarn, glue and paper for the children to make their own designs.

7. Record Player Designs

Punch a hole in the middle of a paper plate and place on the turntable of a record player. Turn the record player on. As the turntable spins around, the children can apply color by holding a yellow felt-tip marker on the paper plate. Interesting designs can be made.

Sensory:

1. Shaving Cream Fun

Spray the contents of one can of shaving cream in the sensory table. Color the shaving cream by adding yellow food coloring.

2. Corn Kernels

Place corn kernels in the sensory table.

3. Yellow Goop

In the sensory table, mix one cup cornstarch, one cup water and yellow food coloring. Mix together well.

4. Water Toys

Add yellow food coloring to three inches of water in the sensory table. Provide water toys as accessories to encourage play during self-selected play activites.

Field Trips/Resource People:

1. Paint Store

Visit a paint store and observe the different shades of yellow. Collect samples of paint for use in the art area. If possible, also observe the manager mix yellow paint.

2. Yellow In Our World

Take a walk and look for yellow objects. When you return to the classroom prepare a language experience chart.

3. Greenhouse

Visit a greenhouse and observe the different kinds of yellow flowers.

Math:

Sorting Shapes

Cut circles, triangles and rectangles out of yellow tagboard. Place on the math table. The children can sort the yellow shapes into groups. For younger children, the objects can be cut from different colors. Then the objects can be sorted by color.

Social Studies:

Tasting Party

Cut a banana, a pineapple, a lemon and a piece of yellow cheese into small pieces. Let the children sample each during snack time. The concept of color, texture and taste can all be discussed.

Group Time (games, language):

Guessing Game: What's Missing?

Use any yellow familiar objects or toys that can be easily handled. The number will depend upon developmental appropriateness. For two year olds choose only two objects. On the other hand several objects can be used for five year olds. Spread them out on the floor and ask children to name each item. Then ask the group to close their eyes. Remove one item. When the group opens their eyes, ask them to tell you which item is missing.

Cooking:

1. Banana Bobs

Cut bananas into chunks and dip into honey. Next roll in wheat germ and use large toothpicks for serving.

2. Carribean Banana Salad

3 green (unripe) bananas, peeled
2 cups water
1 teaspoon salt
2 medium carrots, shredded
1 small cucumber, sliced
1 medium tomato, chopped
1 avocado, cubed
1 stalk clery, sliced
vinaigrette dressing

Heat bananas, water and salt to boiling; reduce heat. Cover and simmer until bananas are tender, about 5 minutes. Drain and cool. Cut bananas crosswise into 1/2-inch slices. Toss bananas and remaining ingredients with vinaigrette dressing.

Source: *Betty Crocker's International Cookbook.* (New York: Random House, 1980).

3. Corn Bread

1 cup flour
1 cup cornmeal
2 tablespoons sugar
4 teaspoons baking powder
1 teaspoon salt
1 cup milk
1/4 cup cooking oil or melted shortening
1 egg, slightly beaten

Preheat oven to 425 degrees. Grease (not oil) an 8- or 9-inch square pan. In medium mixing bowl, combine the dry ingredients. Stir in the remaining ingredients, beating by hand until just smooth. Pour batter into prepared pan. Bake for 20 to 25 minutes or until toothpick inserted in center comes out clean.

Records:

The following records can be found in preschool educational catalogs:

1. **Learning Basic Skills Through Music—Volume 1.** "Colors." Hap Palmer.

2. **Color Me a Rainbow.** Jerry Caspell.

3. **There's Music in the Colors.** Kimbo Records.

Books and Stories:

The following books and stories can be used to complement the theme:

1. **Is it Red? Is it Yellow? Is it Blue?** Tana Hoban. (New York: William Morrow and Company, 1978).

2. **Little Blue and Little Yellow.** Leo Lionni. (New York: Irian Obslensky, Inc., 1959).

3. **See What I Am.** Roger Duvoisin. (New York: Lothrop, Lee and Shepard Company, 1974).

4. **Adventures with Color.** Seymour Reit. (New York: The Bobbs Merrill Company, Inc., 1970).

5. **Yellow, Yellow.** Frank Asch. (New York: McGraw Hill, 1971).

Puzzles:

The following puzzles can be found in preschool educational catalogs:

1. **"Great Big Yellow School Bus"** 19 pieces. Judy/Instructo.

2. **"Three Ducks"** 3 pieces. Childcraft.

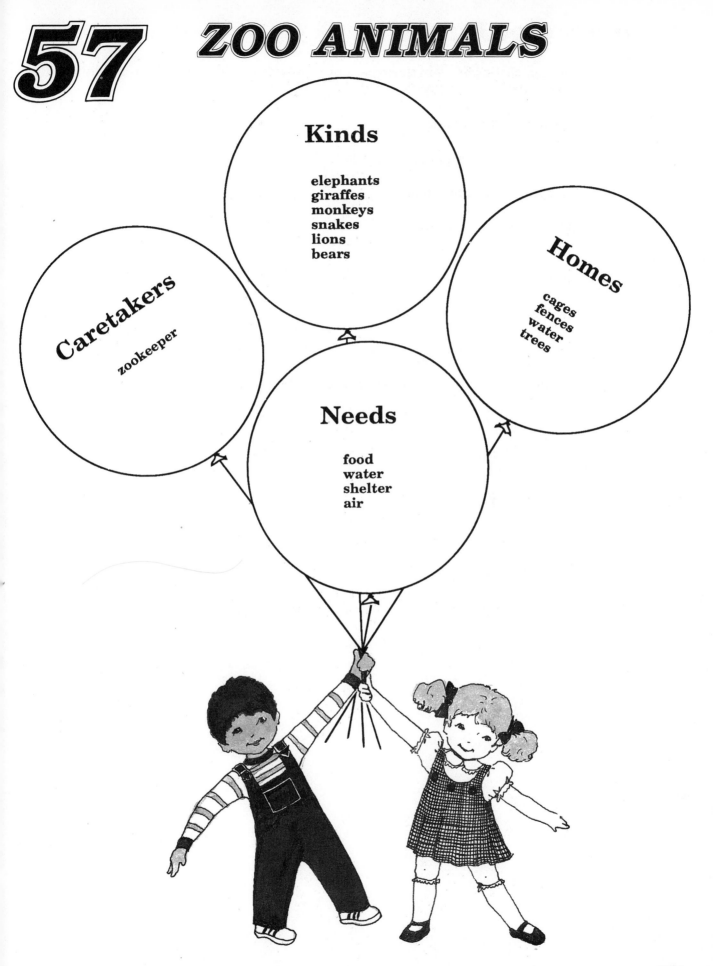

Kinds

elephants
giraffes
monkeys
snakes
lions
bears

Caretakers

zookeeper

Homes

cages
fences
water
trees

Needs

food
water
shelter
air

Theme Goals:

Through participating in the experiences provided by this theme, the children may learn:

1. Names of zoo animals.

2. Needs of zoo animals.

3. Types of animal homes.

4. The caretaker's role.

Concepts for the Children to Learn:

1. A zoo is a place for animals.

2. Zoo animals are kept in cages, fences, water or in trees.

3. Elephants, giraffes, monkeys, snakes, lions and bears are zoo animals.

4. A zookeeper feeds and takes care of the animals.

5. Zoo animals need food, water and shelter.

Vocabulary:

1. **zoo**—a place to look at animals.

2. **cage**—a home for animals.

3. **zookeeper**—a person who feeds the zoo animals.

4. **veterinarian**—an animal doctor.

Bulletin Board

The purpose of this bulletin board is to encourage the children to place the correct amount of balls above each seal corresponding to the numeral on the drum. To prepare the bulletin board, construct seals sitting on a drum as illustrated. Place a numeral on each drum with the corresponding number of dots. Construct colored balls from tagboard. Laminate. Staple the seal figures and drums to bulletin board. Place a magnetic strip above each seal. Also adhere a magnetic strip on the back of each ball.

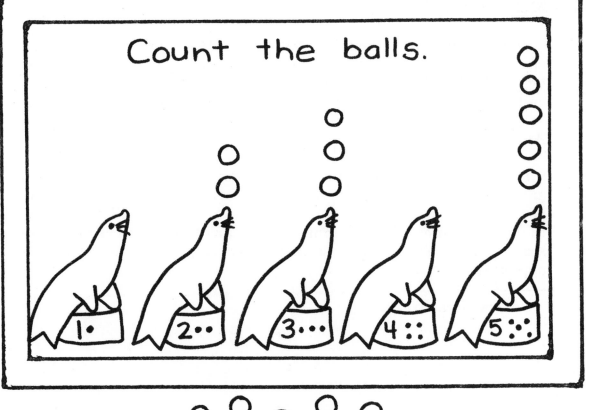

Parent Letter

Dear Parents,

Our theme for this week is zoo animals. This is an appropriate theme to introduce to the children because they are fascinated by the zoo and the animals that live there. Through our study of zoo animals, the children will become familiar with the names of many familiar zoo animals. They will also be introduced to new occupations: the zookeeper and the veterinarian.

At School This Week

Some of the experiences planned for the week include:

* looking at peek-a-boo pictures of zoo animals.
* using zoo animal-shaped cookie cutters with playdough at the art table.
* pretending to be caged zoo animals using boxes as cages in the dramatic play area.

Field Trip

Our class will be taking a field trip to the Dunn County Reserve Park on Friday. There we can see some unusual animals. Please let me know by Wednesday if you are interested in accompanying the group. We will be leaving the center at 9:30 and be returning by 11:30.

At Home

To develop observation skills, you can show your child pictures of zoo animals from books or magazines. Plan a family trip to a zoo. Many opportunities for learning present themselves at the zoo. Children can actually see different kinds of animals and many times, such as in petting zoos, are able to touch and feed them. What a great way to develop an appreciation for and respect of animal life.

Have a Great Week!

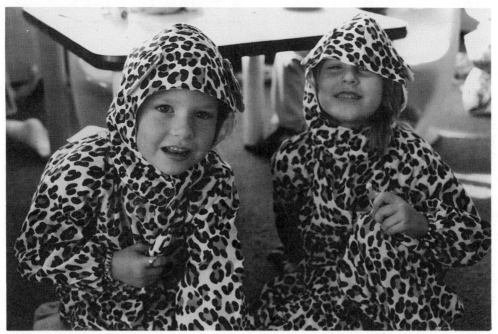

FIGURE 57 Leopards and other animals can be found in a zoo.

Music:

1. "Zoo Animals"
(Sing to the tune of "Muffin Man")

Do you know the kangaroo
The kangaroo, the kangaroo?
Oh, do you know the kangaroo
That lives in the zoo?

Adapt this song and use other zoo animals
such as the monkey, elephant, giraffe,
lion, turtle, bear, snake, etc.)

2. "One Elephant"

One elephant went out to play
On a spider web one day.
He had such enormous fun
That he called for another elephant to come.

(Makes a nice flannel story or chose   one
child as an "elephant." Add another
"elephant" with each verse.)

3. "Animals at the Zoo"
(Sing to the tune of "Frere Jacque")

See the animals, see the animals
At the zoo, at the zoo.
Elephants and tigers, lions and seals
Monkeys too, monkeys too.

Fingerplays:

LION

I knew a little lion who went roar, roar, roar.
  (make sounds)
Who walked around on all fours.
  (walk on both hands and feet)
He had a tail we could see behind the bars
  (point to tail)
And when we visit we should stand back far.
  (move backwards)

ALLIGATOR

The alligator likes to swim.
  (two hands flat on top of the other)
Sometimes his mouth opens wide.
  (hands open and shut)
But when he sees me on the shore,
Down under the water he'll hide.

THE MONKEY

The monkey claps, claps, claps his hands.
  (clap hands)
The monkey claps, claps, claps his hands.
  (clap hands)
Monkey see, monkey do.
The monkey does the same as you.
  (use pointer finger)
  (change actions)

ZOO ANIMALS

This is the way the elephant goes.
  (clasp hands together, extend arms, move
  back and forth)
With a curly trunk instead of a nose.
The buffalo, all shaggy and fat.
Has two sharp horns in place of a hat.
  (point to forehead)
The hippo with his mouth so wide—
Let's see what's inside.
  (hands together and open wide and close
  them)
The wiggly snake upon the ground
Crawls along without a sound.
  (weave hands back and forth)
But monkey see and monkey do is the
funniest animal in the zoo.
  (place thumbs in ears and wiggle fingers)

THE ZOO

The zoo holds many animals inside
  (make a circle with your hands and peer
  inside)
So unlatch the doors and open them wide.
  (open your hands wide)
Elephants, tigers, zebras and bears
  (hold up one finger for each animal)
Are some of the animals you'll find there.

Science:

1. Animal Skins

Place a piece of snake skin, a patch of
animal hide and animal fur out on the
science table. The children can look and
feel the differences. These skins can usually
be borrowed from the Department of
Natural Resources.

2. Habitat

On the science table, place a bowl of
water, a tray of dirt and a pile of hay or
grass on the table. Also, include many
small toy zoo animals. The children can
place the animals in their correct habitat.

Dramatic Play:

1. The Zoo

Collect large appliance boxes. Cut slits to
resemble cages. Old fur coats or blankets
can be added. The children may use the
fur pieces pretending to be animals in the
zoo.

2. Pet Store

Cages and many small stuffed animals can
be added to the dramatic play area.

3. Block Play

Set out many blocks and rubber, plastic or
wooden models of zoo animals.

Arts and Crafts:

1. Paper Plate Lions

Collect paper plates, sandwich bags and
yellow cotton. Color the cottonballs by
pouring powdered tempera paint into the
sandwich bag and shaking. The children
can trim the cut side of the paper plate
with the yellow cotton to represent a
mane. Facial features can also be added.
This activity is for older children.

2. Cookie Cutters

Playdough and zoo animal-shaped cookie
cutters can be placed on a table in the art
area.

Sensory:

Additions to the sensory table include:

* sand and zoo animal models
* seeds and measuring scoops
* corn and scales
* hay
* water

Large Muscle:

1. Walk Like the Animals

Walk Like the Animals is played like Simon Says. Say, "The zookeeper says to walk like a giraffe." The children can walk as they believe that particular zoo animal would walk. Repeat using different animals such as monkeys, elephants, lions, tigers, bears, etc. This activity can also be used for transition.

2. Zookeeper, May I?

Designate one child to be the zookeeper. This child should stand about six feet in front of the remainder of the children. The zookeeper provides directions for the other children. To illustrate, they may say take three elephant steps, one kangaroo hop, two alligator glides, etc. Once the children reach the zookeeper, the zookeeper chooses a child as his successor.

Field Trips/Resource People:

1. Zoo

Visit a local zoo if available. Observe the animals that are of particular interest to the children such as the elephants, giraffes, bears and monkeys.

2. Reserve Park

If your community has a reserve park, or an area where wild animals are caged in a natural environment, take the children to visit. Plan a picnic snack to take along.

Math:

1. Animal Sort

Collect pictures of elephants, lions, giraffes, monkeys and other zoo animals from magazines, calendars or coloring books. Encourage the children to sort the pictures into labeled baskets. For example, one basket may be for large animals and another for small animals.

2. Which is Bigger?

Collect many toy models of zoo animals in various sizes. Encourage the children to order from smallest to biggest, etc.

3. Animal Sets

Cut and mount pictures of zoo animals. The children can classify the pictures by sorting. Examples might include birds, four legged animals, furry animals, etc.

Social Studies:

Helpful Zoo Animals

Discuss how some animals can be useful during large group. Show the children pictures of various helping animals and discuss their uses. Examples include:

* camel (transportation in some countries).
* elephant (often used to pull things).
* dogs (seeing-eye dogs, sled dogs).
* goats (used for milk).

Group Time (games, language):

What Am I?

Give the children verbal clues in which you describe an animal and the children guess which zoo animal you are talking about. An example is, "I am very large, gray colored and have a long nose that looks like a hose. What zoo animal am I?"

Cooking:

1. Animals on Grass

Take a graham cracker and spread either peanut butter or green-tinted cream cheese on the top. Stand an animal cracker on the top of the graham cracker.

2. Peanut Butter Log

1/2 cup peanut butter
1/2 cup raisins
2 1/2 tablespoons dry milk
2 tablespoons honey

Mix together, roll into log 1 inch × 10 inches long. Chill and slice.

Records:

The following records can be found in preschool educational catalogs.

1. **Animal Antics.** Hap Palmer.

2. **What's New at the Zoo.** Kimbo Records.

3. **Walk Like the Animals.** Kimbo Records.

4. **Animal Walks.** Kimbo Records.

Books and Stories:

The following books and stories can be used to complement the theme:

1. **Let's Go To a Zoo.** Laura Sootin and Robert Doremus. (New York: G.P. Putnam's Sons, 1959).

2. **Animals in the Zoo.** Feodor Rojankovsky. (New York: Knopf, 1962).

3. **Who Is It?** Zhenya Gay. (New York: Viking Press, 1965).

4. **The Zoo that Grew.** Lise Stitch. (New York: Platt and Munk Publishing, 1968).

5. **Zoo Babies.** Donna Grusvernor. (Washington, DC: National Geographic Society, 1978).

6. **Zoo Pets.** William Bridges. (New York: William Morrow, 1953).

7. **Zoo Babies.** William Bridges. (New York: William Morrow, 1955).

8. **Animal Doctors: What Do They Do?** Carla Greene. (New York: Harper and Row, 1967).

9. **Zoo.** Bruno Munari. (Cleveland OH: Collins, Williams and World, 1963).

10. **I Want to be a Zoo Keeper.** Carla Greene. (Chicago: Childrens Press, 1957).

11. **1-2-3 to the Zoo.** Eric Carle. (Cleveland, OH: Collins, William and World, 1968).

12. **Curious George Visits the Zoo.** Margaret Rey and Alan J. Shalleck. (Boston: Houghton Mifflin Co., 1985).

13. **A Children's Zoo.** Tara Hoban. (New York: Greenwillow Books, 1985).

14. **What Happens At the Zoo?** Judith E. Rinard. (Washington, DC: National Geographic Society, 1984).

15. A Visit to the Zoo. Sylvia Root Tester. (Chicago: Childrens Press, 1987).

Puzzles:

The following puzzles can be found in preschool educational catalogs:

1. **"Zoo Animals"** 5 pieces. Judy/Instructo.

2. **"Gorilla"** 17 pieces. Judy/Instructo.

3. **"Giraffe"** 7 pieces. Judy/Instructo.

4. **"Elephant"** 12 pieces. Judy/Instructo.

5. **"Panda and Cub"** 10 pieces. Judy/Instructo.

6. **"Monkey and Baby"** 6 pieces. Judy/Instructo.

7. **"Elephants"** Floor puzzle. 18 pieces. Judy/Instructo.

8. **"Tigers"** Floor puzzle. 24 pieces. Judy/Instructo.

9. **"Koalas"** Floor puzzle. 21 pieces. Judy/Instructo.

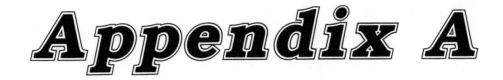

Appendix A

Name Tag
Theme #1
Apples

Cubby Tag
Theme #1
Apples

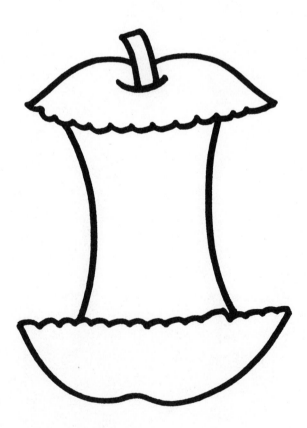

A2

Name Tag
Theme #2
Art

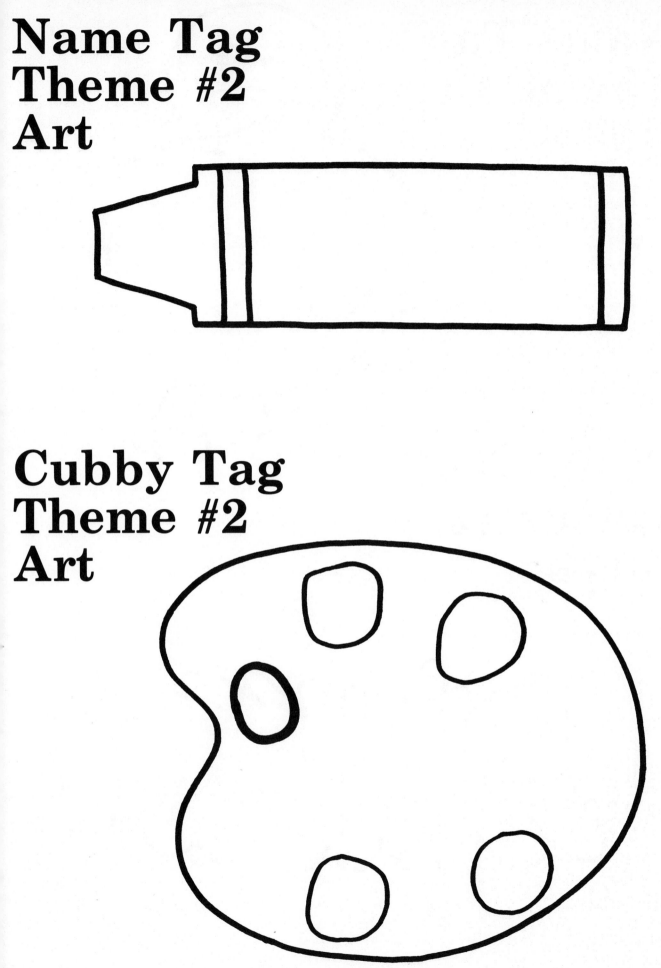

Cubby Tag
Theme #2
Art

A3

Name Tag
Theme #3
Birds

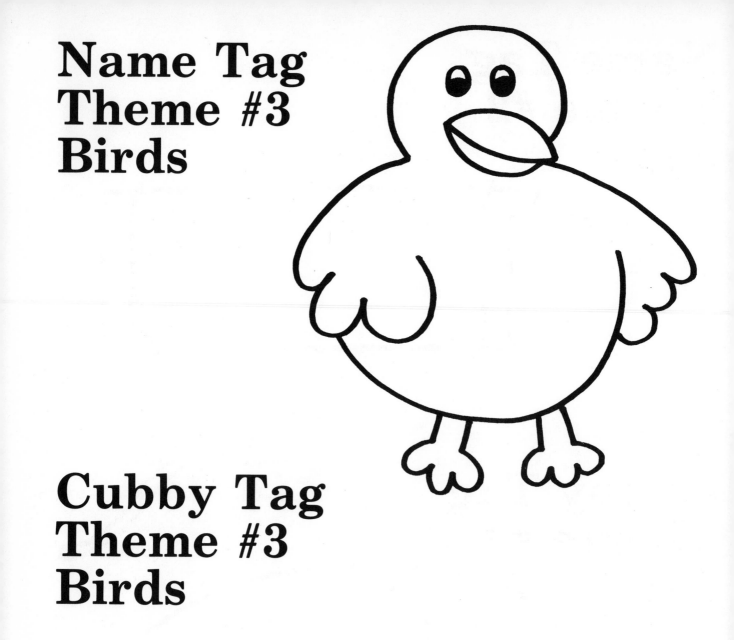

Cubby Tag
Theme #3
Birds

A4

Name Tag
Theme #4
Blue

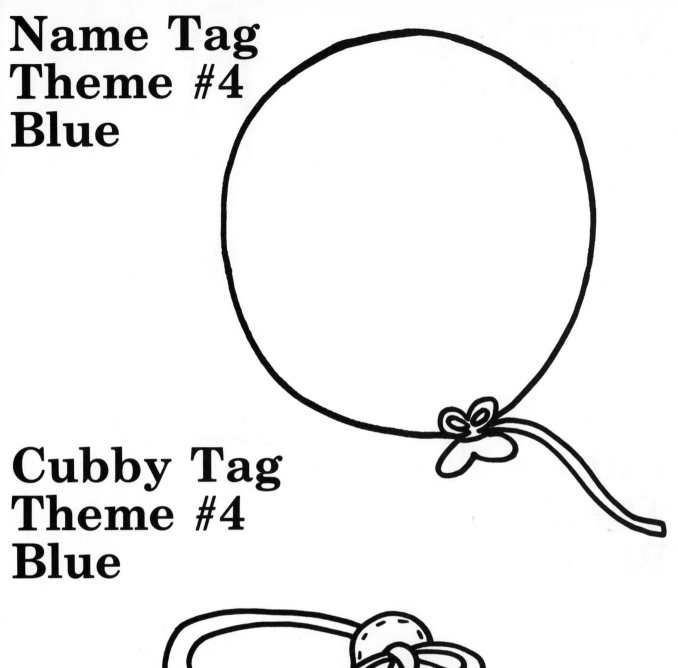

Cubby Tag
Theme #4
Blue

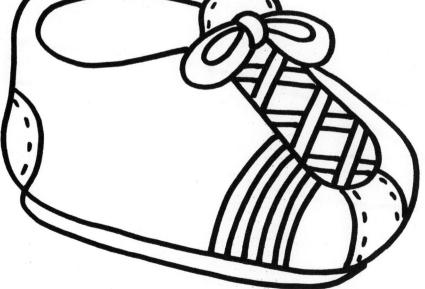

Name Tag
Theme #5
Brushes

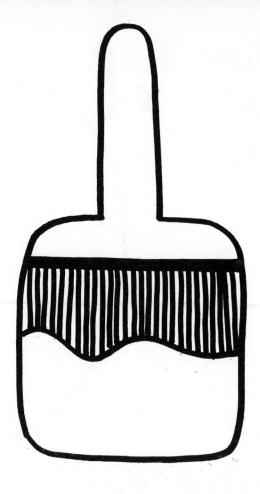

Cubby Tag
Theme #5
Brushes

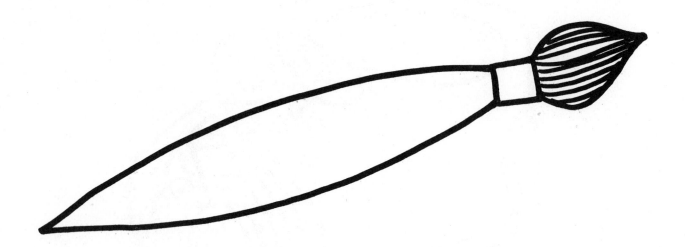

Name Tag
Theme #6
Buildings

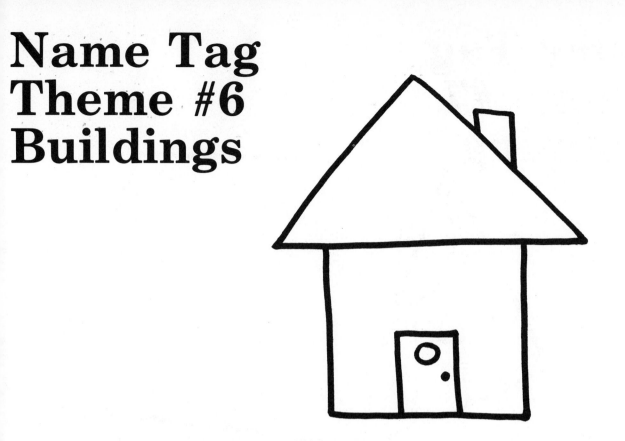

Cubby Tag
Theme #6
Buildings

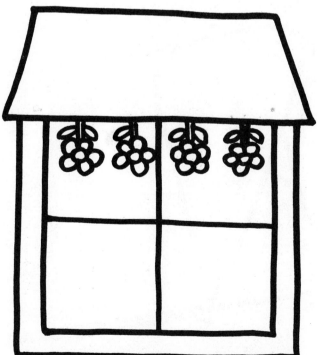

Name Tag
Theme #7
Camping

Cubby Tag
Theme #7
Camping

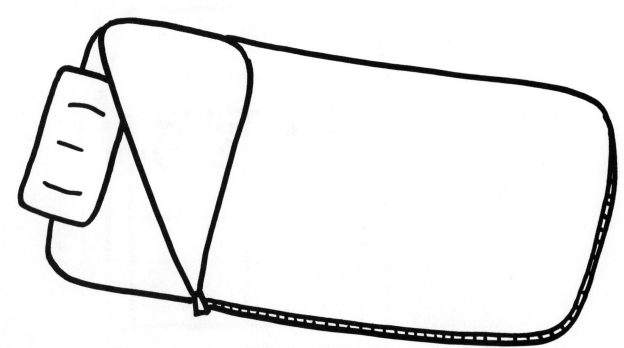

Name Tag
Theme #8
Cars, Trucks
and Buses

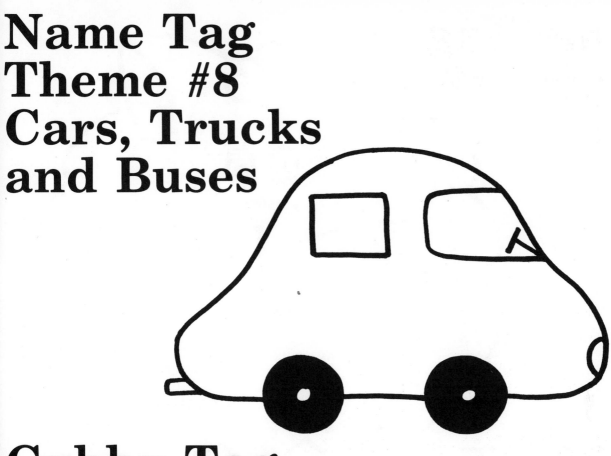

Cubby Tag
Theme #8
Cars, Trucks
and Buses

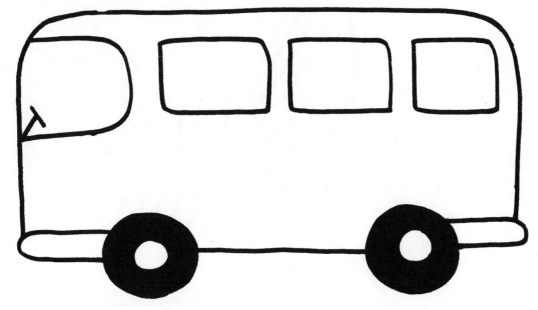

Name Tag
Theme #9
Cats

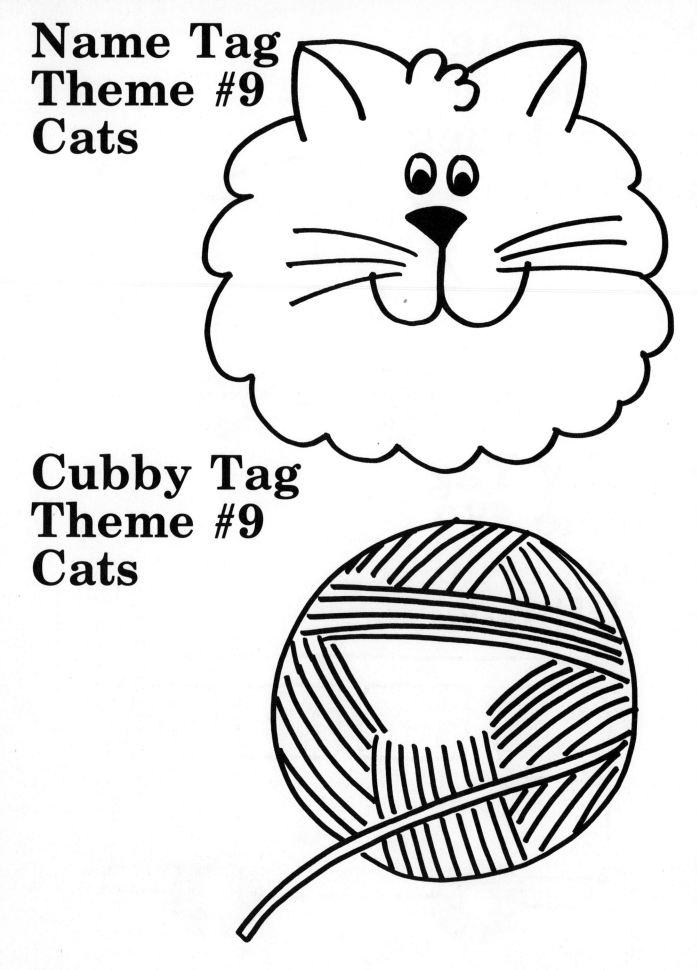

Cubby Tag
Theme #9
Cats

Name Tag
Theme #10
Christmas

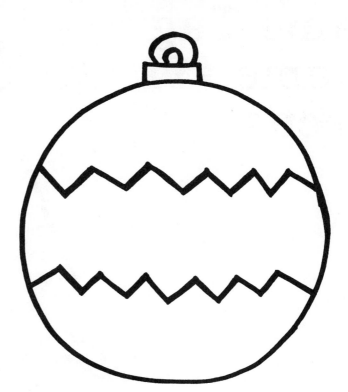

Cubby Tag
Theme #10
Christmas

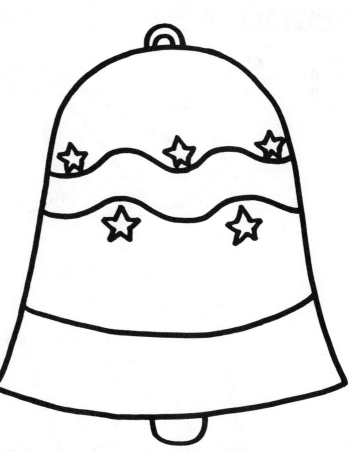

Name Tag
Theme #11
Circus

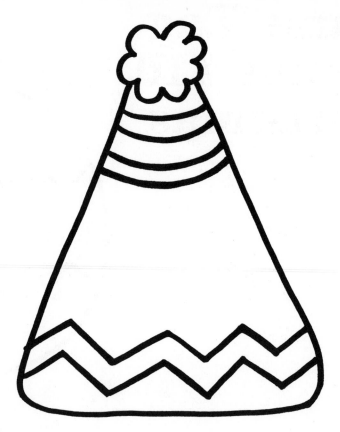

Cubby Tag
Theme #11
Circus

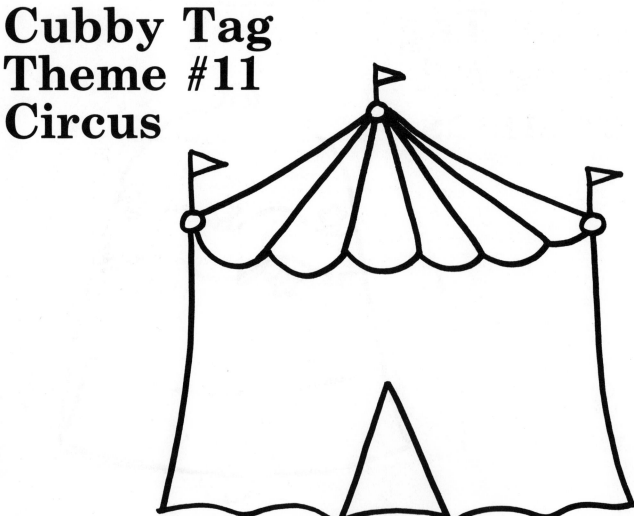

A12

Name Tag
Theme #12
Clothes

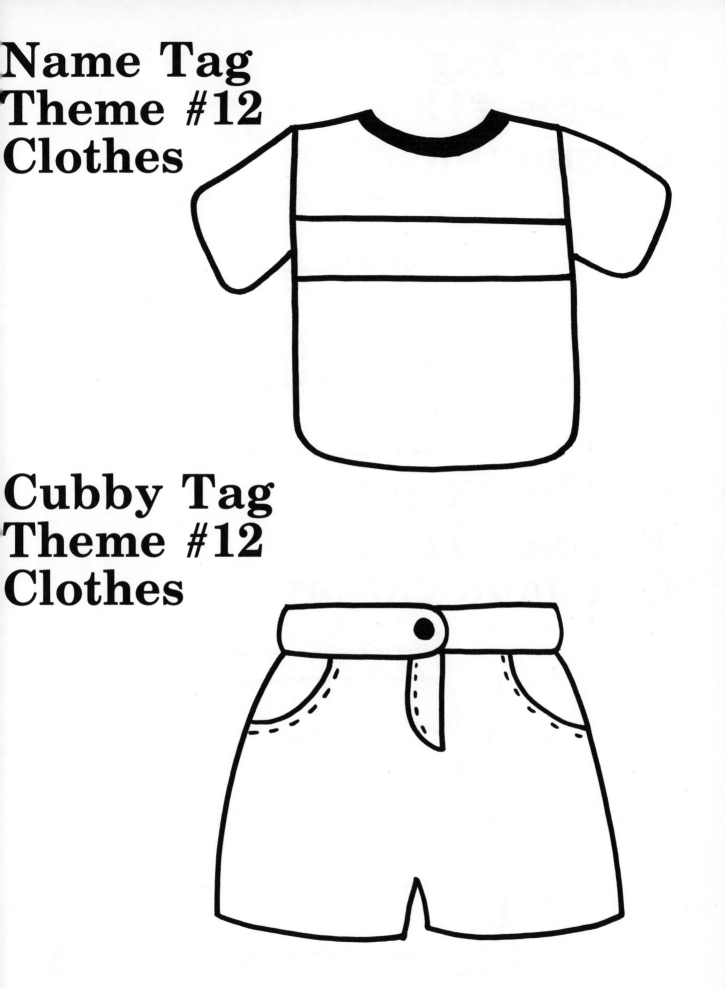

Cubby Tag
Theme #12
Clothes

Name Tag
Theme #13
Communication

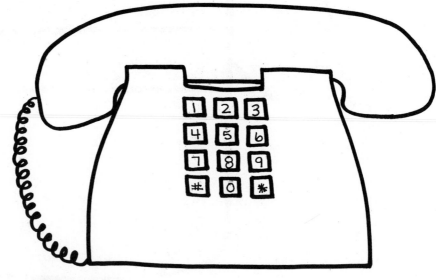

Cubby Tag
Theme #13
Communication

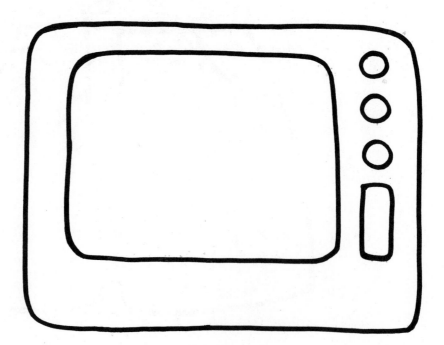

Name Tag
Theme #14
Construction
Tools

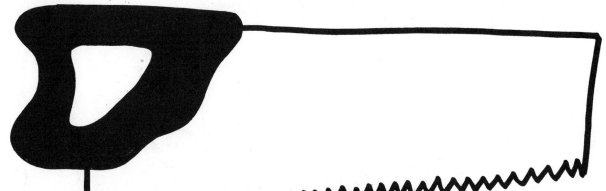

Cubby Tag
Theme #14
Construction
Tools

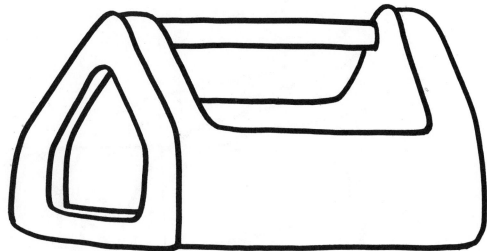

Name Tag
Theme #15
Creative
Movement

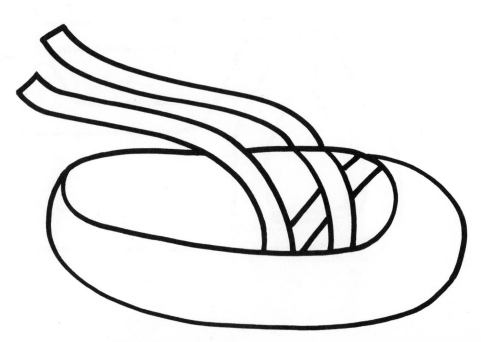

Cubby Tag
Theme #15
Creative
Movement

Name Tag
Theme #16
Dentist

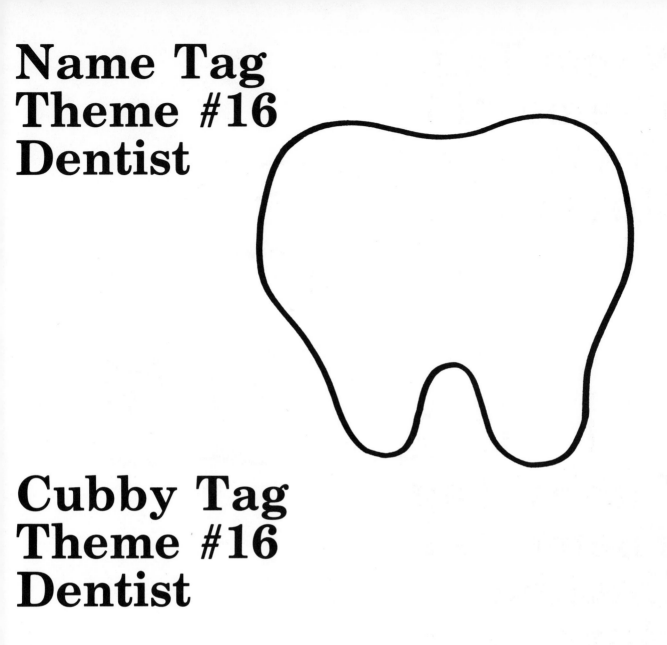

Cubby Tag
Theme #16
Dentist

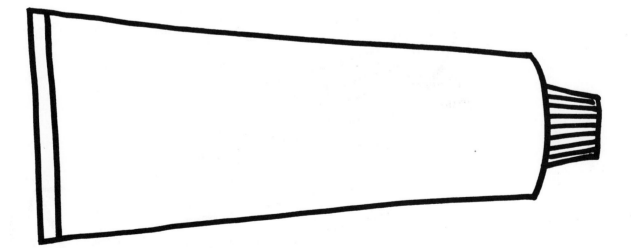

Name Tag
Theme #17
Doctors and
Nurses

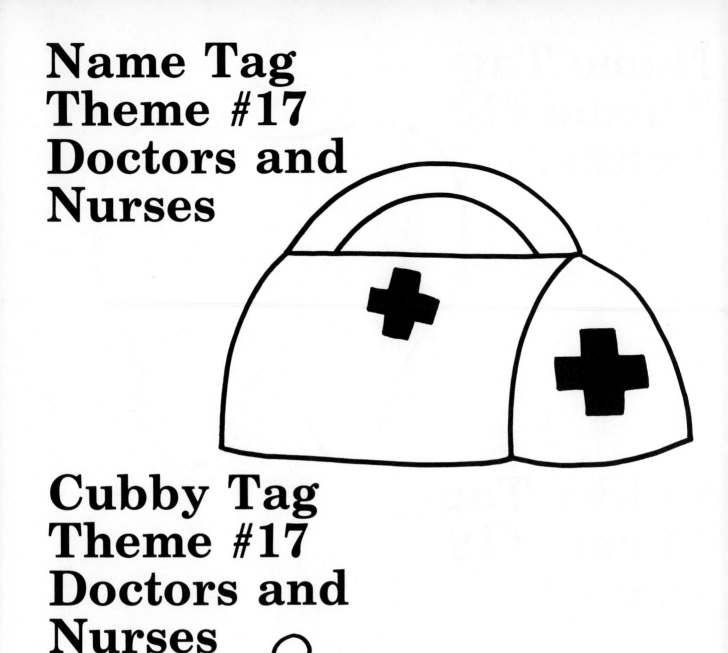

Cubby Tag
Theme #17
Doctors and
Nurses

Name Tag
Theme #18
Dogs

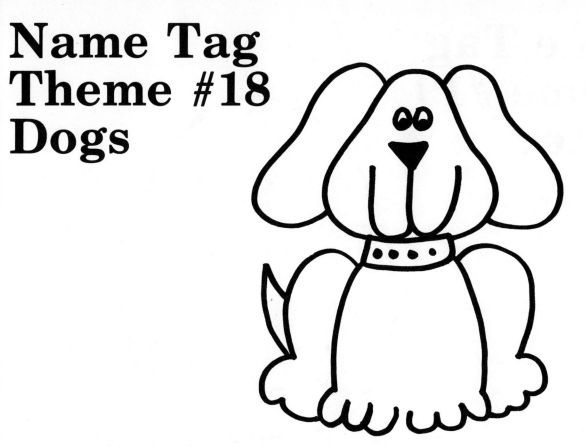

Cubby Tag
Theme #18
Dogs

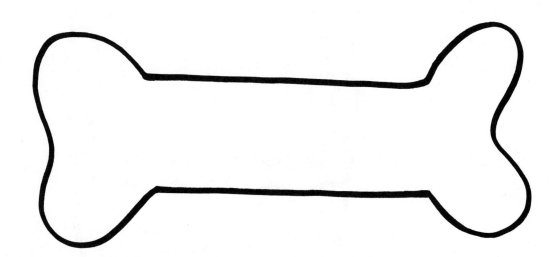

Name Tag
Theme #19
Easter

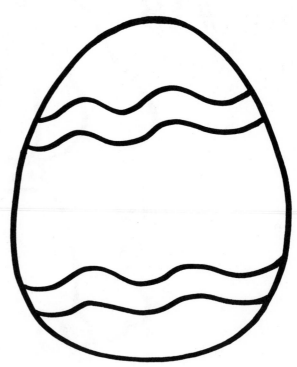

Cubby Tag
Theme #19
Easter

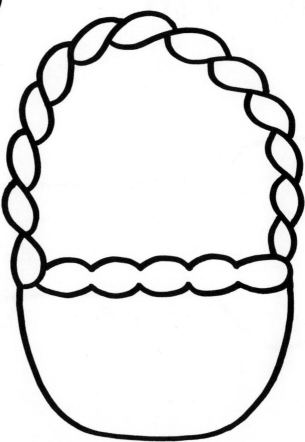

A20

Name Tag
Theme #20
Fall

Cubby Tag
Theme #20
Fall

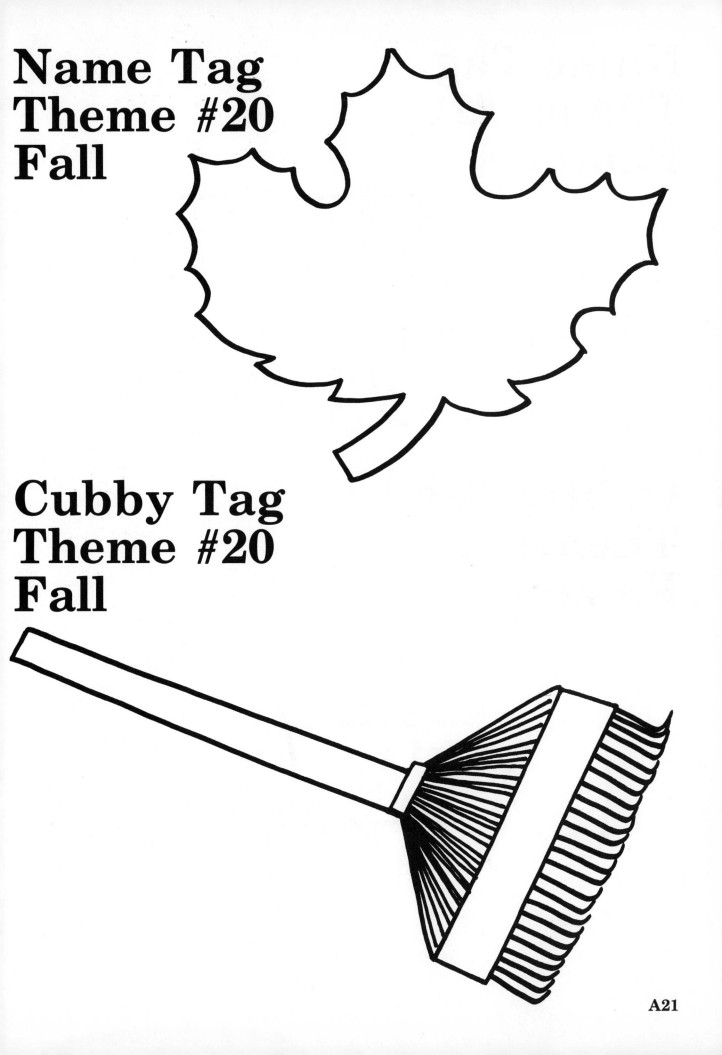

Name Tag
Theme #21
Families

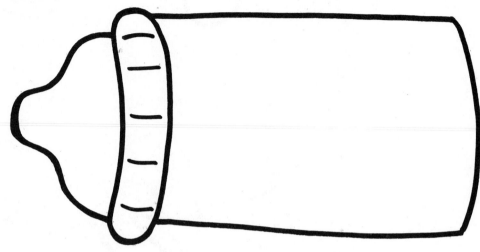

Cubby Tag
Theme #21
Families

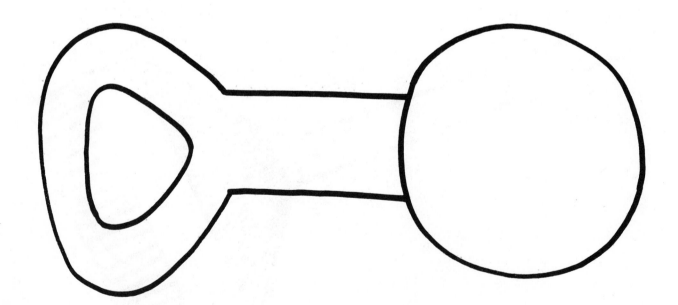

Name Tag
Theme #22
Farm Animals

Cubby Tag
Theme #22
Farm Animals

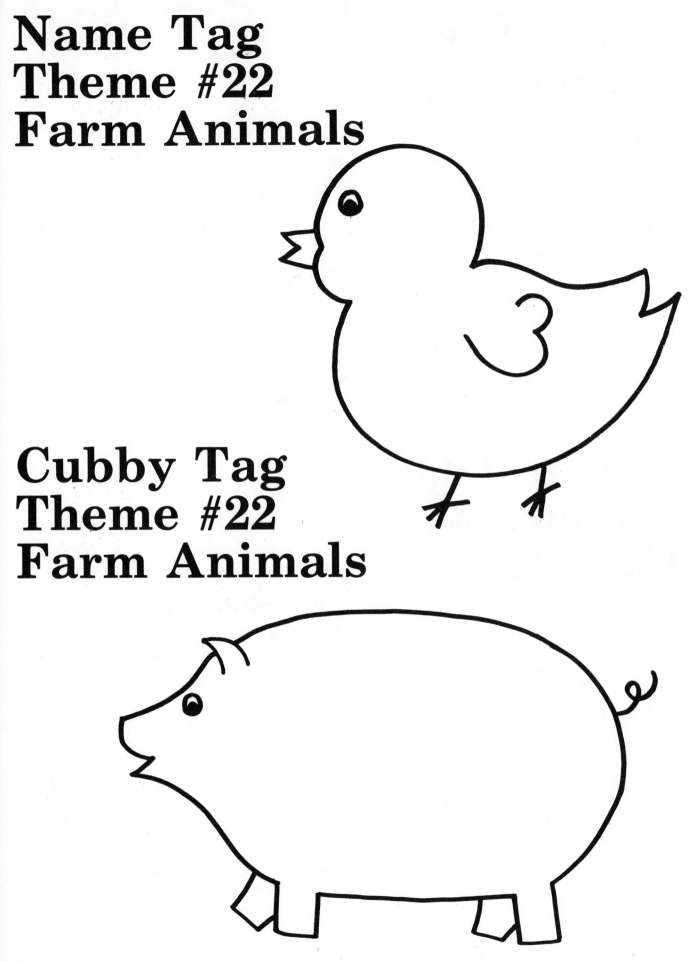

A23

Name Tag
Theme #23
Feelings

Cubby Tag
Theme #23
Feelings

Name Tag
Theme #24
Fire
Fighters

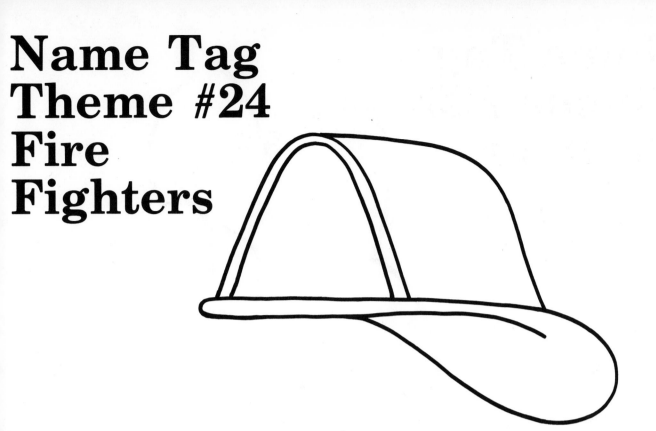

Cubby Tag
Theme #24
Fire
Fighters

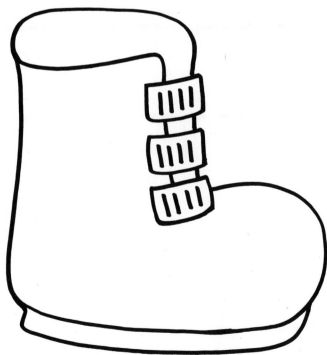

Name Tag
Theme #25
Flowers

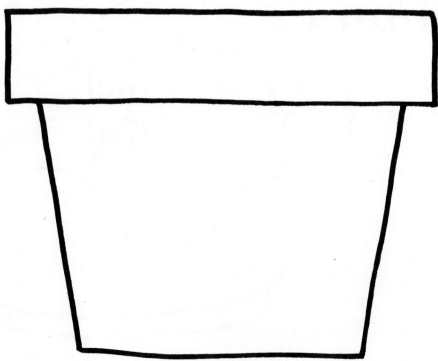

Cubby Tag
Theme #25
Flowers

Name Tag
Theme #26
Friends

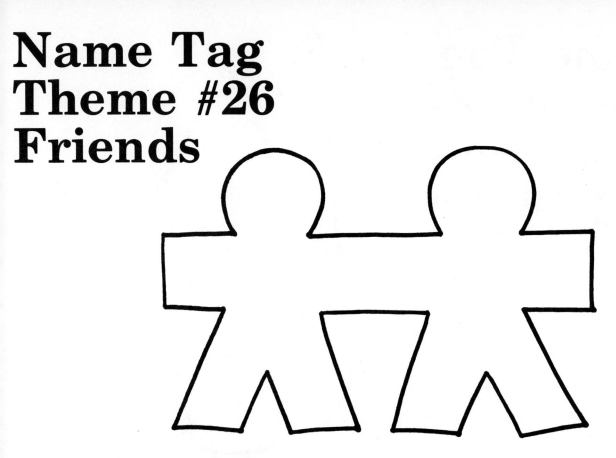

Cubby Tag
Theme #26
Friends

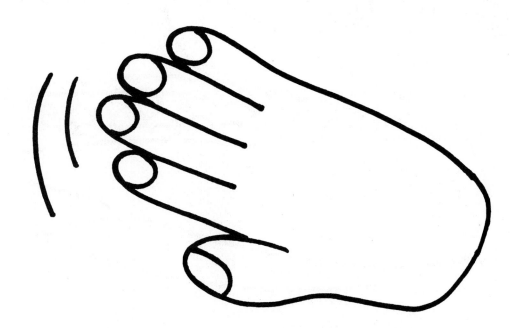

Name Tag
Theme #27
Fruits and
Vegetables

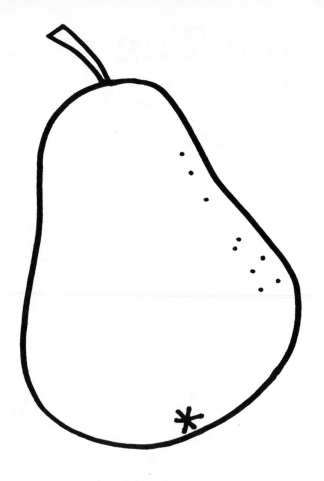

Cubby Tag
Theme #27
Fruits and
Vegetables

A28

Name Tag
Theme #28
Gardens

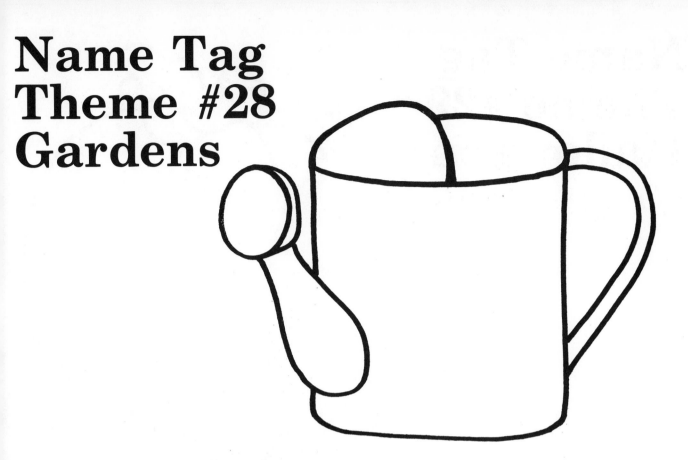

Cubby Tag
Theme #28
Gardens

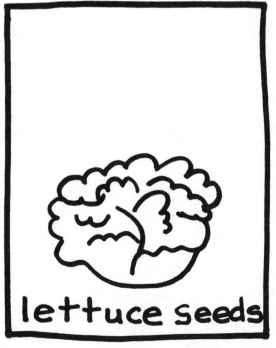

lettuce seeds

Name Tag
Theme #29
Halloween

Cubby Tag
Theme #29
Halloween

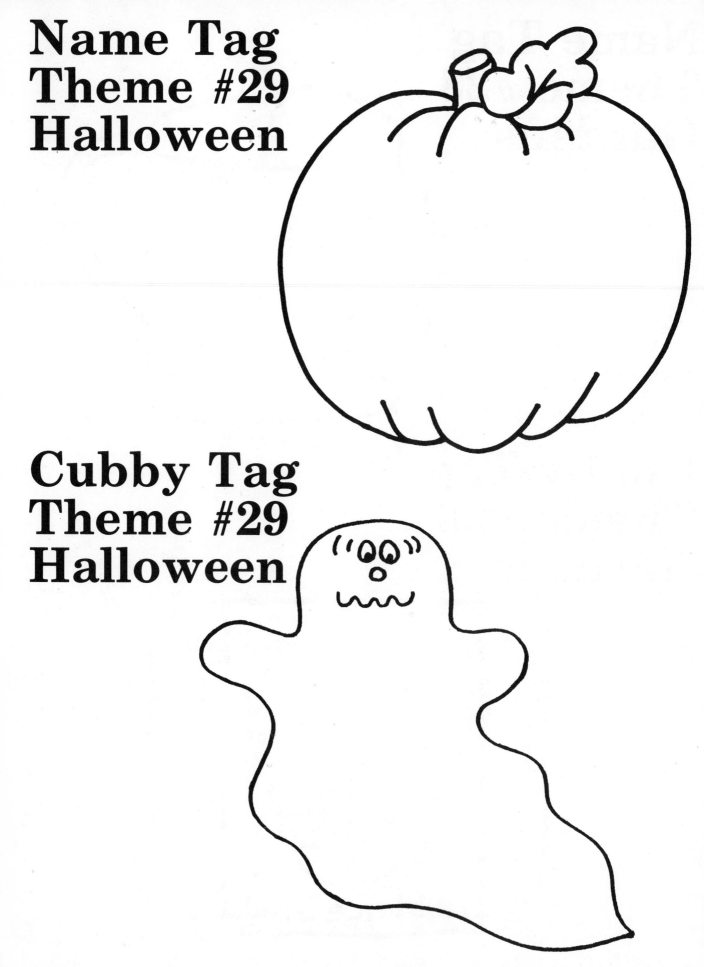

A30

Name Tag
Theme #30
Hanukkah

Cubby Tag
Theme #30
Hanukkah

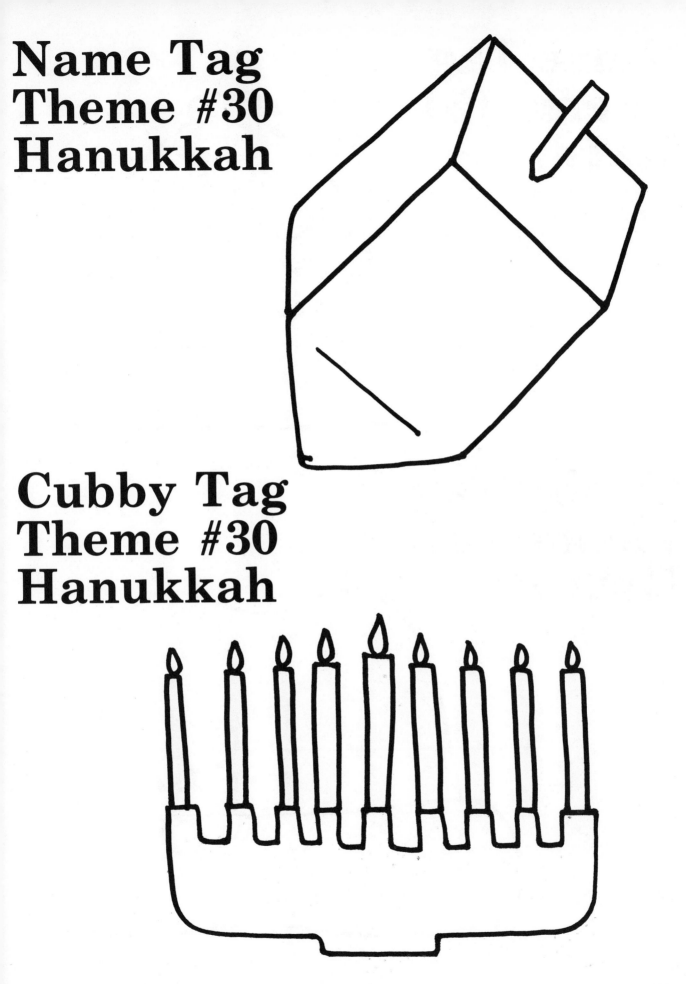

Name Tag
Theme #31
Hats

Cubby Tag
Theme #31
Hats

Name Tag
Theme #32
Health

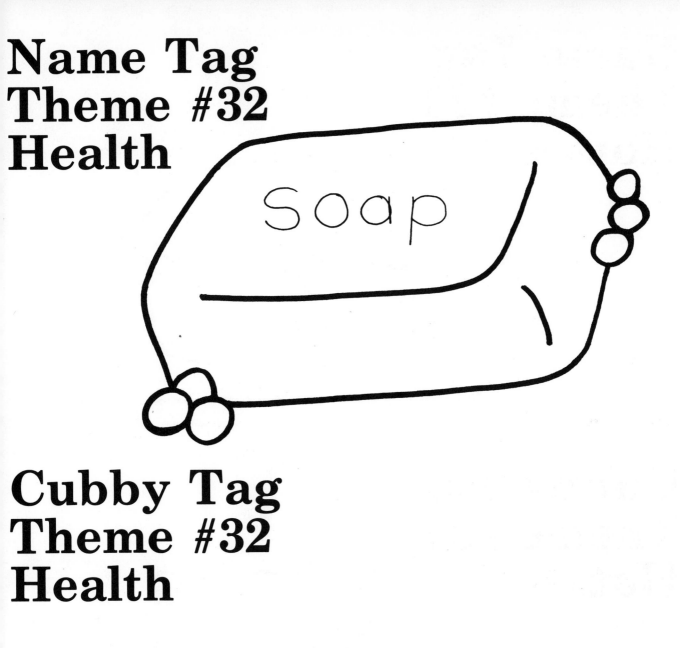

Soap

Cubby Tag
Theme #32
Health

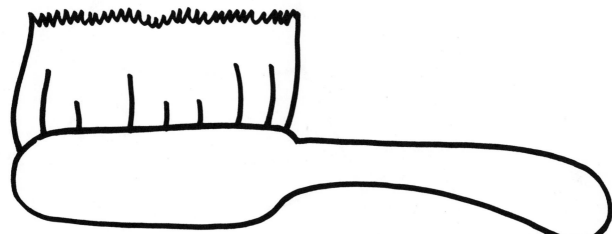

Name Tag
Theme #33
Homes

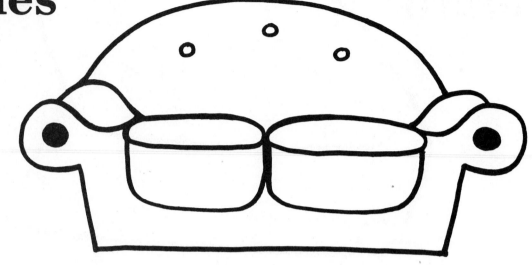

Cubby Tag
Theme #33
Homes

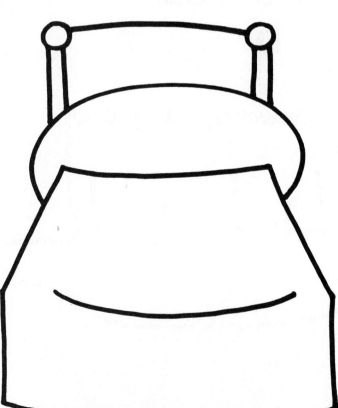

Name Tag
Theme #34
Insects and
Spiders

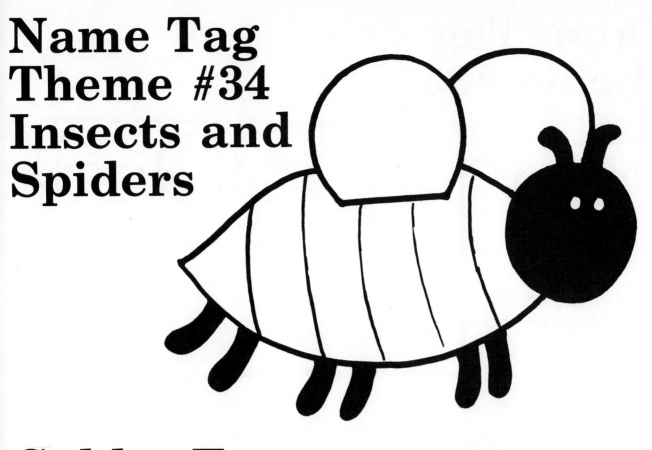

Cubby Tag
Theme #34
Insects and
Spiders

Name Tag
Theme #35
Mail
Carrier

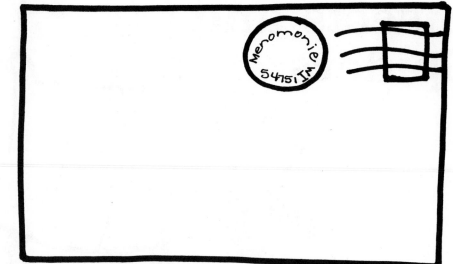

Cubby Tag
Theme #35
Mail
Carrier

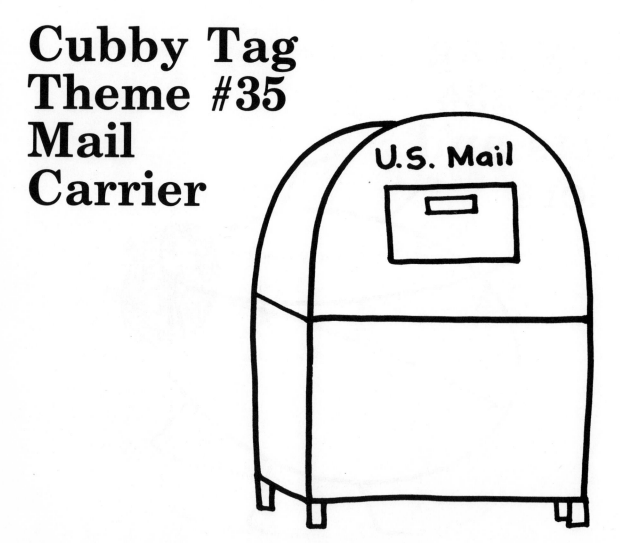

Name Tag
Theme #36
Music

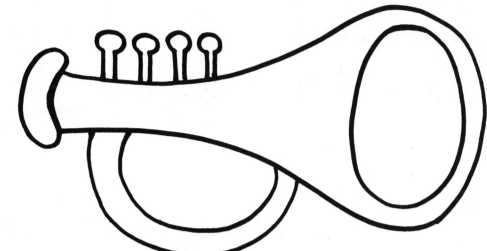

Cubby Tag
Theme #36
Music

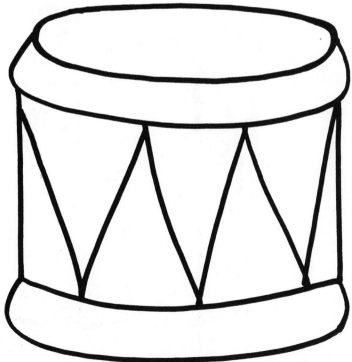

A37

Name Tag
Theme #37
Numbers

(Note: The number of each child's name tag is determined by his/her age)

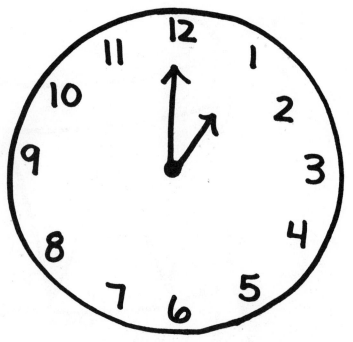

Cubby Tag
Theme #37
Numbers

Name Tag
Theme #38
Nursery
Rhymes

Cubby Tag
Theme #38
Nursery
Rhymes

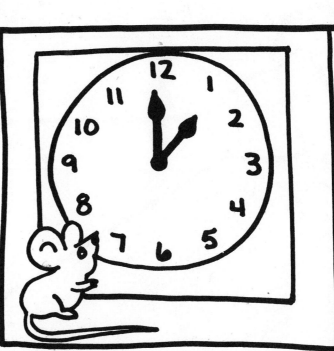

A39

Name Tag
Theme #39
Occupations

Cubby Tag
Theme #39
Occupations

Name Tag
Theme #40
Pets

Cubby Tag
Theme #40
Pets

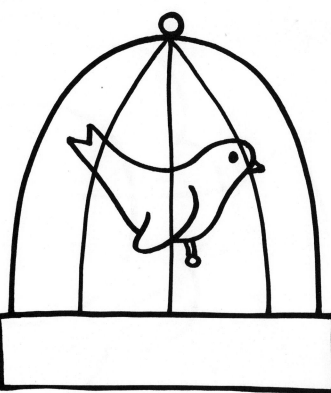

Name Tag
Theme #41
Plants

Cubby Tag
Theme #41
Plants

A42

Name Tag
Theme #42
Puppets

Cubby Tag
Theme #42
Puppets

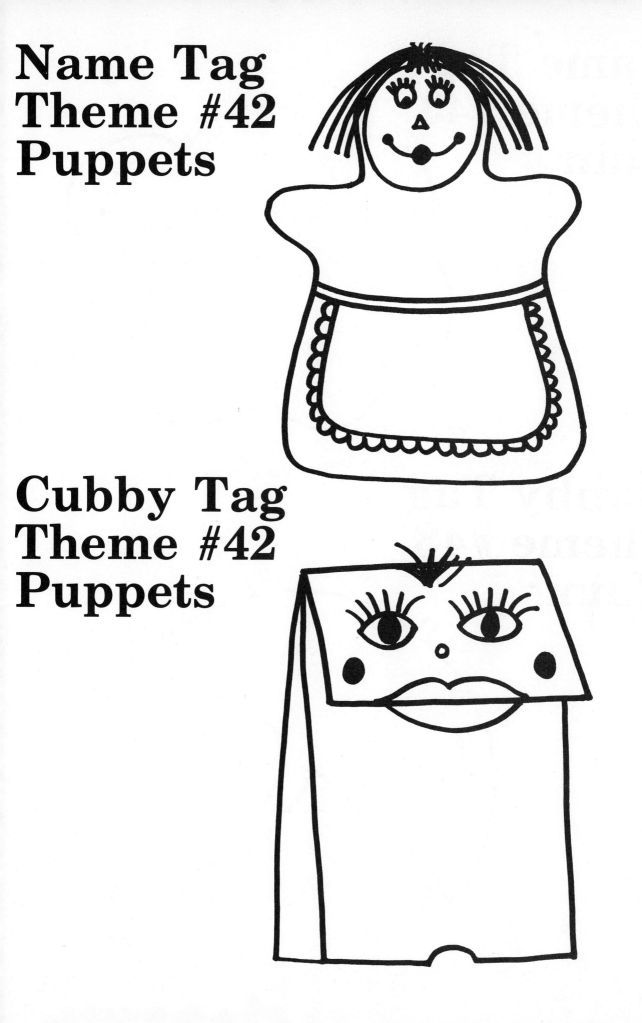

Name Tag
Theme #43
Rain

Cubby Tag
Theme #43
Rain

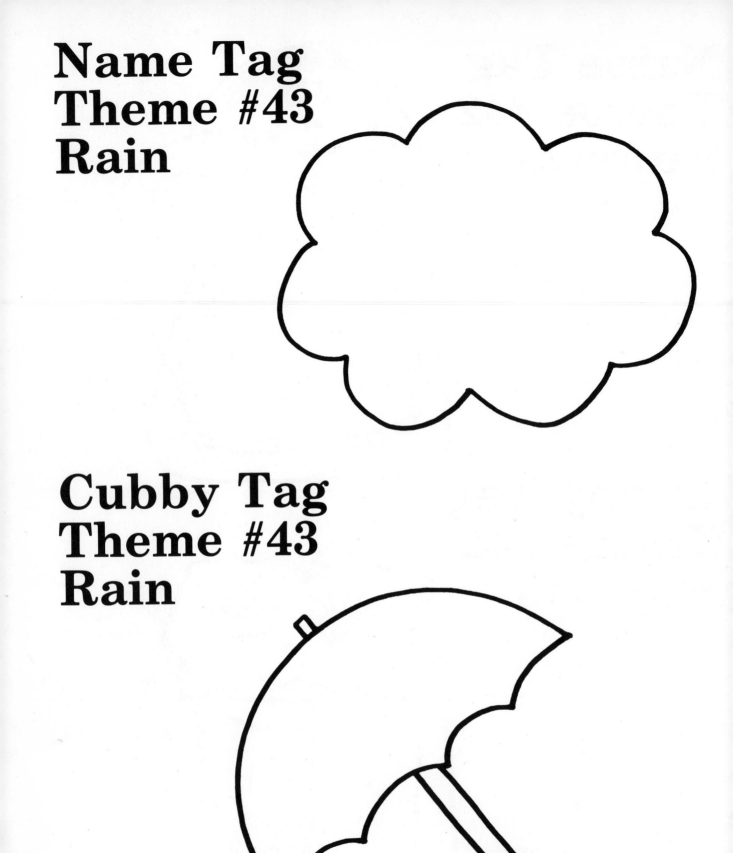

A44

Name Tag
Theme #44
Red

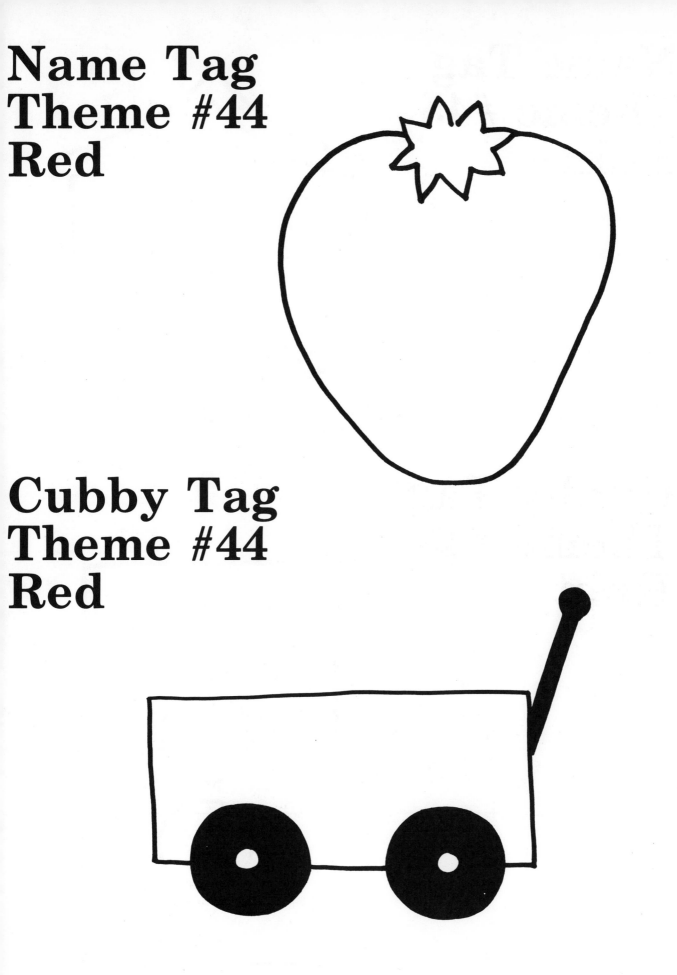

Cubby Tag
Theme #44
Red

Name Tag
Theme #45
Safety

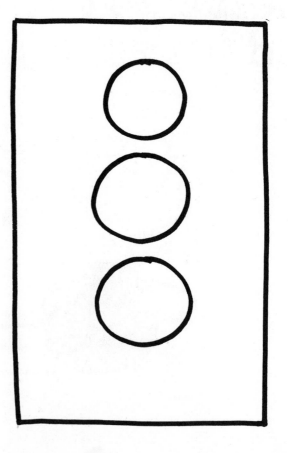

Cubby Tag
Theme #45
Safety

Name Tag
Theme #46
Scissors

Cubby Tag
Theme #46
Scissors

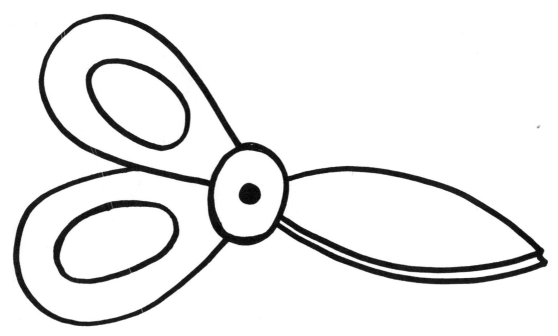

A47

Name Tag
Theme #47
Shapes

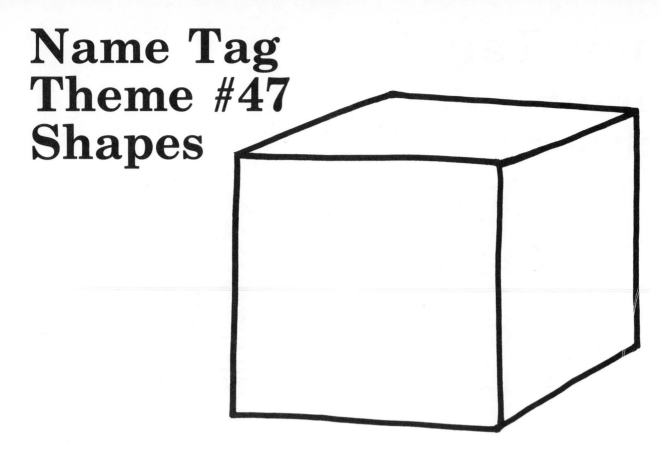

Cubby Tag
Theme #47
Shapes

Name Tag
Theme #48
Sports

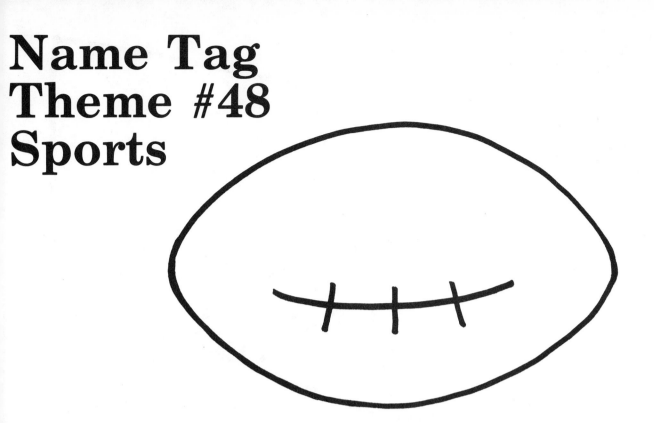

Cubby Tag
Theme #48
Sports

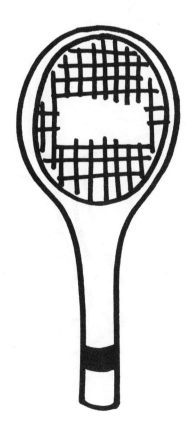

Name Tag
Theme #49
Spring

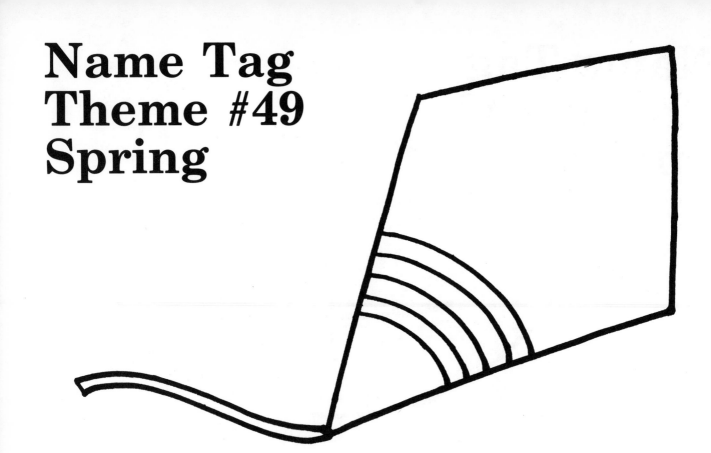

Cubby Tag
Theme #49
Spring

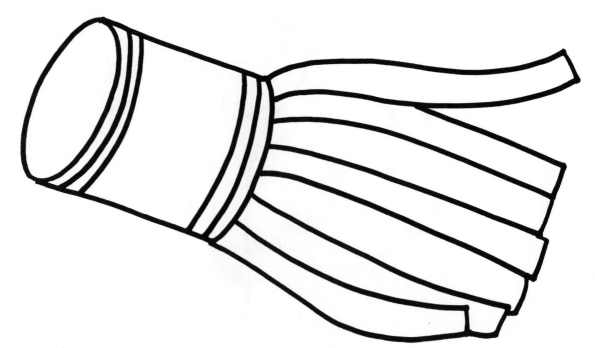

A50

Name Tag
Theme #50
Summer

Cubby Tag
Theme #50
Summer

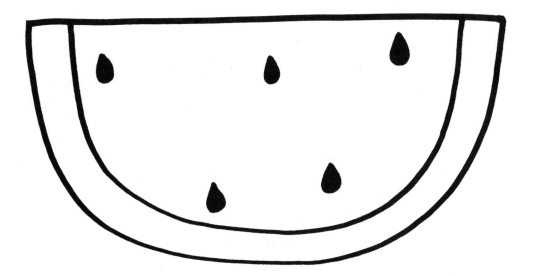

Name Tag
Theme #51
Thanksgiving

Cubby Tag
Theme #51
Thanksgiving

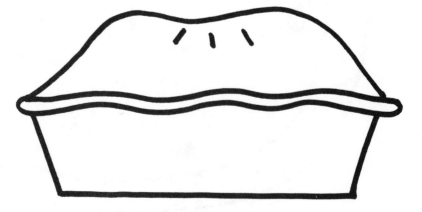

Name Tag
Theme #52
Valentine's
Day

Cubby Tag
Theme #52
Valentine's
Day

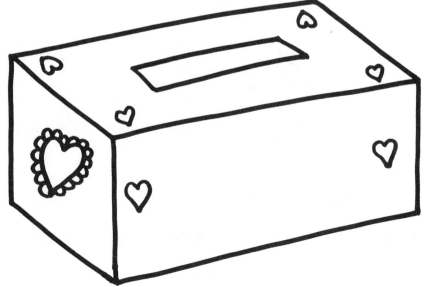

Name Tag
Theme #53
Water

Cubby Tag
Theme #53
Water

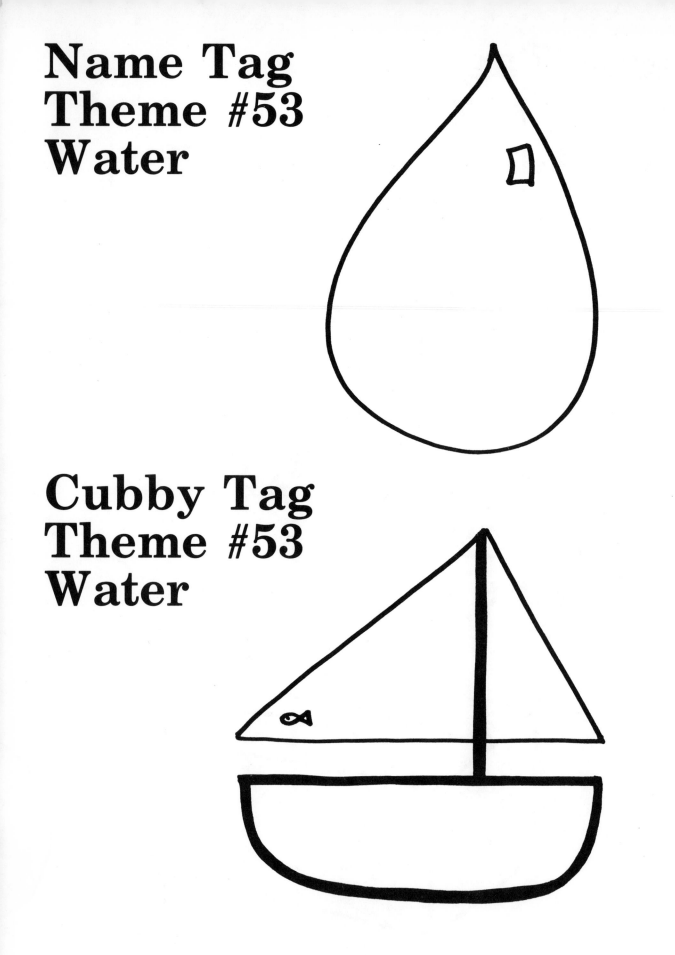

Name Tag
Theme #54
Wheels

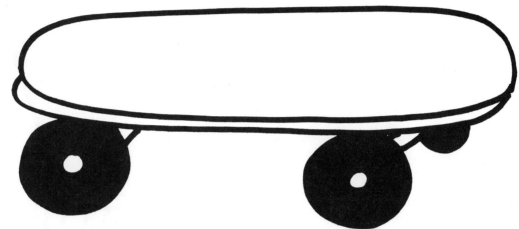

Cubby Tag
Theme #54
Wheels

Name Tag
Theme #55
Winter

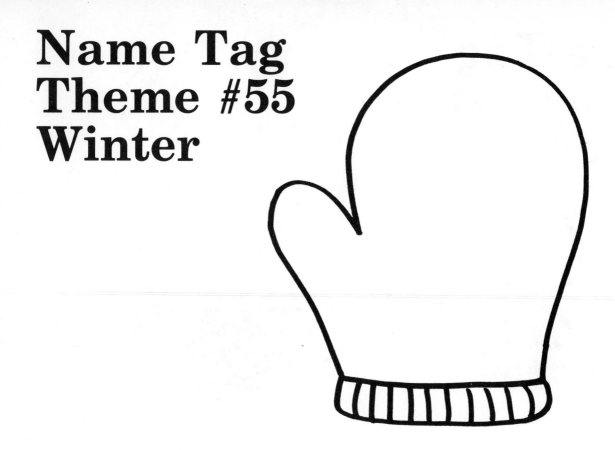

Cubby Tag
Theme #55
Winter

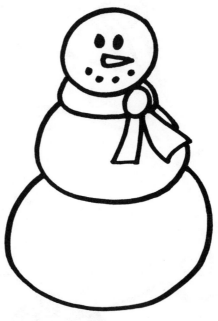

A56

Name Tag
Theme #56
Yellow

Cubby Tag
Theme #56
Yellow

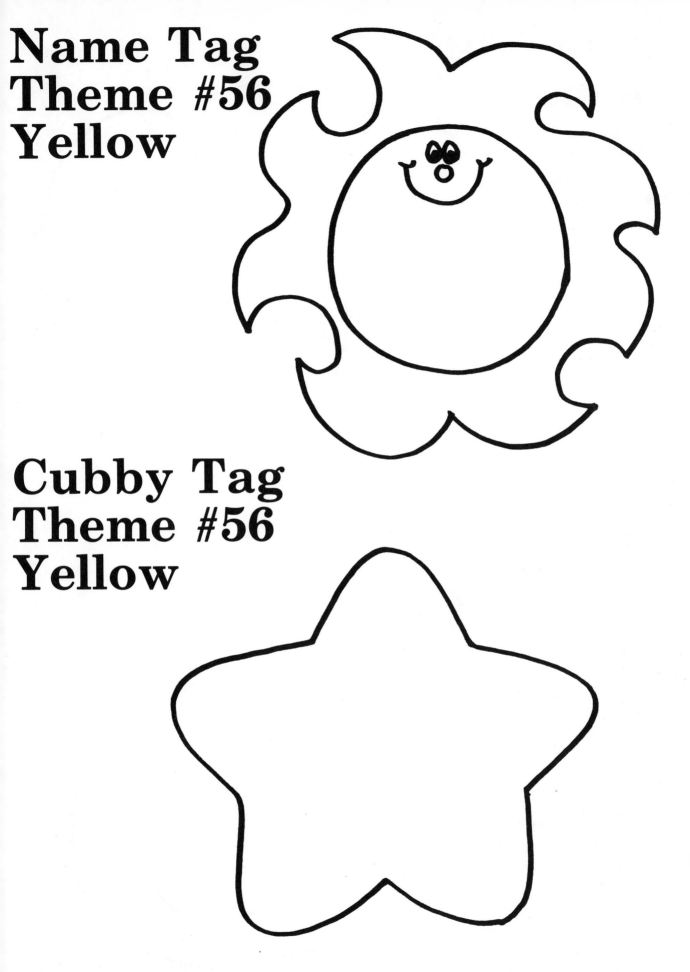

Name Tag
Theme #57
Zoo
Animals

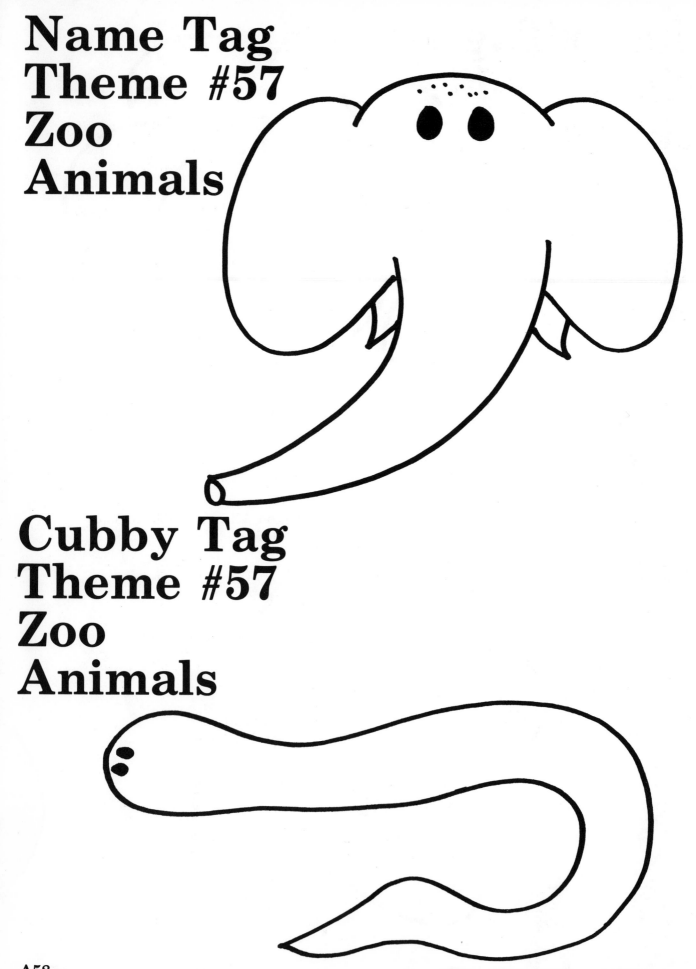

Cubby Tag
Theme #57
Zoo
Animals

A58

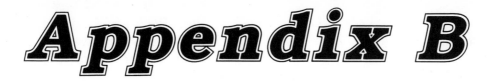

Appendix B

EARLY CHILDHOOD COMMERCIAL SUPPLIERS

ABC School Supply, Inc.
6500 Peachtree Industrial Boulevard
P.O. Box 4750
Norcross, Georgia 30091
(404) 447-5000

American Guidance Service
Publisher's Building
Circle Pines, Minnesota 55014

Beckley Cardy
One East First Street
Duluth, Minnesota 55802
1-800-227-1178

Childcraft Educational Corporation
20 Kilmer Road
P.O. Box 3081
Edison, New Jersey 08818-3081
1-800-631-5652

Children's Book and Music Center
2500 Santa Monica Boulevard
Santa Monica, California 90404
1-800-443-1856

Childrens Press
5440 North Cumberland Avenue
Chicago, Illinois 60656
1-800-621-1115

Community Playthings
Route 213
Rifton, New York 12471
(914) 658-3141

Constructive Playthings
1227 East 119th Street
Grandview, Missouri 64030-1117
1-800-832-0224

Cuisenaire Company of America, Inc.
12 Church Street, Box D
New Rochelle, New York 10802
1-800-237-3142

Delmar Publishers Inc
2 Computer Drive, West
Box 15-015
Albany, New York 12212
(518) 459-1150

Didax Educational Resources
6 Doulton Place
Peabody, Massachusetts 01960

Educational Teaching Aids
199 Carpenter Avenue
Wheeling, Illinois 60090
(312) 520-2500

Environments, Inc.
P.O. Box 1348
Beaufort Industrial Park
Beaufort, South Carolina 29901-1348

The Highsmith Co., Inc.
W5527 Highway 106
P.O. Box 800
Fort Atkinson, Wisconsin 53538-0800
1-800-558-2110

Judy/Instructo
4325 Hiawatha Avenue
Minneapolis, Minnesota 55406

Kaplan School Supply Corporation
P.O. Box 609
Lewisville, North Carolina 27023-0609
1-800-334-2014

Kimbo Educational
10 North Third Avenue
Long Branch, New Jersey 07740
1-800-631-2187

Latta's School and Office Supplies
2218 Main street
Cedar Falls, Iowa 50613
(319) 266-3501

Nasco
901 Janesville Avenue
Fort Atkinson, Wisconsin 53538
1-800-558-9595

Play Thinks
201 Old Town Road
P.O. Box 2628
Setauket, New York 11733
(516) 751-2421

Primary Educator
1200 Keystone Avenue
P.O. Box 24155
Lansing, Michigan 48909-4155
1-800-444-1773

Scholastic, Inc.
P.O. Box 7502
Jefferson City, Missouri 65102
1-800-392-2179

St. Paul Book and Stationery
1233 West County Road E
St. Paul, Minnesota 55112
1-800-338-SPBS (7727)

Valley School Supply
1000 North Bluemound Drive
P.O. Box 1579
Appleton, Wisconsin 54913
1-800-242-3433

Walter's Child Care Supplies
P.O. Box 14260
Madison, Wisconsin 53714
1-800-433-6252